PHARMACEUTICAL CHEMISTRY

Dr. Aarushi Singh

ALLIED HEALTH PRESS

Pharmaceutical Chemistry

Author: **Dr. Aarushi Singh**

Allied Health Press
4164 Lakeshore Road
Burlington ON L7L 1A4
Canada
www.alliedhealthpress.com
Email: orders@arclereducation.com

ISBN: 978-1-77956-274-6

ABOUT THE AUTHOR

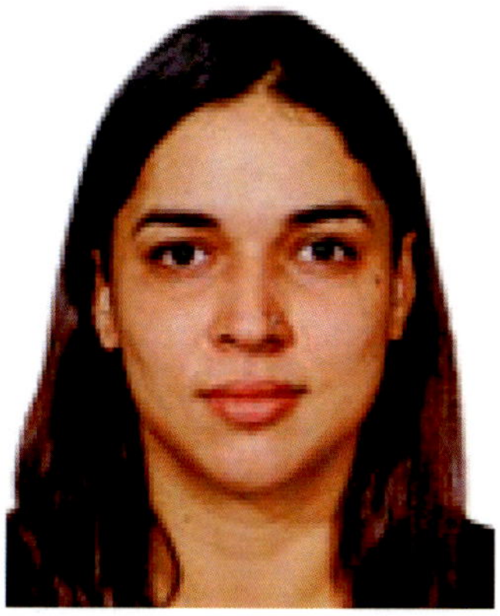

Dr. Aarushi Singh is an accomplished chemist currently serving as an Assistant Professor in the Department of Chemistry at Ramjas College, University of Delhi. She embarked on her academic journey with a B.Sc. in Chemistry from Ramjas College in 2011, followed by a Master's in Chemistry from the University of Delhi in 2013. Driven by a passion for research, Dr. Singh pursued her Ph.D. at the same institution, completing it in 2021. Her doctoral thesis, conducted under the mentorship of Prof. Ramesh Chandra and Dr. Rakeshwar Bandichhor, focused on the synthesis of biologically active Pyrazinoindoles and their mechanistic interaction studies.

Dr. Singh has accumulated significant research experience through various prestigious roles and projects. She worked as a Senior Research Fellow at the Indian Council of Medical Research (ICMR), where she developed inhalable nanomicelles for lung cancer treatment. She has also held positions as a Research Associate at the University of Alberta, Canada, focusing on the synthesis of Piperidinyl allylboronates, and at the Max Planck Institute for Multidisciplinary Sciences in Germany, where she synthesized magnetic resonance contrast agents.

Her international experience includes a stint as a Visiting Scientist at Humboldt Universität zu Berlin, Germany, and as a Ph.D. Exchange Student at the Japan Advanced Institute of Science and Technology (JAIST), where she studied the inhibition of protein aggregation by zwitterionic polymers. These experiences were supported by several prestigious fellowships, including the Shastri Research Student Fellowship and the JASSO Fellowship.

Dr. Singh's research interests are broad and interdisciplinary, encompassing multi-step organic synthesis, heterocyclic synthesis, and the development of biologically active compounds. Dr. Singh has authored one book and published over 15 original scientific research papers in internationally recognized journals. In addition to her research, Dr. Singh is dedicated to teaching and mentoring the next generation of chemists. Her diverse background and international collaborations enrich her teaching, providing students with a global perspective on chemical research and applications.

Dr. Aarushi Singh continues to contribute to the field of chemistry through her innovative research, dedicated teaching, and active participation in the scientific community. Her work aims to bridge the gap between advanced research and practical applications, making complex chemical concepts accessible and impactful.

Word Roots, Prefixes, and Suffixes by Chapter

Chapter 1 Introduction to Pharmaceutical Chemistry

-asone: betamethasone; dexamethasone; diflorasone; fluticasone; mometasone

-afil:avanafil; sildenafil; tadalafil; vardenafil

-asone: betamethasone; dexamethasone; diflorasone; fluticasone; mometasone

-bicin: doxorubicin; epirubicin; idarubicin; valrubicin

-bital: butabarbital; butalbital; phenobarbital; secobarbital

Chapter 2 Drug Design and Molecular Modeling

-caine: bupivacaine; lidocaine; mepivacaine; prilocaine; proparacaine

cef-, ceph-: cefaclor; cefdinir; cefixime; cefprozil; cephalexin

-cillin: amoxicillin; ampicillin; dicloxacillin; nafcillin; oxacillin

Cort: clocortolone; fludrocortisone; hydrocortisone

-cycline: demeclocycline; doxycycline; minocycline; tetracycline

-dazole: albendazole; mebendazole; metronidazole; tinidazole

Chapter 3 Drug Delivery Systems

-dazole: albendazole; mebendazole; metronidazole; tinidazole

-dipine: amlodipine; felodipine; nifedipine; nimodipine; nisoldipine

-dronate: alendronate; etidronate; ibandronate; risedronate

-eprazole: esomeprazole; omeprazole; rabeprazole

-fenac: bromfenac; diclofenac; nepafenac

-floxacin: besifloxacin; ciprofloxacin; levofloxacin; moxifloxacin; ofloxacin

Chapter 4 Pharmacokinetics and Pharmacodynamics

-caine: lidocaine

-azole: omeprazole

-mycin,-floxacin: levofloxacin

-arin: warfarin

Chapter 5 Chemotherapy and Drug Action

-oxetine,-ipramine: fluoxetine

-dine,-mine: diphenhydramine

-one: cortisone

-azine,-apine: olanzapine

-olol: metoprolol

Chapter 6 Medicinal Chemistry of Central Nervous System (CNS) Drugs

-terol: albuterol

-soneor–solone: prednisone

-semide,-thiazide: furosemide

-ide: glipizide

-statin: atorvastatin

Chapter 7 Drug Metabolism and Toxicology

-bicin: antineoplastic; cytotoxic agent

-caine: local anesthetic

cef-, ceph-: cephalosporin antibiotic

-cillin: penicillin antibiotic

cort: corticosteroid

-floxacin: quinolone antibiotic

-olol: beta blocker

-olone: corticosteroid

-phylline: xanthine derivative (bronchodilator)

-vudine: antiviral; nucleoside analogs

-zepam: benzodiazepine

Chapter 8 Natural Products and Herbal Medicines

-azine: promethazine

-caine: local anesthetic

-cillin: penicillin antibiotic

-cycline: tetracycline antibiotic

-prazole: lansoprazole

-terol: levalbuterol

-phylline: theophylline

Chapter 9 Analytical Techniques in Pharmaceutical Chemistry

A-, An-: Anemia

Andr/o-: Androgen

Anti-: Anticholinergic drugs

Auto-: Autocrine

Bio-: Biology

Chem/o: Chemotherapy

Contra-: Contraceptionac

Chapter 10 Regulatory Affairs and Drug Development

adversus: adverse effect

alb(i/o)-: albumin, albinism

ex-: extraction, edentatus

trans-: transfer, transaminase

par(a)-: parapsychology, parallel

pharmaco-: pharmacology, pharmaceutic

Table of Contents

5 Chemotherapy and Drug Action 173

6 Medicinal Chemistry of Central Nervous System (CNS) Drugs 213

LIST OF FIGURES

LIST OF TABLES

PREFACE

The International Union for Pure and Applied Chemistry (IUPAC) defines medicinal chemistry as a multidisciplinary field deeply rooted in chemistry, incorporating key elements from biology, medicine, and pharmaceutical sciences. This field is dedicated to the innovative processes of creating, discovering, designing, identifying, and preparing biologically active compounds. Additionally, medicinal chemistry explores the metabolism of these compounds, examines their mechanisms of action at the molecular level, and develops structure-activity relationships to understand how variations in chemical structure impact biological function.

In Brazil, this branch of chemistry is commonly referred to as pharmaceutical chemistry, reflecting a broader perspective that emphasizes the direct impact on patient care rather than purely chemical analysis. Within the pharmacy profession in Brazil, pharmaceutical chemistry is distinguished because it underscores the pharmacist's role as a therapeutic consultant—a pivotal figure in healthcare—beyond just a traditional chemist. This distinction is particularly critical for pharmacy students who aspire to roles in clinical pharmacy, as it emphasizes the importance of a comprehensive understanding of medicinal chemistry in their education.

Studying pharmaceutical chemistry not only prepares students to develop life-saving treatments but also enhances the speed at which new medications can be brought to market, thereby contributing significantly to healthcare. It empowers pharmacy students to become integral players in the medical field, aiding in the design and delivery of treatments that can save lives and improve patient outcomes. Additionally, the scope of pharmaceutical chemistry extends beyond its core areas to include specialized subjects such as pharmacokinetics, pharmacodynamics, and drug metabolism. These fields study the absorption, distribution, metabolism, and excretion of drugs, as well as their biochemical and physiological effects, and how these effects are correlated with their chemical structures. This comprehensive approach ensures that students are well-equipped to tackle a variety of challenges in drug research, development, and implementation, enhancing their ability to contribute effectively in diverse healthcare settings.

This book is written as a comprehensive guide to pharmaceutical chemistry, aiming to bridge the gap between basic chemistry and its application in the field of pharmacy. The primary objective is to provide an in-depth exploration of the principles of medicinal chemistry and their practical applications in drug development, emphasizing the roles of pharmacokinetics, pharmacodynamics, and drug metabolism in the design of new therapeutic agents.

Pharmaceutical chemistry encompasses a wide range of topics, and this book aims to cover all the critical aspects, starting with the fundamental concepts of chemistry and progressing to the more complex applications in pharmaceutical development. The text will systematically explore the structure, properties, and synthesis of biologically active compounds, offering detailed explanations of how these compounds interact with biological systems at the molecular level. It will cover the mechanisms by which drugs act in the human body and the factors affecting their efficacy and safety, providing a thorough grounding in the methods used for the design, synthesis, and optimization of drug candidates.

The book also intends to cover modern technological advancements in drug discovery, including computational methods for drug design, and the role of biomarkers in drug development. It will discuss the ethical, regulatory, and economic aspects that play crucial roles in the pharmaceutical industry, preparing readers to navigate the complexities of the field. Additionally, the text will provide practical insights into the challenges and strategies involved in the formulation and delivery of drugs, including the development of resistant forms and the consideration of patient-specific factors. The book will also address the global impact of pharmaceutical chemistry, discussing both global health challenges and the role of pharmacists as healthcare providers and therapeutic consultants.

The book is intended for a diverse audience, including students of pharmacy and medicinal chemistry, pharmaceutical science researchers, practicing pharmacists, and other healthcare professionals involved in drug therapy. It is also suitable for professionals in the pharmaceutical industry, from those involved in drug design and development to those focusing on regulatory affairs and drug approval processes. The book aims to serve as both an educational resource for students and a reference for professionals, providing updates on the latest research and developments in the field. This dual focus makes it an essential addition to academic libraries and pharmaceutical research institutions, as well as a valuable resource for personal and professional development in the pharmaceutical and healthcare sectors.

Chapter

INTRODUCTION TO PHARMACEUTICAL CHEMISTRY

1

Contents

Introduction

A branch of chemistry and pharmacology is known as medicinal or pharmaceutical chemistry. The study of medicinal chemistry aims to understand the chemical characteristics of pharmaceuticals as well as their synthesis and manufacture. Organic chemistry is generally thought of as having a specialization in medicinal chemistry. Drug development is a part of the study of pharmaceutical chemistry. This covers the development, delivery, absorption, metabolism, and other aspects of drugs. Pharmacology, pharmacokinetics, pharmacodynamics, and biomedical analysis are all included. Work in pharmaceutical chemistry is typically conducted in a lab environment.

Pharmaceutical chemistry includes drug chemistry, pharmacology, metabolism, quality control, and methods for treating and curing illnesses. Many students studying pharmaceutical chemistry will go on to work in a lab. Careers in drug development, biotechnology, pharmaceutical firms, research facilities, and other fields can be attained through a degree in pharmaceutical chemistry. Students can improve the speed at which new medications are delivered, contribute to the development of life-saving treatments, and assist others by studying pharmaceutical chemistry. Other fields of study like drug metabolism, pharmacokinetics, and pharmacodynamics are also included in pharmaceutical chemistry. These are crucial to understanding how drugs affect the body.

Orientation and Directional Terms

Term	Definition	Illustration
Pharmacokinetics	Branch of pharmacology dedicated to describing how the body affects a specific substance after administration. The substances of interest include any chemical xenobiotics such as pharmaceutical drugs, pesticides, food additives, cosmetics, etc.	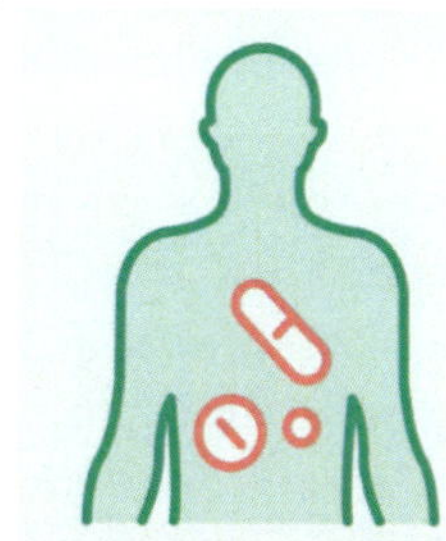
Pharmacodynamics	The study of the biochemical and physiologic effects of drugs. The effects can include those manifested within animals, microorganisms, or combinations of organisms.	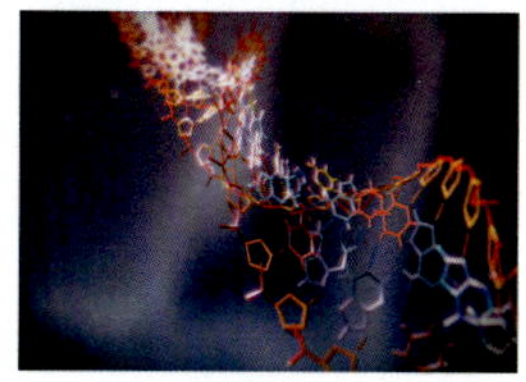
Drug metabolism	The metabolic breakdown of drugs by living organisms, usually through specialized enzymatic systems.	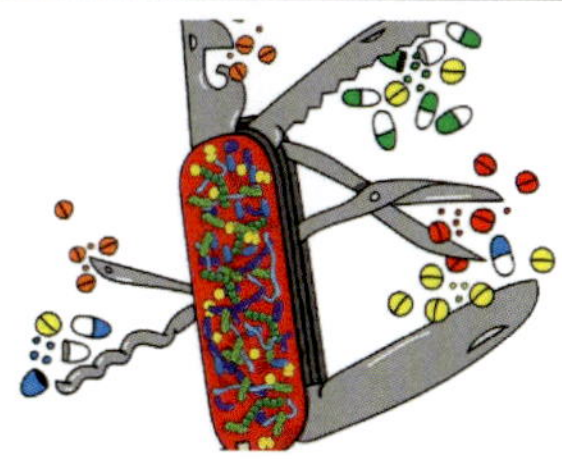
Nuclear chemistry	The sub-field of chemistry dealing with radioactivity, nuclear processes, and transformations in the nuclei of atoms, such as nuclear transmutation and nuclear properties.	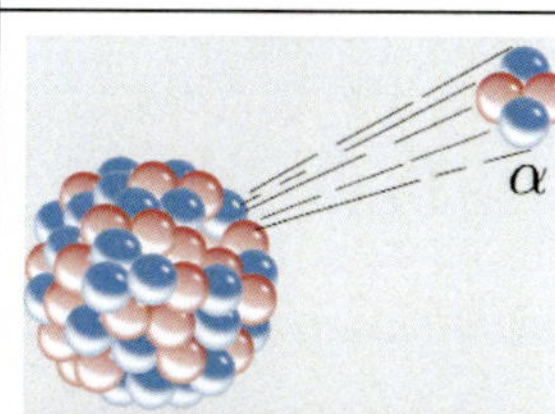
Chemotherapy	A type of cancer treatment that uses one or more anti-cancer drugs as part of a standardized chemotherapy regimen. Chemotherapy may be given with a curative intent or it may aim to prolong life or to reduce symptoms.	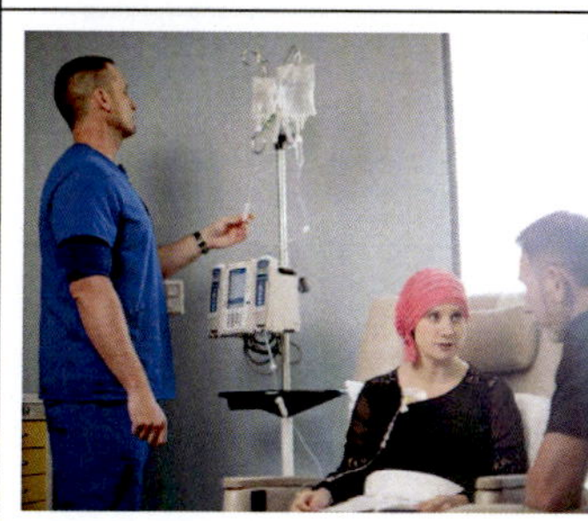

1.1. Definition and Scope of Pharmaceutical Chemistry

The creation of medications and their synthesis are the main topics of pharmaceutical (medical) chemistry. The objective is to acquire novel chemical compounds that may facilitate the identification of novel pharmaceuticals or enhance the existing drug structures, consequently broadening the range of chemical drugs. While organic chemistry is important, only highly skilled pharmaceutical chemists can function well in an extremely interdisciplinary setting and collaborate with researchers in other fields, including toxicology, molecular biology, structural biology, pharmacology, physical chemistry, biochemistry, pharmacokinetics, pharmaceutical technology, and pharmacology.

Not long after World War II, the term "pharmaceutical" chemistry made its literary debut. All chemical compound's biological activity could be expressed using quantifiable molecular properties (g. $_{p}A_2$, EC_{50}, and IC_{50}) thanks to advancements in molecular pharmacology. Subsequently, scientists started methodically creating new drugs and started referring to this process as drug design. Structure-activity relationships, or SARs, and quantitative SARs, or QSARs, are studies of the relationship between a molecule's chemical structure and biological activity. These studies were made possible by the introduction of computer technology and programming. Although the observation of chance or adverse effects still plays a significant role in the development of new drugs, these rational methods are preferred these days for designing new drugs.

In the years that have followed, radioactive drug and metabolite labeling has significantly sped up the process of developing new medications by allowing researchers to pinpoint novel therapeutic targets. Pharmacokinetics—the study of how a drug and its metabolites behave in the body—and pharmacodynamics—the study of how drugs work at the molecular level—were completely transformed by the advent of molecular biology. The breadth and application of pharmaceutical chemistry have been greatly increased by developments in the analytical assessment of novel molecules, computer technology, and their applications in molecular modeling techniques. These developments have also raised the possibility of producing a wider variety of novel drugs with novel therapeutic potential. New molecules with an ever-increasing structural diversity have been developed at the start of the twenty-first century by pharmaceutical (medical) chemistry. Pharmaceutical chemists concentrate on the creation of altered peptides and proteins, biological agents (such as) in addition to natural products and tiny synthetic ligands. G. synthetic vaccines, multifunctional molecular complexes, and monoclonal antibodies.

1.1.1. Demystifying a Rapidly Evolving Discipline

Over the past few decades, medicinal chemistry has advanced quickly as a scientific field. The early understanding of medicinal chemistry as "synthesizing bioactive molecules" has become the connecting link between several related scientific disciplines, made possible by technological advancement.

1.1.1.1. Past

The idea that chemicals could be used to treat illnesses dates back to ancient times, even though the term "medical chemistry" was first used after World War II. Without any explanation for how they could so magically cure the body, ancient people observed the therapeutic effects of some herbs, which we now know contain natural products with medicinal properties. Opium was used by the Sumerians as early as 2100 BCE. 3 Since 3000 BCE, fevers have been treated with the ancient Chinese herb ma huang, or ephedra. To create chemical medicines during the Renaissance, Paracelsus pushed the early alchemists to identify the chemical essence, particularly for inorganic components like antimony and mercury, which gave rise to the rudimentary concept of "active ingredients.". Before Louis XIV's antimony purge healed him of his chronic digestive issues, the French courts had forbidden the use of chemistry in medicine. A pivotal moment in the development of medicinal chemistry was the Second World War. Following World War II, the biological activity of a compound could be expressed as measurable molecular properties thanks to advances in our understanding of pharmacology at the molecular level. An IC50, for instance, shows how well a drug inhibits a target. When rational drug design first emerged, scientists would progressively alter different molecular components and track how these modifications affected the molecules' biological properties. This made it possible for researchers to identify the essential structural components of a molecule that support its biological activity. Later on, this assay gave rise to the well-known and educational structure-activity relationship studies, which are still widely used in drug discovery and development processes today and are frequently mistaken for medicinal chemistry itself.

1.1.1.2. Present

In addition to creating new bioactive compounds, medicinal chemists nowadays are also enhancing already-available medications. The process involves refining the structure and consequently, the properties of molecules to enhance their interactions with target(s), metabolism, toxicities, and drug delivery dynamics. The end result is the development of selective medicines with minimal side effects. The biological target of a compound can be clarified thanks to our expanding knowledge of the different biological pathways. We can now better understand how drugs enter, circulate through, and leave the human body thanks to the development of analytical techniques. Automated robotic advancement and microliter-scale reactions are combined in the emergence of high-throughput screens to enable the screening of hundreds of thousands of compounds with incredibly small sample sizes. By doing this, we are able to increase the drug screening process's scientific and financial efficiency and expand the pool of possible candidates. The drug bedaquiline, which was just approved to treat multidrug-resistant tuberculosis, was initially found in a high-throughput screen.

We now have access to biologics, which were previously thought to be extremely complex medications, in our pool of possible drug candidates, rather than just small molecules. These consist of biological probes and linkers, antibody-drug conjugates, and protein therapy, among others. Multi-protein complexes or interactions have also been shown to be necessary for certain pathologies. A new frontier in medicinal chemistry has emerged in these situations: the development of novel classes of molecules that either facilitate or inhibit the formation of multi-protein complexes. Aside from using chemical probes to investigate biochemically significant processes, alternative approaches like using natural product biosynthesis give us access to molecules that are relevant to medicine and are produced by a variety of organisms. Chemical mixing is no longer the only method used by medicinal chemists to create new medications. By using nature's power, they are producing new compounds through chemoenzymatic synthesis. Medicinal chemistry has developed into the hub of a wide range of related scientific disciplines, even though the majority of people still view it as the design and synthesis of biologically active molecules. Joining the communities of analytical, computational, biochemical, molecular, cell, structural, microbiological, pharmacological, toxicological, and translational medicine specialists is the responsibility of medicinal chemists. They assign the medicinal chemistry orchestra to work together to create a harmonious composition that creates answers for health-related issues.

While chemists have been a part of history, there are now many different subfields in chemistry, including theoretical, analytical, material, biological, physical, and nuclear chemistry. All these can produce active molecules, but only a medicinal chemist can turn an active ingredient into a medication (Garneau-Tsodikova). To proceed with the development of a drug product from a molecule exhibiting in vitro activity, medicinal chemists possess supplementary training and expertise (Garcia). In fact, the inventiveness and inventiveness of scientists have been stimulated by the development of new technologies, which have enabled the realization of previously unthinkable possibilities. Nonetheless, it is important to remember that, even in the age of omics, a molecule's structure—which is designed and synthesized—is ultimately what determines its activity, side effects, and attrition—or lack thereof—in clinical states (Bottegoni). Experts from a variety of disciplines are united by medicinal chemistry to fight for the welfare of humans. Although there are still problems and opportunities for development, we work together and with inventiveness to find solutions. For example, it can be challenging to target a particular molecule due to the intricate network of interconnected biological pathways in human biology, which can lead to undesired off-target effects. Nevertheless, even these unintended consequences may help in the creation of novel treatments. Researchers noticed a common side effect, which was later used to treat erectile dysfunction in patients, even though the original purpose of Viagra was to control blood pressure. Furthermore, the advancement of computational chemistry has produced effective medications like Gleevec, a treatment for a particular kind of leukemia, and has given essential direction to rational drug design. Even so, there aren't many of these cases, so more and better computer models must be created.

1.1.1.3. Future

Emerging generations are inspired to innovate and work together by the challenges in medicinal chemistry. The line separating the possible from the impossible has become more hazy with the rate of technological advancements in this day and age. We work to reduce undesired side effects as our understanding of biology grows. Furthermore, the field of personalized medicine will persist in its leadership role in drug development, offering customized care to patients based on their unique biological makeup. In the fields of cancer and infectious diseases, this approach is still in its infancy but has generated a lot of interest in joint ventures. We will be able to give each patient individualized care in other areas and the best possible outcome for that particular patient. To reduce the workload for medicinal chemists and increase synthesis efficiency and cost, automated synthesis and purification are also in the works. The discovery of novel therapeutic targets, which is still desperately needed and will be crucial to the direction of medicinal chemistry, cannot be overlooked. The field of medicinal chemistry relies heavily on data and is a precise science. The precision of earlier discoveries, which have given modern medicinal chemists access to a wealth of invaluable data and databases as a strong basis for advancement, is essential for producing excellent medicinal chemistry. To paint the right picture, a medicinal chemist must combine a subtle blend of knowledge, experimental learning, inventiveness, intuition, audacity, and serendipity (Jung and Radi). In search of improving our quality of life, medicinal chemistry is a treasure hunt and an adventure. Frequently, the hidden gem is what's inside the box. Medicinal chemists are the front-line soldiers with an optimistic outlook, and medicinal chemistry is hope for those battling diseases (Arai).

1.1.2. Classification of Drugs Based on Chemical Structure and Therapeutic Use

Chemistry is incredibly important to daily living. Even though we occasionally have a tendency to ignore them, the concepts of chemistry have greatly improved human life. Chemicals are used to process all textiles. Our clothing—some of which are entirely synthetic—involves dyes, fibers, chemicals, and processes. Think about hygiene. We have an abundance of detergents, soaps, bleaches, toothpaste varieties, etc., in our home. Furthermore, a number of chemicals are present in even the food that we eat on a daily basis. Fuels, explosives, rocket propellants, building materials, electronic materials, etc., are all regarded as chemicals. The impact of chemistry on daily life is so great that it is easy to forget that chemicals are around us all the time, that humans are magnificent chemical beings, and that chemicals govern every action. People use medications, which are once more chemicals, to treat illnesses and diseases. Drugs are substances with a low molecular mass (~100 to 500u) that, when ingested, change or affect the physiology of a living system. The way these medications interact with macromolecular targets results in a biological response. We use them as medicines for disease diagnosis, prevention, and treatment if the biological response is beneficial and therapeutic. Drugs that are legally given by doctors in very small doses when necessary are known as medicines. Higher dosages have the potential to be poisonous and deadly. To elicit the necessary biological response, the majority of these interact with the nervous system, primarily the brain. Chemotherapy is the term for the application of chemicals for medical purposes. Drugs are categorized according to their chemical structure, molecular targets, pharmacological effect, and drug action. To guarantee that the medications are prescribed and used effectively, this classification is carried out.

Let's discuss each of these classifications in detail:

1. **Based on their Pharmacological Effect:** Pharmacological effect refers to the effect that the drug has on the body. Based on this effect, drugs are classified into various categories:

i **Analgesics**: Medications known as analgesics reduce pain without making you unconscious. They are divided into two additional groups: non-narcotic analgesics (e.g., ibuprofen, acetaminophen) and opioid analgesics (e.g., codeine, morphine).

ii. **Antacids:** Antacids are drugs that neutralize stomach acid and relieve heartburn, acid indigestion, and upset stomach. Examples include calcium carbonate, magnesium hydroxide, and aluminum hydroxide.

iii. **Anti-anxiety drugs:** Anti-anxiety drugs, also known as anxiolytics, are drugs that reduce anxiety and nervousness. Examples include diazepam, lorazepam, and alprazolam.

iv. **Antibiotics:** Antibiotics are drugs that fight bacterial infections. Examples include penicillin, tetracycline, and erythromycin.

v. **Antidepressants:** Antidepressants are drugs that treat depression and other mood disorders. Examples include fluoxetine, sertraline, and paroxetine.

vi. **Antihistamines:** Antihistamines are medications that prevent the effects of histamine, which is a substance the body releases in reaction to allergens. They are applied to alleviate allergy symptoms, including itching and sneezing. Loratadine, cetirizine, and diphenhydramine are a few examples.

vii. **Anti-inflammatory drugs:** Anti-inflammatory drugs are drugs that reduce inflammation and swelling. They are used to treat conditions such as arthritis and asthma. Examples include aspirin, ibuprofen, and naproxen.

viii. **Antipsychotics**: Antipsychotics are drugs that treat psychotic disorders such as schizophrenia. Examples include haloperidol, chlorpromazine, and clozapine.

ix. **Bronchodilators:** Drugs known as bronchodilators ease breathing by relaxing the muscles surrounding the lungs' airways. They are employed in the management of ailments like chronic obstructive pulmonary disease (COPD) and asthma. Ipratropium, salmeterol, and albuterol are a few examples.

2. **Based on their Drug Action:** Drug action refers to how a drug works in the body to produce a therapeutic effect. Based on this action, drugs are classified into the following categories:

i. **Agonists:** Agonists are drugs that activate receptors in the body and produce a therapeutic effect. Examples include morphine (an opioid agonist) and albuterol (a beta-2 agonist).

ii. **Antagonists:** Antagonists are drugs that block the action of agonists. Examples include naloxone (an opioid antagonist) and flumazenil (a benzodiazepine antagonist).

iii. **Enzyme inhibitors:** Medication called an enzyme inhibitor prevents the body's enzymes from doing their job. Acetylcholinesterase inhibitors, which are used to treat Alzheimer's disease, and angiotensin-converting enzyme (ACE) inhibitors, which are used to treat hypertension, are two examples.

iv. **Ion channel blockers:** Ion channel blockers are medications that prevent ions from entering the body through ion channels. Calcium channel blockers, which are used to treat hypertension, and sodium channel blockers, which are used to treat epilepsy, are two examples.

3. **Based On Chemical Structure:** Chemical structure-based drug classification is

the categorization of drugs according to their chemical makeup and structure. This categorization scheme is especially helpful in comprehending the chemical and physical characteristics of medications, in addition to their modes of action and possible adverse effects.

Here are some common classes of drugs based on their chemical structure:

i. **Alcohols:** Compounds with a hydroxyl (-OH) group bonded to a carbon atom are known as alcohols. The main component of alcoholic drinks, ethanol, is one type of alcohol that is used in medicine as an antiseptic and solvent.

ii. **Amines:** Amines are compounds that contain a nitrogen atom that is bonded to one or more carbon atoms. Many drugs, including antidepressants, antihistamines, and muscle relaxants, are amines.

iii. **Carboxylic acids:** Carboxylic acids are compounds that contain a carboxyl (-COOH) group attached to a carbon atom. Aspirin, a popular pain reliever and anti-inflammatory drug, is an example of a carboxylic acid.

iv. **Esters:** Esters are compounds that are formed when an alcohol reacts with a carboxylic acid. Many drugs, including aspirin, are esters.

v. **Phenols**: Phenols are compounds that contain a hydroxyl (-OH) group attached to an aromatic ring. Many drugs, including antiseptics, disinfectants, and anesthetics, are phenols.

4. **Base on Molecular Targets:** Drugs are categorized according to how they specifically interact with target molecules in the body, such as enzymes, ion channels, and receptors, in a process known as molecular targets drug classification. Comprehending these interplays can aid in the creation of novel pharmaceuticals as well as the detection of possible drug interactions and adverse effects. G protein-coupled receptor (GPCR) agonists and antagonists: GPCRs are a family of cell surface receptors that mediate numerous physiological responses in the body, such as neurotransmission, hormone secretion, and immune response. These are some of the commonly recognized categories of drugs based on molecular targets. GPCR-inhibiting or -activating medications can have important therapeutic effects, such as reducing inflammation or relieving pain. GPCR agonists include drugs like morphine, which is used to treat severe pain, and epinephrine, which is used to treat asthma. GPCR antagonists include, for example, antihistamines (used to treat allergies) and beta blockers (used to

treat hypertension). Enzyme inhibitors: Enzymes are biochemical reaction catalysts in the body, and they have the ability to stop or alter the progression of certain diseases. There are two types of enzyme inhibitors: reversible inhibitors and irreversible inhibitors. Reversible inhibitors can bind to the enzyme non-covalently and competitively or non-competitively, whereas irreversible inhibitors bind covalently. Protease inhibitors, which are used to treat HIV, and acetylcholinesterase inhibitors, which are used to treat Alzheimer's disease, are two examples of enzyme inhibitors.

1.1.3. Importance of Pharmaceutical Chemistry in Healthcare

Since pharmaceutical chemistry is the foundation for drug discovery, development, and optimization, it plays a crucial role in the healthcare industry. The design, synthesis, characterization, and analysis of compounds with potential therapeutic value are the fundamental concerns of pharmaceutical chemistry. Its capacity to lay the groundwork for the development of novel medications that treat illnesses and enhance patient outcomes accounts for its significance in the healthcare industry. Finding new drug candidates is one of pharmaceutical chemistry's main contributions to medicine. Pharmaceutical chemists find and create compounds with the desired biological activity by using chemical principles and techniques. To modify disease pathways, this process entails comprehending the molecular mechanisms underlying those pathways and creating molecules that can interact with particular targets. Pharmaceutical chemistry increases the number of treatments for a variety of illnesses, fills in gaps in the medical field, and improves patient care by finding new drug candidates.

Moreover, pharmaceutical chemistry directs the optimization of lead compounds into secure and efficient drugs, which is a critical aspect of drug development. Pharmacokinetic and pharmacodynamic properties of candidate drugs are assessed by pharmaceutical chemists in collaboration with experts from other fields, including formulation science, toxicology, and pharmacology. Pharmaceutical chemistry makes sure that drugs have the intended therapeutic effects while minimizing side effects by optimizing parameters like potency, selectivity, bioavailability, and metabolic stability. To turn promising compounds into pharmaceuticals with significant clinical value, an iterative approach to drug optimization is necessary. Furthermore, the development of personalized medicine—which adjusts medical interventions to the unique needs of each patient—is facilitated by advances in pharmaceutical chemistry. Pharmaceutical chemists design medications that are more effective and better tolerated by particular patient populations through the use of precision medicine techniques and targeted therapies. Pharmaceutical chemistry facilitates the development of customized treatment regimens that maximize therapeutic outcomes and reduce the risk of adverse reactions by taking into account variables like genetic variability, biomarker expression, and disease heterogeneity. Furthermore, the quality, safety, and effectiveness of pharmaceutical products are greatly dependent on pharmaceutical chemistry. Pharmaceutical chemists ensure that drug substances and formulations are potent, pure, and identified through exacting analytical techniques and quality control procedures. Pharmaceutical chemistry protects public health and fosters patient confidence in pharmaceutical products by following quality assurance procedures and regulatory standards.

1.2. Drug Discovery and Development Process

Any chemical that has an impact on how living things function or how organisms (like bacteria, fungi, and viruses) infect them is considered a drug. All facets of drugs in medicine, such as their mode of action, physical and chemical characteristics, metabolism, therapeutics, and toxicity, are covered by pharmacology, the science of drugs. Drug discovery is a complex process that involves finding and creating new drugs to treat illnesses and enhance human health. Biology, chemistry, pharmacology, and computational sciences are just a few of the scientific disciplines that are integrated in this multidisciplinary approach. The main objective of drug discovery is to find molecules, or "drug candidates," that have therapeutic effects against particular targets or diseases while limiting the possibility of adverse effects. The first step in the procedure is usually target identification, in which scientists identify chemicals, proteins, or biological pathways linked to a specific illness. This may entail looking into the causes of diseases, researching genetics, or using cutting-edge imaging methods to find possible intervention targets. Target validation is the next stage after a target has been identified, when scientists verify that modifying the target's activity can produce the intended therapeutic effect. This frequently entails conducting studies both in vivo and in vitro with cell cultures, animal models, and occasionally human tissues.

The drug discovery process advances to the lead discovery and optimization stage after target validation. Large libraries of synthetic compounds, natural products, or small molecules are screened by researchers to find those that may interact with the target and change its activity. Computational modeling, virtual screening techniques, and high-throughput screening technologies all contribute to reducing the number of potential candidates. The potency, selectivity, and pharmacokinetic qualities of promising lead compounds are then further optimized via medicinal chemistry techniques to lower toxicity. Following optimization, lead compounds are put through preclinical testing in animal models to evaluate their pharmacokinetics, safety, and effectiveness. To assess the compound's overall therapeutic potential, its capacity to reach the target site in the body, and its potential for toxicity, extensive testing is required at this stage. Preclinical study data are used to guide decisions about whether to move forward with human clinical trials.

Phases of clinical trials are carried out to assess the drug candidate's safety, effectiveness, and dosage in human subjects. Phase II and III trials involve larger patient groups to assess efficacy and further evaluate safety, while Phase I trials primarily focus on safety and pharmacokinetics in a small group of healthy volunteers. Regulatory bodies closely monitor clinical trials to guarantee adherence to ethical principles and protect participants' welfare. Following the successful conclusion of clinical trials, the drug candidate is submitted for regulatory approval. To evaluate the safety and effectiveness of a drug, regulatory bodies such as the European Medicines Agency (EMA) in Europe or the Food and Drug Administration (FDA) in the United States examine the accumulated data. The medication can then be marketed and made accessible to patients if it is approved. Despite technological advancements and our growing understanding of biological systems, the drug discovery process in the medical, biotech, and pharmacological domains is all too frequently a protracted, costly, challenging, and ineffective one. Prior to conducting clinical trials, a compound will start the drug development process once testing has demonstrated its value. Peira lowers the expenses related to the drug discovery process's research and development.

Drug discovery and design requires the identification of candidates, synthesis, characterization, screening, and assays for therapeutic efficacy.

The five key steps of the drug discovery process:

1. **Research & Early Development:** The basic research stage of the drug development process is the first one. In this stage, scientists work to identify the fundamental cause or mechanism of a particular illness. Scholars search for novel chemical or molecular entities that exhibit encouraging activity against a specific biological target that is believed to be significant for the illness. At this point, there is no focus on the identified entities' other characteristics (such as toxicity, safety, etc.) or their effects on human metabolism.
2. **Preclinical Research:** Before clinical trials, or testing on humans, can begin, preclinical research must be finished. Important data is gathered on safety, iterative testing, and feasibility during this phase. Finding a product's ultimate safety profile is the primary objective of preclinical research. Products could be medications, gene therapy treatments, or brand-new or improved medical devices.

   Preclinical research can take many forms for any given class of product. Animal testing may be used to test drugs for pharmacodynamic, pharmacokinetic, ADME, and toxicity. Tests conducted in vivo as well as in vitro are usually carried out.
3. **Chemical & Pharmaceutical Development:** The goal of the chemical and pharmaceutical development phase is to create a high-quality product and manufacturing process that will reliably yield the desired product performance. The design space, specifications, and manufacturing controls are established with the help of scientific understanding provided by the data and knowledge gathered from studies and manufacturing experience.
4. **Clinical Research:** Clinical trials are carried out during this stage to gather information on the safety and effectiveness of novel medications. Only after the product's non-clinical safety and quality have been sufficiently established, and the product has received approval from the relevant health authority, can these trials begin. The number of patients is usually increased as evidence of safety and efficacy is obtained. Clinical trials can range in size from single-center studies conducted in a single nation to multi-center trials conducted

in several nations. Following the completion of the clinical trials, the medication will be submitted for regulatory approval, possibly to the European Medicines Agency or the US Food and Drug Administration.

5. **Chemical & Pharmaceutical Production:** A full-scale manufacturing facility will be constructed based on the scientific knowledge obtained during the chemical and pharmaceutical development phase of a new drug's approval by regulatory bodies like the US Food and Drug Administration.

1.2.1. Drug Development

To determine which drug is most effective, the drug development process entails extensive testing and optimization of specific compounds. To investigate metabolism and create a product that is safe and complies with all legal requirements, testing is conducted both in vivo (on animals) and in vitro (on cells). The two main reasons why drugs fail in clinical practice are largely to blame. Two reasons exist for this: first, they should function properly; second, they should be safe. Identifying a target and validating the solution are the two most crucial steps in the drug invention process. Since this protein receptor might be linked to a medical condition, it's critical to understand the disease's cellular, molecular, and genetic causes. The role the target plays in the disease process is the next step to be taken after it has been identified. To determine which compound interacts with the target and either neutralizes or slows down the disease process, the target is tested against a variety of known and novel compounds.

1.2.1.1. Stages of Drug Development

1. Drug Invention
2. Product Characterization
3. Formulation& development
4. Pharmacokinetics and Drug Disposition
5. Preclinical Toxicology Testing and IND Application
6. Bioanalytical Testing
8. Regulatory review
9. Marketing the product or drug
10. Post-marketing monitoring (phase-IV) trials

1. **Drug Invention:** Phenotypic screens as a revitalized approach to drug discovery: Phenotypic-based screening techniques were the cornerstone of pharmaceutical drug discovery long before molecular target-based drug discovery gained popularity. Molecular target-based drug screening has emerged as the predominant paradigm for drug discovery in the pharmaceutical industry and academic translational research centers during the last 25 years. Particular biological delivery: The biologicals era has begun. Numerous novel biological products, including antibodies and their derivatives, siRNA, cytokines, enzymes, and other therapeutic peptides, are currently being developed, even though new chemical entities are still being created and successfully brought to market. In 2011, biological products accounted for one-

third of all new therapeutic products, as opposed to chemical derivatives. Click chemistry is having a growing impact on drug discovery because it is a modular approach that only employs the most dependable and practical chemical transformations. It is finding more and more uses in all areas of drug discovery, from combinatorial chemistry and target-templated in situ chemistry for lead discovery to proteomics and DNA research through the use of bio conjugation reactions. The 1, 2, 3-triazole formation from azides and terminal acetylenes catalyzed by copper (I) is a highly potent linking reaction because of its complete specificity, high degree of reliability, and reactant biocompatibility. Through hydrogen bonds and dipole interactions, the triazole products associate with biological targets more easily than they would with merely being passive linkers.

Targeting drug resistance in cancer-initiating cells is a potential a path to next-generation cancer treatments. Drug resistance in oncology is a factor in treatment failure and relapse of various tumor types. A small number of "cancer-initiating cells," which are able to self-renew and divide asymmetrically, together with cells at different stages of differentiation are present in cancers and are responsible for the genesis of tumors. Cells that cause cancer exhibit a variety of self-defense mechanisms, nearly all of which involve drug resistance. Various molecular pathways and markers found in this malignant subpopulation are being used as targets for monoclonal antibodies and new compounds, which may be taken in addition to traditional medications. These treatments may eradicate drug-resistant cancer-initiating cells, resulting in cancer patients' remission or complete recovery. A novel approach to drug development is the biomarker-guided repurposing of chemotherapeutic drugs for cancer therapy. This research approach, also referred to as drug repositioning or repurposing, offers a quicker route to clinical trials. Our approach to the standard drug repurposing strategy, which we review here, has been modified by us. Specifically, we now concentrate on finding new cancer indications for chemotherapeutic anti-cancer drugs that have already received approval, rather than examining target-promiscuous noncancer drugs for potential anti-cancer activity. This strategy's clinical application often starts with phase II clinical trials, which involve patients who have already received treatment. Such testing must be based on predictive biomarkers because the response rates to any non-standard chemotherapeutic drug will be relatively low in such a patient cohort. This review outlines our approach to biomarker-guided chemotherapeutic drug repurposing for cancer therapy, using Top1 as a potential predictive biomarker and the repurposing of inhibitors of topoisomerase I (Top1) as a case study.

Oncoplastic surgery: For early-stage breast cancers, breast-conserving surgery (lumpectomy or partial mastectomy) is frequently utilized. On the other hand, it can cause breasts of varying shapes and/or sizes in some women. It might not even be feasible for larger tumors; in that case, a mastectomy might be required. As a solution to this issue, some physicians perform oncoplastic surgery, which combines plastic surgery and cancer surgery techniques. To achieve greater symmetry, this usually entails reshaping the breast during the initial surgery and may even require surgery on the other breast. Since this method is still relatively new, not all physicians feel at ease using it.

Potential Use of Scorpion Peptides in the Development of New Drugs: A number of peptides found in scorpion fluids demonstrated a wide range of biological activities with high site specificity. Numerous studies described their strong antimicrobial properties and demonstrated their ability to alter a range of biological processes implicated in immunological, neurological, cardiovascular, and neoplastic disorders. Scorpion-derived peptides are thought to have essential structural and functional diversity, making them potential candidates for novel targeted drug development.

2. **Product Characterization:** Any novel drug molecule that exhibits potential therapeutic activity is identified by its size, shape, strength, weakness, application, toxicity, and biological activity. The earliest phases of pharmacological research are useful for defining the compound's mode of action.

3. **Formulation and Development:** To create a bioavailable, stable, and ideal dosage form for a particular administration route, the physicochemical properties of Active Pharmaceutical Ingredients (APIs) are characterized during the pharmaceutical formulation stage of drug development. The following factors are assessed in preformulation studies:

i. Solubility in different media and solvents

ii. Dissolution of the active pharmaceutical ingredient (API)

iii. Accelerated Stability Services under various conditions

iv. Solid state properties (polymorphs, particle size, particle shape etc.)

v. Formulation Services and Capabilities:

vi. Formulation development of new chemical entities (NCE)

vii. Optimization of existing formulations

viii. Process development for selected dosage forms

ix. Novel formulations for improved delivery of existing dosage forms

x. Controlled release and sustained release formulations

xi. Self-emulsifying drug delivery systems

xii. Colloidal drug delivery systems

xiii. Sub-micron and nano-emulsions

4. **Pharmacokinetics and Drug Disposition:** Pharmacokinetics studies provide useful data for formulation scientists. These studies provide data on parameters like C_{max}, T_{max}, A.U.C, etc.

5. **Preclinical Toxicology Testing and IND Application:** A new compound's toxicity must be tested as part of the drug development process. The in vivo exposure of experimental animals, in vitro studies utilizing cells, and accidental exposure to substances are methods used to observe a substance's toxicity. The no observed adverse effect level can be calculated with the aid of this preclinical toxicity testing. which are required to start the investigational product's clinical evaluation. A typical toxicology profile includes genetic toxicology, acute and subchronic toxicology, reproductive and developmental toxicity, absorption, distribution, metabolism, and excretion (ADME) studies, and a carcinogenic potential assessment.

6. **Bioanalytical Testing:** Bioanalytical Testing supports most of the other activities related to the drug development process. This work is used for proper characterization of the drug molecule, developing optimal methods.

7. **Regulatory Review:** After completion of clinical trials data obtained in clinical trials shows whether there is evidence to support the safety and efficacy of the drug in treating the disease condition. At this stage, the data collected is submitted to the relevant regulatory authorities to obtain approval to market the drug in their jurisdictions.

8. **Marketing the Product:** The last stage in the drug development process is the marketing of the product. Once it has been approved by regulatory authorities, the drug manufacturers submit authorization applications in each country or territory

where they want to sell their product.

9. **Post-Marketing Monitoring (Phase-IV) Trials:** To evaluate a drug's safety in the market, post-marketing trials are conducted. This could involve quality-of-life research, cost-effectiveness analyzes of comparative trials, and reporting and examination of the frequency and severity of uncommon adverse reactions.

1.3. Pharmaceutical Analysis and Techniques

Within the field of analytical chemistry, pharmaceutical analysis focuses on the characterization, quality assurance, and control of pharmaceutical products. It includes a broad range of approaches and procedures used to guarantee the efficacy, safety, and conformity of medications and pharmaceutical formulations with legal requirements. Evaluating active pharmaceutical ingredients (APIs), excipients, and completed dosage forms for identity, purity, potency, and stability is the main objective of pharmaceutical analysis. This process is carried out at every stage of the drug development life cycle, from pre-formulation studies to post-marketing surveillance. Drug characterization, which entails the identification and measurement of the chemical components contained in pharmaceutical formulations, is one of the core areas of pharmaceutical analysis. For this, methods like mass spectrometry, chromatography (HPLC, GC), and spectroscopy (UV-Vis, IR, NMR) are frequently employed. With the aid of these techniques, analysts can identify contaminants and breakdown products in addition to figuring out the concentration, molecular weight, and chemical makeup of the active compounds. Quality assurance (QA) and control (QC) are important components of pharmaceutical analysis. In quality control (QC), raw materials, in-process samples, and final products are tested to make sure they adhere to regulatory standards and specified specifications. Contrarily, quality assurance (QA) entails putting policies and processes in place to preserve and enhance the quality of pharmaceutical products throughout their existence. This entails adhering to Good Manufacturing Practices (GMP) and Good Laboratory Practices (GLP), developing reliable analytical methods, and validating analytical procedures. Additionally, pharmaceutical analysis is essential to the formulation and development of drugs. Through the evaluation of APIs and excipients' physical and chemical characteristics, scientists can optimize formulation parameters like solubility, stability, and bioavailability. This makes it more likely that the finished dosage form will safely and effectively produce the intended therapeutic effect. Furthermore, analytical methods like rheology, particle size analysis, and dissolution testing are used to assess how well pharmaceutical formulations work in different scenarios.

Pharmaceutical analysis is a subfield of practical chemistry that deals with the identification, quantification, and purification of substances as well as the separation of mixture or solution components and the structural analysis of chemical compounds. The substance can come in any dosage form and be either a single compound or a mixture of compounds. Animals, plants, microbes, minerals, and a variety of synthetic materials are used as pharmaceuticals. The sample that needs to be examined is referred to as an analyze. It can be further divided into submicro (0.0001 g to 0.001 g), ultramicro (below 10–4 g), macro (0.1 g or more), semi micro (0.01 g to 0.1 g), micro (0.001 g to 0.01 g), and trace analysis (100 to 10000 ppm) depending on its size. The semi-micro analysis is the most often utilized of all.

1.3.1. Titrimetric Techniques

The middle of the 18th century is when the titrimetric analysis method first emerged. The volumetric method, which is where the term "titration" originated, was created in 1835 by Gay-Lussac. Despite the assay method's age, there are indications of some modernization, i.e., spreading the use of non-aqueous titration, extending the range of acids and bases to which titrimetric methods can be applied, and increasing the precision of the methods through the use of potentiometric end point detection. Titrimetric techniques have proven useful in kinetic measurements, which are then used to determine reaction rates, thanks to the advancement of functional group analysis procedures. These methods offer numerous benefits, such as reduced labor and time requirements, exceptional precision, and the elimination of the need for reference standards. The concentrations of captopril, albendozole, and gabapentin in commercial dosage forms have previously been determined using titrimetric techniques. The non-aqueous titration method was used to measure sparfloxacin. Titrimetry is not only used to estimate drugs but it has also been used in the past to estimate pharmaceutical degradation products.

1.3.2. Chromatographic Techniques

1.3.2.1. Thin Layer Chromatography

The field of pharmaceutical analysis finds extensive use for this technique, despite its age. Typically, a glass, plastic, or aluminum support is used in thin layer chromatography, where a solid phase called the adsorbent is applied in a thin layer. This kind of chromatographic separation is dependent on a number of factors for its efficiency. To achieve a significant difference in the rate of elution, the adsorbent must first exhibit extreme selectivity toward the substances that need to be separated. Adsorbents can have varying degrees of adsorption strength, which can affect how well a mixture separates. The unique benefits of thin layer chromatography, including its low cost, high sample loading capacity, flexible sample distinction, extensive selection of mobile phases, and minimal sample clean-up, make it a popular technique for the analysis of a wide range of organic and inorganic materials. To filter out unidentified substances from bulk medications, TLC is an effective technique. The statement conveys a comparatively high level of certainty regarding the separation of all likely drug constituents. Spot elution followed by spectrophotometric measurement has been used to gain quantitative analytical insight from TLC's high specificity. The levels of noscapine, celecoxib, pioglitazone, and certain steroids have all been determined using TLC. When knowledge of the contaminants and breakdown products in the drug substance and drug product is lacking in the early stages of drug development, TLC is essential. Through the use of TLC, numerous pharmaceutical impurities have been found and identified.

1.3.2.2. High-performance thin Layer Chromatography

High-performance thin layer chromatography (HPTLC) became a crucial tool in drug analysis as the technique developed. HPTLC is a quick separation method with enough flexibility to examine a broad range of materials. Because it is easy to use and takes little time to analyze, this technique is beneficial for both complex and crude sample cleanups. HPTLC analyzes the whole chromatogram without regard to time constraints using a range of parameters. Additionally, multiple independent and simultaneous samples and standards are developed on each plate, increasing the reliability of the results. Drugs like cyproterone, alfuzosin, tramadol, and pentazocine have all been quantified using HPTLC.

1.3.2.3. High-performance Liquid Chromatography (HPLC)

The goal of high-performance liquid chromatography (HPLC) is to better understand the roles of individual molecules by isolating complex mixtures of molecules found in biological and chemical systems. The first time HPLC methods were used for the assay of bulk drug materials was in 1980. This has emerged as the primary method in USP XXVII and, to a lesser extent, as one of the most popular methods. The HPLC method achieves both good specificity and adequate precision at the same time. However, it must be noted that only extensive system suitability testing performed prior to the HPLC analysis can yield astounding specificity, precision, and accuracy. For the same reason high specificity, precision, and accuracy come at a high cost. Throughout the literature review, it was noted that HPLC has been the most popular chromatographic technique. To ensure that every component is detected in liquid chromatography, the detection strategy chosen is essential. The UV detector, which can monitor multiple wavelengths simultaneously when using a multiple wavelength scanning program, is one of the most commonly used detectors in HPLC. A UV detector ensures that every UV-absorbing component is found if it is present in sufficient quantities (Figure 1.1).

A line array of discrete photodiodes on an integrated circuit (IC) chip is called a photodiode array (PDA), and it is used in spectroscopy. It is positioned at the spectrometer's image plane to enable the simultaneous detection of a variety of wavelengths. To ensure that all of the peaks are detected when using a variable wavelength detector (VWD), a sample must be injected multiple times at various wavelengths. When PDA is used, all the compounds that absorb within a given wavelength range can be identified in a single analysis by programming the range. PDA detectors can also match spectra within a peak to analyze peak purity. PDA detectors are used in pharmaceutical companies' method development for iloperidone. When it comes to identifying analytes like polymers, alcohols, sugars, carbs, and fatty acids that have limited or no UV absorption, the refractive index detector is the preferred choice. Low noise ensures decent trace detection performance. Despite having the lowest sensitivity of all the detectors, this one works well at high analyte concentrations. The chemical reaction that occurs at the electrode's surface initiates an electron flow, which is what causes the electrochemical detector to react to either reducible or oxidizable substances. Recently, the glutathione content of human lung adenocarcinoma and prostate cancer cells was examined using this detector.

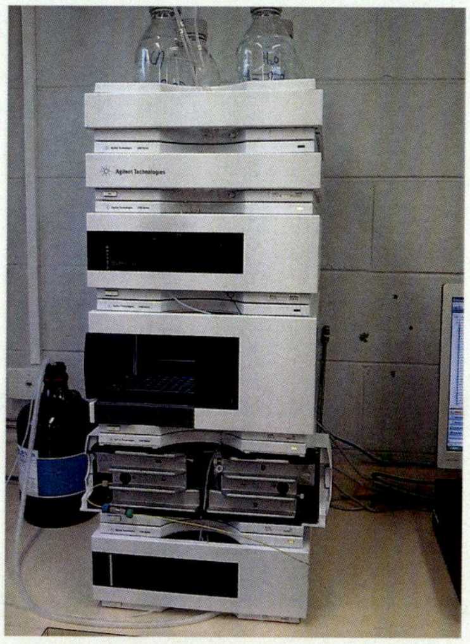

Figure 1.1. *A HPLC unit.*

Source: *By http://en.wikipedia.org/wiki/User:Kommando – Own work. Originally uploaded at http://en.wikipedia.org/wiki/File:HPLC.jpg, CC BY-SA 3.0, https://commons.wikimedia.org/w/index.php?curid=15808573.*

The fluorescence detector is one of the LC detectors with the highest sensitivity. Its sensitivity is typically 10–1000 times higher than the UV detectors for materials that absorb strong UV light, which is advantageous when measuring particular fluorescent species in samples. Pharmaceutical estimation is one of the most significant uses of fluorescence.

When it came to reliability, analysis time, repeatability, and sensitivity, most workers utilized the reversed-phase mode with UV absorbance detection over a certain amount of time. Using HPLC, several medications have been tested in biological fluids and pharmaceutical formulations. Therefore, HPLC plays a significant role in providing answers to numerous inquiries from the pharmaceutical sector. Nevertheless, the cost of columns, solvents, and the proprietary nature of column packing limit HPLC's long-term repeatability. One of the most significant developments of the final ten years of the 20th century is thought to have been the combination of liquid chromatography and mass spectrometry, or LC–MS. It evolved into the preferred technique for analytical support in numerous phases of pharmaceutical industry quality assurance and control. HPLC-MS has been used recently for drug assay. Apart from its use in drug analysis, HPLC has also been applied to analyze pharmaceutical impurities and degradation products, both independently and in conjunction with hyphenated techniques.

1.3.2.4. Gas chromatography

Moving on to a different chromatographic method, gas chromatography is an effective separation method for the identification of volatile organic compounds. When separation and online detection are combined, complex mixtures can be accurately quantified, even with traces of compounds down to parts per trillion in certain circumstances. Pharmacological product analysis heavily relies on gas liquid chromatography. The application of this method is limited to the production of high-molecular mass products like polypeptides or antibiotics that are thermally unstable. Derivatization is essentially required because the primary limitation is the relative non-volatility of the drug substances. Gas chromatography has recently been utilized in the assay of medications like cocaine and isotretinoin, as well as in the measurement of residual solvents in betamethasone valerate. For the analysis of pharmaceutical impurities, gas chromatography is another crucial instrument. The remaining solvents listed as impurities by the International Conference of Harmonization are analyzed by the GC using a variety of detectors. In recent years, GC has been used to estimate the process-related impurities of pharmaceuticals.

1.3.3. Spectroscopic Techniques

1.3.3.1. Spectrophotometry

The spectrophotometric method, which relies on chemical reactions and natural UV absorption, is another significant group of techniques that is included in pharmacopeias. The quantitative measurement of a material's wavelength-dependent transmission or reflection characteristics is called spectrophotometry. These methods' low labor and time consumption are their advantages. These techniques also have very good precision. Over the past few years, there has been a significant increase in the use of UV-Vis spectrophotometry, particularly in the analysis of pharmaceutical dosage forms.

The colorimetric methods are usually based on the following aspects:

- Complex-formation reaction
- Oxidation-reduction process
- A catalytic effect

It is significant to note that bulk material assay frequently employs colorimetric techniques. One method for determining corticosteroid drug formulations is the blue tetrazolium assay. The colorimetric approach is described in European Pharmacopoeia and is also used to determine cardiac glycosides. Several methods for determining the active pharmaceutical ingredients in bulk drugs and formulations have been reported that use spectrophotometry (Table 1.1).

Table 1.1. Quantitative Analysis of Drugs in Pharmaceutical Formulations by UV–Visible Spectrophotometric Procedures

Substance	Accuracy	Statistical Data			
		x_m	SD	Sx_m	RSD, %
Tenoxicam	80%	90.05	2.1753	0.8881	2.42
	100%	100.91	1.9248	0.7858	1.91
	120%	98.82	1.8401	0.7512	1.86
Meloxicam	80%	100.47	2.8261	1.1537	2.81
	100%	97.70	1.8089	0.7385	1.85
	120%	98.37	1.9905	0.8126	2.02
Etoricoxib	80%	99.99	1.5382	0.6279	1.54
	100%	100.51	1.8622	0.76019	1.85
	120%	99.82	2.2460	0.9169	2.25
Celecoxib	80%	100.30	2.4674	1.0073	2.46
	100%	99.99	2.0409	0.8332	2.04
	120%	99.11	1.5011	0.6128	1.51

x_m—arithmetic mean; SD—standard deviation; Sx_m—standard deviation of the mean; RSD,%—relative standard deviation.

Source: Gumułka P, Dąbrowska M, Starek M. Microanalysis of Selected NSAIDs Using the Spectrophotometric Method. Eng. 2020; 1(2):211–221. https://doi.org/10.3390/eng1020014.

For qualitative analysis and estimation, derivative spectroscopy employs first or upper derivatives of absorbance with respect to wavelength. Derivatizing spectral data was first proposed in the 1950s, and its benefits were quickly demonstrated. The difficulty of producing derivative spectra with early UV-visible spectrophotometers, however, prevented much thought from being given to the technique. The use of mathematical techniques to produce derivative spectra quickly, simply, and reliably gained general acceptance with the advent of microcomputers in the late 1970s. The derivative technique was used much more frequently as a result. The derivative method has been applied to infrared, atomic absorption, fluorescence spectrometry, fluorimetry, and UV spectrophotometry. Derivative spectrometry can be useful whenever there are issues with the quantitative analysis of normal spectra and is not just limited to unique situations. A drawback of derivative methods is that they deteriorate the signal-to-noise ratio due to the differential, necessitating the use of smoothing in addition to differentiation.

1.3.3.2. Near Infrared Spectroscopy (NIRS)

Near infrared spectroscopy (NIRS) offers multi-component analysis of nearly any matrix in a quick and non-destructive manner. The pharmaceutical industry has come to value NIR spectroscopy greatly in recent years for process monitoring, product quality control, and raw material testing. The fact that NIR spectroscopy has three main advantages over other analytical techniques—easy sample preparation without the need for pretreatments, the possibility of separating the sample measurement position with the use of fiber optic probes, and the ability to predict chemical and physical sample parameters from a single spectrum—probably explains why the pharmaceutical industry is becoming more and more interested in this technique. NIR techniques have been generally adopted by the major pharmacopeias. When used in conjunction with multivariate data analysis, NIR spectroscopy offers a wealth of intriguing perspectives for pharmaceutical analysis, both qualitative and quantitative. There have been several publications reported that detail quantitative NIR measurements of the active ingredient in intact tablets.

1.3.3.3. Nuclear Magnetic Resonance Spectroscopy (NMR)

NMR-based screening has advanced quickly since the first report detailing its application to drug molecule screening was published in 1996. A multitude of cutting-edge methods have been introduced and widely used in academic and pharmaceutical research in the past few years. Recently, NMR has been used in quantitative analysis to identify drug impurities, characterize drug product composition, and quantify drugs in pharmaceutical formulations and biological fluids. Numerous reviews on the use of NMR in pharmaceuticals have been published.

1.3.3.4. Fluorimetry and Phosphorimetry

The pharmaceutical and micro sample industries are always searching for sensitive analytical methods. Fluorescence spectrometry is a technique that achieves high sensitivity without sacrificing precision or specificity. In the recent past, there has been a noticeable gradual increase in the number of articles on the use of fluorimetry and phosphorimetry in the quantitative analysis of different drugs in dosage forms and biological fluids.

1.3.4. Electrochemical Methods

Over the past few years, there has been a significant increase in the use of electrochemical techniques in the analysis of pharmaceuticals and drugs. More advanced instruments and a deeper comprehension of the methods themselves are partly responsible for the resurgence of interest in electrochemical techniques. (Table 1.2).

Table 1.2. Advantages and Disadvantages of Some Techniques Applied in Fragment-Based Drug Discovery (FBDD)

Techniques	Advantages	Disadvantages
Thermal Shift Assay (TSA)	Low cost and high throughput; Identification of hit compounds which modify the target's thermal stability [**68**].	False positive results are possible.

Techniques	Advantages	Disadvantages
Surface Plasmon Resonance (SPR)	High throughput; Detection of binding interactions in real time and in a label-free manner [**79**].	Targets need to be immobilized; False positive results are possible.
Weak Affinity Chromatography-Mass Spectroscopy (WAC-MS)	High sensitivity; Label free; High efficiency [**80**].	False positive results are possible [**81**,**82**].
X-ray Crystallography	Capable of providing high-resolution and detailed structural information for binding interactions	High quality target crystals are needed.
Micro Scale Thermophoresis (MST)	Low cost; high throughput and high efficiency [**69**].	Fluorescent labeling is needed; False positive results are possible [**69**].
Ligand-observed NMR	No molecular weight limitation for targets; Capable of detecting weak binders.	False positive results are possible due to compound aggregation.
Target-observed NMR	Capable of providing binding site information; Capable of detecting weak binders.	Isotope labeling is needed; Low throughput; Molecular weight limitation for targets.

Source: Shi L, Zhang N. Applications of Solution NMR in Drug Discovery. Molecules. 2021; 26(3):576. https://doi.org/10.3390/molecules26030576.

Furthermore, there are numerous electroanalytical techniques available for pharmaceutical quantification. To measure imipramine, trimipramine, and desipramine, a glassy carbon paste modified with titanium dioxide nanoparticles and amberlite XAD-2 was created. Adsorptive stripping differential pulse voltammetry, electrochemical impedance spectroscopy, chronocoulombometry, and cyclic voltammetry were used to study the electrochemical behavior of these medications. Two electrodes have been developed for the determination of benzocaine and lidocaine: the p-chloranil-modified carbon paste electrode and the capsaicin-modified carbon nanotube-modified basal-plane pyrolitic graphite electrode. A linear decrease in the voltammetric signal corresponding to capsaicin is caused by the electrochemically induced formation of the capsaicin-benzocaine adduct, and this decrease is correlated with the added concentration of benzocaine. A glassy carbon paste electrode modified with copper (II) complex and silver nanoparticles was created and utilized to measure dopamine, levodopa, epinephrine, and norepinephrine.

Chronocoulometry, adsorptive stripping square-wave voltammetry, electrochemical impedance spectroscopy, and cyclic voltammetry were used to investigate the electrochemical behavior of these medications. Using a glassy carbon electrode, cyclic, differential pulse, and square-wave voltammetry were used to examine the electrochemical behavior of clioquinol, a molecule with a wide range of clinical applications, over a broad pH range. The determination of venlafaxine and desvenlafaxine using a Nafion-carbon nanotube composite glassy carbon electrode is possible with the advent of the adsorptive stripping differential pulse voltage method.

For the individual and simultaneous measurement of acetaminophen, aspirin, and caffeine, a carbon nanotube paste electrode modified in situ with Triton X 100 was created. For the subnanomolar determination of bismuth, an electrochemical method based on potentiometric stripping analysis has been proposed, utilizing cryptand and a carbon nanotube-modified paste electrode. Levodopa, bensevazide, and its impurity (R,S)-2-amino-3-hydroxy propanohydrazide in CO-beneldopa pharmaceutical have all been measured quickly and accurately using a novel technique called capillary electrophoresis with amperometric detection. Additionally, a potentiometric stripping analysis of antimony based on a carbon paste electrode modified with rice husk and hexathia crown ether has been reported.

1.3.5. Kinetic Method of Analysis

Though it has been evolving since the 1950s, the kinetic method of analysis is currently experiencing a significant resurgence in activity. The continuous interest in kinetic methods can be attributed to the progress made in data analysis techniques, analytical application, automated instrumentation, chemical and instrumentation understanding, and principles. The literature makes it clear that there are several general benefits to the kinetic approach to analytical chemistry over the more conventional equilibrium approach. Once the sample and reagents have been mixed manually or mechanically, kinetic methods rely on measurements of concentration changes (identified by changes in signal) in a reactant (which could be the analyte itself) over time.

It is clear from reading the literature that initial rate and fixed-time approaches have been employed more frequently to determine the drugs in pharmaceutical formulations. The majority of automatic techniques for kinetic methods are built on open systems; two common examples are the continuous addition of reagent (CAR) technique and the stopped flow system. Using the CAR technique with photometric and fluorimetric detection, several drugs have been identified. It is possible to use catalysts to speed up analytical reactions while maintaining equilibrium and reaction rate estimates. In addition to increasing the rate of reaction through micellar catalysis, the use of micellar media in kinetic methods has been promoted recently. This can also enhance sensitivity and selectivity, reducing the amount of time needed to analyze the analyte. In the field of pharmaceutical research, multicomponent kinetic estimations—more popularly known as differential rate methods—are also finding widespread acceptance. Two novel strategies, i.e., to handle overlapping component spectra in binary mixtures, two methods have been proposed: the kinetic wavelength pair method and the H-point standard addition method.

1.3.6. Electrophoretic Methods

Capillary electrophoresis (CE) is another crucial tool for the analysis of pharmaceuticals. CE is a relatively new analytical method that uses an electric field to separate charged analytes through a tiny capillary. With this method, solutes are seen as peaks as they move through the detector; each peak's area corresponds to its concentration, enabling quantitative estimations. It finds use in inorganic ion analysis and biopolymer analysis in addition to pharmaceutical research. In general, CE analysis is more efficient, can be completed more quickly, only needs a small amount, less than nanoliter injection volumes, and is typically carried out in aqueous conditions. Numerous pharmaceutical applications have demonstrated the benefits of these four CE characteristics. Numerous articles about the use of this method in standard drug analysis have surfaced. Numerous capillary electrophoresis techniques, including affinity capillary electrophoresis, capillary zone electrophoresis, microgel electrokinetic chromatography, isotachophoresis, capillary gel electrophoresis, and isoelectric focusing, have been developed and used in pharmaceutical purity testing and drug bioanalysis.

1.3.7. Flow Injection and Sequential Injection Analysis

In the latter half of the 20th century, laboratory automation was revolutionized by the development of the flow injection analysis (FIA) technique. Scientists such as Steward in the U.S. and Ruzicka and Hansen in Denmark were instrumental in creating this automated method for chemical procedures. FIA changed the way automation was viewed in chemical analysis by allowing instrumental measurements to be performed without the need for physical and chemical equilibria. In FIA, a liquid sample is injected into a continuous flow of liquid, creating a zone that is then transported to a detector. This detector records changes in absorbance, electrode potential, or other physical parameters as the sample material moves through the flow cell. The process of flow injection analysis is depicted in Figure 1.2.

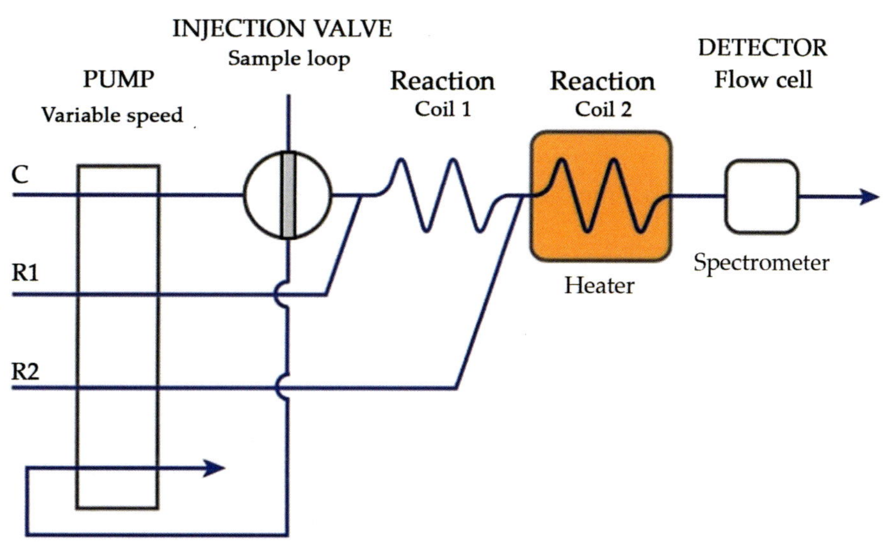

Figure 1.2. *Stages of flow injection analysis.*

Source: https://upload.wikimedia.org/wikipedia/commons/3/38/Diagram_of_Flow_Injection_Analysis.jpg.

A second generation of flow analysis known as sequential injection analysis (SIA) emerged after computers were widely used in everyday laboratory operations. This arrangement of continuous flow is non-segmented and operates on the same principle as the FIA—controlled dispersion and repeatable manipulation of the FIA perception—but it is based on the theory of programmable flow.

1.4. Pharmaceuticals Production from Microorganisms

A vast array of pharmaceutical products are produced by pharmaceutical biotechnology, which uses microorganisms like yeast, fungus, and bacteria. Due to their ease of growth, capacity to generate large amounts of the desired product, and ability to be modified to produce particular molecules, microorganisms are used.

Here are some examples of pharmaceutical products that can be produced from microorganisms:

- **Antibiotics:** Microorganisms produce substances known as antibiotics that have the ability to either kill or stop the growth of bacteria. Antibiotics derived from microorganisms encompass penicillin and erythromycin, as instances.
- **Vaccines:** Microorganisms produce proteins called enzymes, which can catalyze chemical reactions. Microorganism-derived enzymes are employed in numerous pharmaceutical procedures, including the synthesis of insulin.
- **Enzymes:** Microorganisms produce enzymes, which are proteins with the ability to catalyze chemical reactions. Microorganism-derived enzymes are employed in numerous pharmaceutical procedures, including the synthesis of insulin.
- **Recombinant Proteins:** Microorganisms that have had certain genes inserted into their DNA are able to produce recombinant proteins. Recombinant proteins made from microorganisms include erythropoietin and human growth hormone.

The synthesis of pharmaceuticals from microorganisms usually entails multiple stages, such as the selection of strains, fermentation, downstream processing, and purification. To guarantee the ultimate product's quality, purity, and safety, the production process needs to be closely regulated. Pharmaceutical biotechnology is a field that is constantly researching and developing new strains of production, enhancing fermentation conditions, and refining downstream processing and purification techniques to improve the manufacturing of pharmaceuticals from microorganisms.

1.4.1. Microbial Strain Selection for Pharmaceutical Production

The process of producing pharmaceuticals from microorganisms involves a critical step called microbial strain selection. To guarantee the effective and successful production of the intended pharmaceutical product, a suitable microbe possessing the required traits must be chosen. A variety of factors, such as a microbial strain's capacity to generate a target compound, growth rate, and resistance to particular environmental conditions, can be taken into consideration when choosing one. Large-scale screening of microorganisms may be part of the selection process, which is then followed by a more thorough examination of a smaller subset of strains that meet the desired criteria. Potential microbial strains can be found in soil, water, and plant or animal tissues, and identifying them is the first step in the selection process. Upon identification of potential strains, their capacity to yield the intended pharmaceutical compound is assessed. For the purpose of microbial strain screening, a number of techniques are available, such as metagenomics, targeted screening, and high-throughput screening. With robotic systems and automated assays, a large number of microorganisms are tested concurrently in high-throughput screening. Microorganisms are chosen for targeted screening based on their demonstrated capacity to produce the target compound or related compounds. Toidentify possible microorganisms that might produce the desired compound, metagenomics entails the direct sequencing of environmental DNA (Figure 1.3).

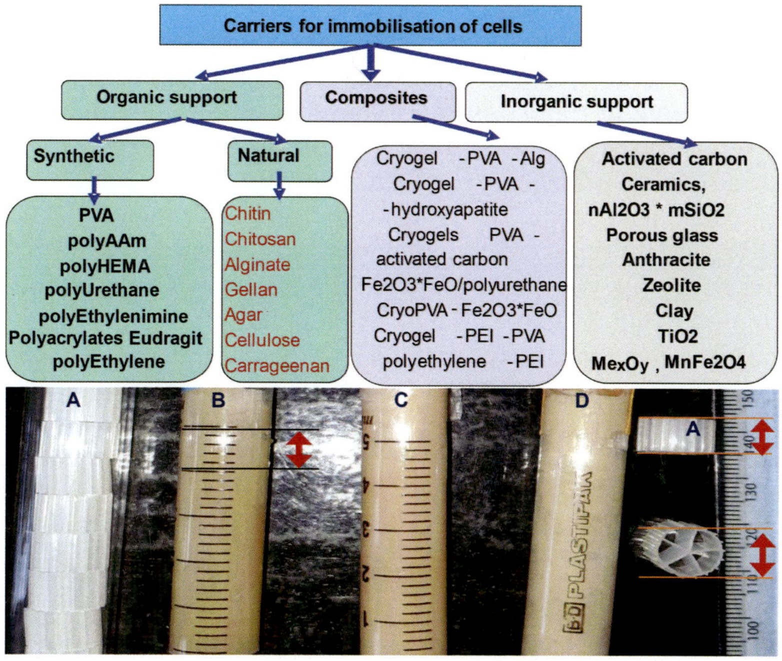

Figure 1.3. *Microbial immobilization for the removal of pharmaceutical pollutants.*

Source: Berillo D, Al-Jwaid A, Caplin J. Polymeric Materials Used for Immobilization of Bacteria for the Bioremediation of Contaminants in Water. Polymers. 2021; 13(7):1073. https://doi.org/10.3390/polym13071073.

Further in-depth genetic and phenotypic characterization can be done after a group of promising strains has been identified. To determine the genes and proteins involved in the synthesis of the desired compound, this may entail transcriptomics, proteomics, and genomic sequencing. The productivity of particular strains can also be increased by applying strain improvement strategies like directed evolution, metabolic engineering, and mutagenesis. These methods entail altering the microorganism's DNA to maximize its potential for the intended pharmaceutical production. Optimizing growth conditions and choosing the right equipment for large-scale production are key components of scaling up microbial strains for pharmaceutical production. The selection of microbial strains for pharmaceutical production should also take quality control factors, such as regulatory approval, product safety, and adherence to Good Manufacturing Practice (GMP) guidelines, into account. A variety of factors, such as strain screening techniques, genetic and phenotypic characterization, strain improvement techniques, and quality control considerations, must be carefully taken into account during the complex process of selecting microbial strains for pharmaceutical production. Technological developments like synthetic biology, CRISPR-Cas9 gene editing, and high-throughput screening should lead to even more improvements.

1.4.2. Fermentation Optimization for Pharmaceutical Production

Being able to produce substances like enzymes, vitamins, and antibiotics on a large scale makes fermentation an essential step in the process of turning microorganisms into pharmaceuticals. To produce these compounds as effectively and economically as possible, fermentation optimization is a vital step. Adjusting different aspects of the fermentation process to increase the amount of the target product is known as fermentation optimization. Choosing the right microbial strain, planning the fermentation process, and optimizing process variables like pH, temperature, and nutrient availability are some of these considerations. To successfully optimize fermentation, the right microbial strain must be chosen. The capacity of the strain to produce the desired compound, its rate of growth, and its resistance to particular environmental conditions are all important considerations when choosing a strain. An important aspect of fermentation is its design. The size of the fermentation vessel, its type, and the agitation and aeration conditions are all important considerations when designing the process. It is possible to greatly influence the yield of the intended product by optimizing process parameters like pH, temperature, and nutrient availability. A higher yield of the intended product, for instance, may result from increasing the availability of a crucial nutrient like glucose. The availability of nutrients must be balanced, though, with other elements like the microorganism's rate of growth and the buildup of byproducts.

Fermentation processes can be optimized with sophisticated tools like machine learning, statistical analysis, and mathematical modeling. These instruments facilitate the expeditious examination of extensive datasets and the determination of the ideal conditions for the fermentation procedure. For the intended product to be recovered effectively and economically, downstream processing is just as crucial as fermentation process optimization. The product is separated from the fermentation broth and then purified and formulated during downstream processing. An essential step in the synthesis of pharmaceuticals from microorganisms is fermentation optimization. The design of the fermentation process, the optimization of process parameters, and the choice of a suitable microbial strain are crucial elements in guaranteeing the productive and economical production of these compounds. Fermentation optimization can be made even more efficient by utilizing cutting-edge techniques like machine learning and mathematical modeling.

1.4.3. Downstream Processing and Purification of Microbial-Produced Pharmaceuticals

The final product must be obtained by processing and purifying the microbial broth containing the desired product, once fermentation has finished. Pharmaceuticals produced by microbes must undergo a sequence of downstream processing and purification procedures to extract the desired product from the fermentation broth, eliminate contaminants, and produce a highly concentrated and pure form of the product.

The downstream processing of microbial-produced pharmaceuticals typically includes the following steps:

1. **Separation:** The first step is to separate the microbial cells from the fermentation broth. This can be achieved by centrifugation, filtration, or sedimentation. The separated cells can be recycled or used for other purposes.

2. **Concentration:** The next step is to concentrate the target product from the fermentation broth. This can be achieved by techniques such as ultrafiltration, evaporation, or precipitation.
3. **Purification:** The purification step involves the removal of impurities from the concentrated product. This can be achieved by techniques such as chromatography, ion exchange, or affinity purification.
4. **Formulation: The** final step involves the formulation of the purified product into a suitable form for use. This can include lyophilization, freeze-drying, or formulation into tablets, capsules, or injectable forms.

The type of product, the production volume, and the required level of purity all influence the downstream processing and purification methods selected. For the ultimate product to have the highest possible yield, purity, and quality, the downstream processing and purification techniques need to be meticulously tuned. The creation of new downstream processing and purification techniques that are more effective, economical, and environmentally sustainable has received more attention in recent years. For instance, membrane-based separation technologies have been developed that, with minimal energy consumption and waste production, can efficiently separate and concentrate pharmaceuticals produced by microorganisms. Essential stages in the manufacturing process for pharmaceuticals made by microbes are downstream processing and purification. Product type and intended final product purity determine which downstream processing and purification techniques are used. To increase the production process's effectiveness, economy, and sustainability, new and creative techniques for downstream processing and purification are continuously being developed.

1.4.4. Genetic Engineering of Microorganisms for Pharmaceutical Production

Microorganisms can be genetically engineered to produce powerful pharmaceuticals. Through the introduction of foreign genes into microbial hosts, pathways that result in complex molecules possessing therapeutic properties can be engineered. The following procedures are commonly involved in the genetic engineering of microorganisms for pharmaceutical production:

1. **Identification of the Target Molecule:** The first step is to identify the target molecule that is to be produced. This can be a naturally occurring molecule or a modified form of a natural molecule.
2. **Identification of the Host Organism:** The next step is to identify a suitable host organism that can be genetically engineered to produce the target molecule. This can be a bacterium, yeast, or fungus that is capable of producing and secreting the target molecule.
3. **Genetic Modification of the Host Organism:** The target genes that encode the enzymes required for the synthesis of the target molecule are introduced into the host organism. This is typically achieved using recombinant DNA technology.
4. **Screening and Selection:** The genetically modified organisms are screened and selected for their ability to produce the target molecule. This can involve the use of high-throughput screening methods or selection based on the expression level of the target genes.

5. **Optimization of Production:** The final step involves the optimization of the production process to achieve maximum yield and purity of the target molecule. This can involve the optimization of fermentation conditions, downstream processing, and purification methods.

There are several benefits to using genetic engineering to produce pharmaceuticals over conventional chemical synthesis techniques. Complex molecules that are difficult or impossible to synthesize chemically can be produced thanks to it. Moreover, compared to conventional chemical synthesis techniques, it may be less expensive to produce the target molecule in large quantities. But there are a number of difficulties involved in using genetic engineering to produce pharmaceuticals using microorganisms. These include the potential for unethical outcomes, regulatory difficulties related to the use of genetically modified organisms, and the possibility of unforeseen effects on the host organism. A potent technique for producing pharmaceuticals is the genetic engineering of microorganisms. It has the potential to produce complex molecules more cheaply than conventional chemical synthesis techniques. However, using genetically modified organisms to produce pharmaceuticals comes with many issues that need to be properly considered.

1.4.5. Microbial Biosynthesis of Natural Products for Drug Discovery

A key strategy for drug discovery is the microbial biosynthesis of natural products. Bioactive compounds found in natural products have been utilized for centuries in medicine. It can be costly and time-consuming to separate and extract natural products from their natural sources, though. Further impeding the development of certain natural products as therapeutics has been their limited availability. One possible alternative strategy for drug discovery is the microbial biosynthesis of natural products. To create bioactive compounds, genetically modified microorganisms are used in the process of microbial biosynthesis of natural products.

The process typically involves the following steps:

1. **Identification of the Target Natural Product:** The first step is to identify the natural product of interest. This can be a compound with known therapeutic properties or a new compound with potential therapeutic activity.
2. **Identification of the Biosynthetic Pathway:** The biosynthetic pathway for the natural product is identified. This involves the identification and characterization of the genes and enzymes involved in the biosynthesis of the natural product.
3. **Genetic Engineering of the Host Organism:** The genes encoding the enzymes required for the biosynthesis of the natural product are introduced into a suitable host organism. This can be a bacterium, yeast, or fungus.
4. **Optimization of Production:** The production process is optimized to achieve maximum yield and purity of the natural product. This can involve the optimization of fermentation conditions, downstream processing, and purification methods.

There are various benefits to using microbial biosynthesis of natural products for drug discovery in comparison to conventional methods. It makes it possible to produce intricate natural products that are hard or impossible to make chemically. In comparison to conventional isolation and extraction techniques, it also presents the possibility of producing the natural product in large quantities at a reduced cost. Nonetheless, the microbial biosynthesis of natural products poses many difficulties for drug discovery. These include the potential for the synthesis of toxic compounds, the identification and characterization of the biosynthetic pathway, and the process optimization. The microbial biosynthesis of natural products has become a significant drug discovery strategy. It is superior to conventional methods in a number of ways and could transform drug discovery in the future. But this strategy also comes with several drawbacks that need to be properly considered.

1.4.6. Microbial Production of Therapeutic Enzymes

A significant area of biotechnology is the microbial production of therapeutic enzymes, which uses genetically modified microorganisms to produce therapeutic-grade enzymes. Proteins called enzymes are essential for numerous physiological processes because they catalyze particular biochemical reactions in the body. Enzymes that are used to treat a variety of medical conditions, including immune deficiencies, metabolic diseases, and genetic disorders, are known as therapeutic enzymes.

Microbial production of therapeutic enzymes involves the following steps:

1. **Identification of the Target Enzyme:** The first step is to identify the enzyme of interest that has therapeutic applications.
2. **Genetic Engineering of the Host Organism:** The genes encoding the enzyme of interest are introduced into a suitable host organism. This can be a bacterium, yeast, or fungus.
3. **Optimization of Production:** The production process is optimized to achieve maximum yield and purity of the enzyme. This can involve the optimization of fermentation conditions, downstream processing, and purification methods.
4. **Characterization of the Enzyme:** The enzyme is characterized to ensure that it has the desired therapeutic properties and is safe for use in humans.

Using microbial production of therapeutic enzymes has a number of benefits. Compared to conventional methods of extraction and isolation, it enables the production of the enzyme in large quantities at a lower cost. It also provides the chance to produce altered enzymes with better medicinal qualities. The microbial synthesis of therapeutic enzymes is not without its difficulties, though. These consist of identifying and characterizing the enzyme, streamlining the manufacturing procedure, and checking for the possibility of hazardous byproducts or contaminants being produced. One significant area of biotechnology that has the potential to completely transform the way that many medical conditions are treated is the microbial production of therapeutic enzymes. It has the potential to raise millions of people's standards of living globally and has several advantages over conventional methods. To guarantee the efficacy and safety of the therapeutic enzymes, there are a few additional issues with this strategy that need to be properly resolved.

1.4.7. Quality Control and Regulatory Considerations in Microbial Pharmaceutical Production

Quality control and regulatory considerations are critical aspects of microbial pharmaceutical production that ensure the safety, efficacy, and quality of the final product. The following are some key considerations in this regard:

1. **Good Manufacturing Practices (GMP):** The GMP guidelines outline standards for producing and overseeing pharmaceutical products, including those produced using microbial organisms. These regulations address every stage of the production process, from facility layout to equipment testing, staff training, and record-keeping.
2. **Quality Control:** Quality control procedures guarantee that the finished product satisfies all necessary requirements and is safe for use. To guarantee the consistency and purity of the product, this entails using batch release testing, in-process testing, and validated analytical methods.
3. **Contamination Control:** In the microbial pharmaceutical production process, contamination control is essential because it can impact the final product's safety and effectiveness. This includes using efficient cleaning and sterilization techniques, keeping an eye on the surroundings, and using the right personal protective equipment (PPE) to avoid contamination.
4. **Regulatory Compliance:** Ensuring that a product satisfies safety, efficacy, and quality regulations is crucial to the production of microbiological pharmaceuticals. To comply with pertinent regulations, such as those set forth by the Food and Drug Administration (FDA) in the United States, regulatory filings must be submitted.
5. **Process Validation:** To guarantee that the production process is dependable, consistent, and capable of yielding a safe and effective product, process validation is an essential component of the manufacturing of microorganism-based pharmaceuticals. This entails assessing the crucial components of the production process—equipment, supplies, and labor—using process validation protocols.

To guarantee the final product's safety, effectiveness, and quality, quality control and regulatory considerations are essential components of the microbial pharmaceutical production process. The application of GMP guidelines, quality control, contamination control, regulatory compliance, and process validation are some of these factors to take into account. Manufacturers can comply with these considerations.

1.4.8. Scale-up of Microbial Pharmaceutical Production

Scale-up of microbial pharmaceutical production is the process of increasing the production of a microbial-based drug from the laboratory or pilot scale to the commercial scale. The following are some key considerations in this regard:

1. **Process Optimization:** Before increasing the microbial pharmaceutical production process's scale, the pilot or laboratory scale version of the process needs to be optimized. Assessing critical process parameters (CPPs) and critical quality attributes (CQAs) is necessary to determine the ideal circumstances for achieving the highest possible yield and quality.
2. **Equipment Design:** Because equipment must hold the higher material volumes needed at the commercial scale, equipment design is essential to the process of scaling up microbial pharmaceutical production. Equipment needs

to be built with consistency, dependability, and safety in mind, along with a lower chance of contamination.

3. **Validation:** Ensuring the reliability and consistency of microbial pharmaceutical production at different scales is crucial for scaling up. This requires conducting validation studies at both pilot and commercial scales to confirm the process can consistently produce a safe and effective product.
4. **Regulatory Compliance:** Regulatory compliance is critical in scaling up microbial pharmaceutical production as it ensures that the product meets the regulatory requirements for safety, efficacy, and quality. This involves compliance with relevant regulations such as those issued by the FDA in the United States.
5. **Risk Assessment:** Risk assessment is critical in scaling up microbial pharmaceutical production as it helps identify potential risks associated with the production process and develop strategies to mitigate those risks. This involves evaluating potential hazards such as contamination, equipment failure, and product variability.

Risk assessment, equipment design, validation, regulatory compliance, and process optimization must all be carefully taken into account when scaling up microbial pharmaceutical production. Manufacturers can guarantee the safety and efficacy of their pharmaceuticals produced using microorganisms on a commercial scale by taking these factors into account.

1.4.9. Emerging Technologies in Microbial Pharmaceutical Production

Emerging technologies are changing the way microbial pharmaceuticals are produced, making the process more efficient, cost-effective, and sustainable. Here are some of the emerging technologies in microbial pharmaceutical production:

1. **Synthetic Biology:** Synthetic biology involves the design and construction of new biological systems and devices, often using genetic engineering techniques. This technology is being used to engineer microorganisms for the production of pharmaceuticals, such as insulin and vaccines.
2. **CRISPR/Cas9 Gene Editing:** CRISPR/Cas9 gene editing is a powerful tool for precise genome editing. This technology is being used to engineer microbial strains for the production of pharmaceuticals, as well as to improve their performance and yield.
3. **Metabolic Engineering:** By optimizing microorganisms' metabolic pathways, metabolic engineering can increase the yield of targeted products. With the aid of this technology, microorganisms are being engineered to produce drugs like antibiotics and antivirals.

4. **Continuous Bioprocessing:** Continuous bioprocessing involves the use of continuous processes rather than batch processes for the production of pharmaceuticals. This technology is more efficient and cost-effective than traditional batch processes and is being used to produce microbial-based pharmaceuticals such as enzymes and monoclonal antibodies.
5. **High-throughput Screening:** High-throughput screening involves the rapid screening of large numbers of microbial strains for desirable traits, such as high productivity and yield. This technology is being used to identify new microbial strains for the production of pharmaceuticals, as well as to optimize the performance of existing strains.
6. **Omics technologies:** Omics technologies, such as genomics, proteomics, and metabolomics, involve the large-scale analysis of biological data to understand the molecular mechanisms involved in microbial pharmaceutical production. These technologies are being used to identify new drug targets, optimize production pathways, and improve product quality.

Emerging technologies are changing the way microbial pharmaceuticals are produced, making the process more efficient, cost-effective, and sustainable. By leveraging these technologies, manufacturers can improve the production of microbial-based pharmaceuticals and accelerate the development of new drugs.

1.4.10. Industrial Applications of Microbial Pharmaceutical Production

Microbial pharmaceutical production has become an important field in the pharmaceutical industry due to the numerous benefits that microorganisms offer as a platform for drug production. Here are some of the industrial applications of microbial pharmaceutical production:

1. **Production of Therapeutic Proteins:** Microorganisms, such as bacteria and yeast, can be engineered to produce therapeutic proteins, such as insulin, growth hormones, and cytokines, which are used in the treatment of various diseases.
2. **Antibiotic Production:** Many antibiotics are produced by microorganisms, such as bacteria and fungi, and can be mass-produced using fermentation technology. Examples include penicillin, streptomycin, and tetracycline.
3. **Vaccine Production:** Microorganisms can also be used to produce vaccines, such as the hepatitis B vaccine and the human papillomavirus vaccine, which are used to prevent infectious diseases.
4. **Enzyme Production:** Microorganisms are used to produce enzymes, such as amylase, lipase, and protease, which are used in various industries, including food, textiles, and paper.

5. **Biofuel Production:** Microorganisms are also being used to produce biofuels, such as ethanol and butanol, which are renewable and more environmentally friendly alternatives to fossil fuels.
6. **Bioremediation:** Microorganisms are being used to clean up environmental pollutants, such as oil spills, by breaking down the pollutants into harmless substances.
7. Microbial pharmaceutical production has numerous industrial applications and has become an important tool in drug development. Microorganisms offer a scalable, cost-effective, and sustainable platform for the production of various drugs and other industrial products.

A Closer Look

Structure-Activity Relationship (SAR) Studies

Biological activity can be predicted from molecular structure using Structure-Activity Relationships (SAR). This potent technology is employed in the drug discovery process to direct the procurement or synthesis of novel, desirable compounds and to provide additional characterization for already existing molecules. A novel chemical compound's biological effects can frequently be inferred from its molecular structure by utilizing information about other compounds that are similar to it. This is due to the possibility that related compounds will share biological and physical characteristics. The Structure Activity Relationship (SAR) principle states that there is a connection between the biological activity of molecules and their molecular structures.

Using correlation analysis and model building, SAR tools are able to assess novel chemical structures and forecast their biological activity. After that, they can be used to create and describe new, desirable compounds. SAR can be used to further assess existing compounds for potential side-effect activities. The identification of the structural properties that are correlated with chemical and biological reactivity is essential to SAR. Therefore, conclusions about an unknown compound can only be made based on the structural features that can be described and the database of molecules that the unknown compound can be compared. When similarities are discovered, SAR can be a useful tool for determining the functional implications when used in conjunction with appropriate professional judgment. For instance, information from the most sensitive toxicological endpoints, such as cardiotoxicity or carcinogenicity, should be incorporated into the analysis when assessing the risk of uncharacterized compounds.

An SAR table, or Structure Activity Relationship, is the standard table format used for evaluation. SAR tables include the compounds along with their physical characteristics and functions. To identify potential relationships, experts sort, graph, and even scan structural features in the table.

Summary

- Pharmaceutical chemistry or medicinal chemistry is a discipline of chemistry and pharmacology. Medicinal chemistry is interested in finding out about the chemical properties of drugs have and about the synthesis and production of drugs.
- Pharmaceutical chemistry involves cures and remedies for disease, analytical techniques, pharmacology, metabolism, quality assurance, and drug chemistry. Many pharmaceutical chemistry students will later work in a lab.
- Pharmaceutical (medicinal) chemistry is concerned with the design (drug design) and synthesis of biologically active molecules. The aim is to gain new chemical molecules that could enable the discovery of new pharmaceuticals or optimize already-known drug structures, thereby expanding the portfolio of chemical drugs.
- Medicinal chemists today are not only making new bioactive molecules but also improving existing pharmaceuticals. They optimize the structure and, hence, properties of molecules to improve their interactions with target(s) as well as their metabolism, toxicities, and drug delivery dynamics to create medicines that are selective and have limited side effects (George).
- Drug classification based on molecular targets refers to categorizing drugs based on their specific interactions with target molecules in the body, such as receptors, enzymes, and ion channels.
- Drug discovery is the intricate process of identifying and developing new medications to treat diseases and improve human health. It involves a multidisciplinary approach that integrates various scientific fields, including biology, chemistry, pharmacology, and computational sciences.
- The drug development process involves rigorous testing and optimization of selected compounds to identify the most effective drug. This testing is done in cells (in vitro) and in animals (in vivo) to study the metabolism and to produce a product that is safe and has passed all regulatory requirements.
- Biomarker-guided repurposing of chemotherapeutic drugs for cancer therapy: a novel strategy for drug development: This research strategy is commonly known as drug repurposing or drug repositioning and provides a faster path to the clinics.
- Pharmaceutical formulation is a stage of drug development during which the physicochemical properties of Active Pharmaceutical Ingredients (APIs) are characterized to produce a bioavailable, stable and optimal dosage form for a specific administration route.
- Pharmaceutical analysis is a branch of analytical chemistry that focuses specifically on the quality control, quality assurance, and characterization of pharmaceutical products.
- Near-infrared spectroscopy (NIRS) is a rapid and non-destructive procedure that provides multi-component analysis of almost any matrix. In recent years, NIR spectroscopy has gained a wide appreciation within the pharmaceutical industry for raw material testing, product quality control and process monitoring.

References

1. Dunne, S., Shannon, B., Dunne, C., & Cullen, W. (2013). A review of the differences and similarities between generic drugs and their originator counterparts, including economic benefits associated with usage of generic medicines using Ireland as a case study. *BMC Pharmacology and Toxicology, 14*, 1.
2. Keshavarz-Moore, E., Kay, J., & Edmondson, R. (2013). Pharmaceutical biotechnology: Challenges and opportunities. *Advanced Drug Delivery Reviews, 65*(15), 1981–1982. https://doi.org/10.1016/j.addr.2013.11.007.
3. Lee, J. W., Kim, D. H., Lee, J. S., & Park, J. H. (2008). Recent developments in the production of recombinant therapeutic proteins in Escherichia coli. *Journal of Microbiology and Biotechnology, 18*(5), 835–851.
4. Parasuraman, S. (2011). Toxicological screening. *Journal of Pharmacology and Pharmacotherapeutics, 2*, 74–79.
5. Shukla, A. A., & Thömmes, J. (2010). Recent advances in large-scale production of monoclonal antibodies and related proteins. *Trends in Biotechnology, 28*(5), 253–261. https://doi.org/10.1016/j.tibtech.2010.02.005.
6. Smales, C. M., & James, D. C. (2013). Advances in mammalian cell line development technologies for recombinant protein production. *Pharmaceuticals (Basel), 6*(5), 579–603. https://doi.org/10.3390/ph6050579.
7. Stenvang, J., Kümler, I., Nygård, S. B., Smith, D. H., & Nielsen, D. (2013). Biomarker-guided repurposing of chemotherapeutic drugs for cancer therapy: A novel strategy in drug development. *Frontiers in Oncology, 3*, 313.
8. Walsh, G. (2014). Biopharmaceutical benchmarks 2014. *Nature Biotechnology, 32*(10), 992–1000. https://doi.org/10.1038/nbt.3040.

Chapter

2

DRUG DESIGN AND MOLECULAR MODELING

Contents

Introduction

To develop and improve therapeutic interventions, drug design and molecular modeling are essential components of contemporary pharmaceutical research. The complex process of finding and creating compounds that can interact with biological targets to produce desired pharmacological effects while minimizing adverse reactions is at the core of drug design. An essential tool in this endeavor is molecular modeling, which simulates and analyzes the behavior of molecules at the atomic level using computational techniques, providing important insights into the structure, interactions, and function of molecules. Target identification is the first step in the drug design process, in which particular molecules or biological pathways involved in disease processes are identified for potential intervention. Clarifying the structure and function of important proteins, receptors, enzymes, or nucleic acids involved in the development of disease may be one way to do this. Following the identification of a target, the next stage entails investigating chemical compounds, either synthetic or natural, that may be able to alter the target's activity. At this stage, rational drug design strategies based on the target's structure and function understanding are often used, or high-throughput screening of large compound libraries is required.

Throughout the drug design process, molecular modeling is essential because it offers comprehensive insights into the dynamics, energetics, and interactions of molecules. Utilizing computational methods like molecular docking, molecular dynamics simulations, and quantitative structure-activity relationship (QSAR) modeling, one can forecast the interactions between potential compounds and target molecules as well as evaluate the binding affinity and specificity of these compounds. To help identify possible lead compounds, molecular docking, for example, predicts the preferred orientation and conformation of a small molecule within the binding site of a target protein. Molecular dynamics simulations, on the other hand, provide dynamic information about the behavior of the drug-target complex under physiological conditions by simulating the movement of atoms and molecules over time.

Moreover, lead compounds can be optimized to improve their potency, selectivity, and pharmacokinetic characteristics with the help of molecular modeling. By employing structure-based drug design methodologies, including fragment-based drug design, ligand-based drug design, and de novo design, scientists can methodically alter and enhance chemical structures to maximize therapeutic efficacy and reduce toxicity and off-target effects. When combined with experimental validation, this iterative computational modeling process shortens the timeframe for drug discovery and development and makes it possible to find novel drug candidates that may be able to treat unmet medical needs. At the forefront of pharmaceutical research, drug design and molecular modeling are complementary fields that work together to drive innovation and improvements in therapeutic interventions. Researchers can accelerate the discovery and development of safe and effective medications to combat various diseases and improve patient outcomes by utilizing computational techniques to clarify molecular interactions and optimize drug candidates.

Orientation and Directional Terms

Term	Definition	Illustration
Pharmacology	Pharmacology is the science of medical drugs and medications, including a substance's origin, composition, pharmacokinetics, therapeutic use, and toxicology.	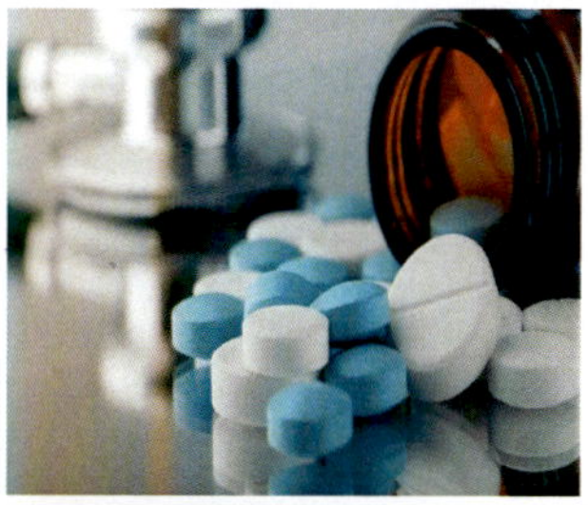
Biomolecular target	A biological target is anything within a living organism to which some other entity (like an endogenous ligand or a drug) is directed and/or binds, resulting in a change in its behavior or function.	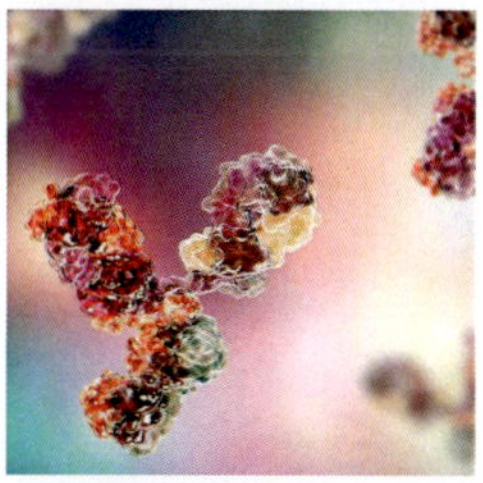
Drug discovery	It is the process by which new candidate medications are discovered.	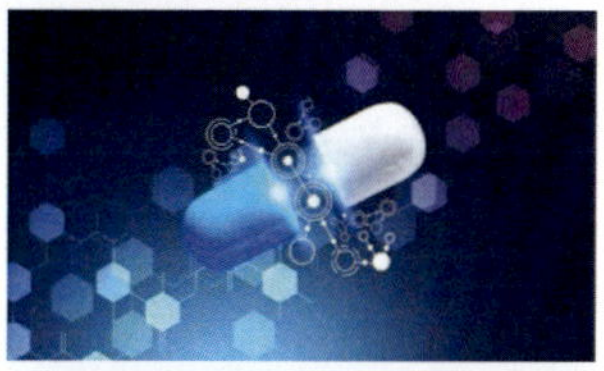
Quantitative structure-activity relationship	QSAR is a technique that tries to predict the activity, reactivity, and properties of an unknown set of molecules based on analysis of an equation connecting the structures of molecules to their respective measured activity and property.	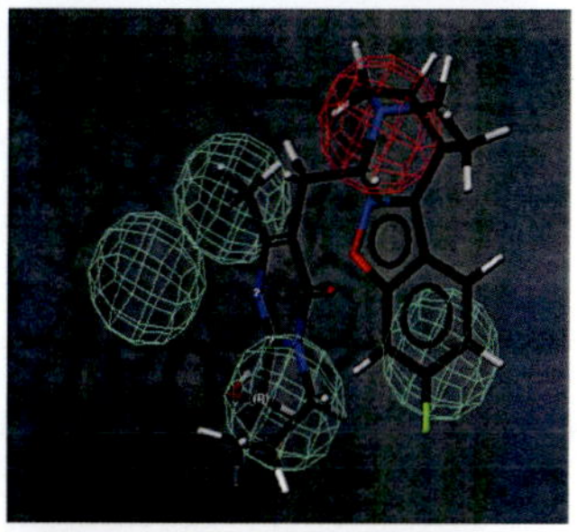
Phenotypic	The phenotype is the set of observable characteristics or traits of an organism.	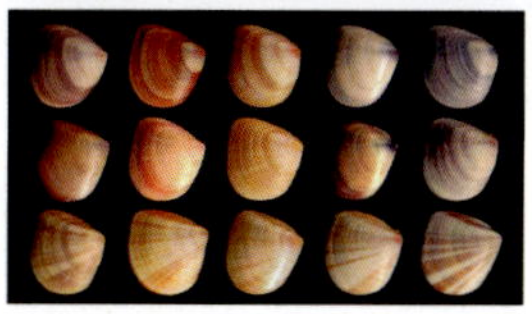

2.1. Basic Concept of Drug Design

Drug design is the creative process of developing novel pharmaceuticals based on the understanding of a biological target. It is also sometimes referred to as rational drug design or just rational design. Usually an organic small molecule, the drug acts by either activating or inhibiting the function of a biomolecule, like a protein, thereby providing the patient with a therapeutic benefit. Drug design, in its most basic form, is the design of molecules that, to interact with a biomolecular target, are complementary to it in shape and charge. The design of drugs often, though not always, depends on computer modeling methods. Computer-aided drug design is another term for this kind of modeling. Lastly, structure-based drug design refers to drug design that makes use of knowledge about the three-dimensional structure of the biomolecular target. Apart from small molecules, biopharmaceuticals, which comprise peptides and therapeutic antibodies in particular, are becoming a significant class of drugs. Computational techniques have been developed to enhance the stability, selectivity, and affinity of these protein-based therapeutics.

2.1.1. Definition

The terms "drug design" and "ligand design" (i.e., creation of a molecule with a strong binding to its target). While the design techniques for predicting binding affinity are fairly successful, before a ligand can become a safe and effective drug, many other properties like bioavailability, metabolic half-life, and side effects need to be optimized. Using logical design techniques, it is frequently challenging to predict these additional features.

A greater emphasis is being placed early in the drug design process on selecting candidate drugs whose physicochemical properties are predicted to result in fewer complications during development and, therefore, more likely to lead to an approved, marketed drug, due to high attrition rates, particularly during clinical phases of drug development. Additionally, early drug discovery is using more and more in vitro experiments combined with computational methods to choose compounds that have better ADME (absorption, distribution, metabolism, and excretion) and toxicological profiles.

2.1.1.1. Drug Targets

A biomolecular target is a critical molecule involved in a specific metabolic or signaling pathway that is linked to a particular disease condition or pathology, or to the infectivity or survival of a microbial pathogen. These targets are most frequently proteins or nucleic acids. Potential therapeutic targets must, by definition, be modifying diseases rather than causing them. Sometimes, the goal of tiny molecules is to either improve or block the target function in a particular disease-modifying pathway. Small molecules that are complementary to the target's binding site will be created, such as agonists, antagonists, inverse agonists, or modulators of receptors; activators or inhibitors of enzymes; and openers or blockers of ion channels. Since drug interactions with off-target molecules can result in undesired side effects, small molecules (drugs) can be engineered to not affect any other significant off-target molecules (often referred to as antitargets). Sequence homology has identified closely related targets with the highest potential for side effects due to their similar binding sites, which increase the likelihood of cross-reactivity.

Drugs are typically organic small molecules made by chemical synthesis, but biopolymer-based medications, or biopharmaceuticals, made by biological processes are also becoming more and more popular. Furthermore, therapeutic uses for mRNA-based gene silencing technologies may exist. For instance, mRNA-based nanomedicines can simplify and speed up the drug development process by allowing immunostimulatory molecules to be expressed transiently and locally. Delivery of in vitro transcribed (IVT) mRNA to different cell types that are accessible can occur through the blood or other routes. The main goal of using IVT mRNA is to transfer particular genetic information into an individual's cells to prevent or modify a specific disease.

2.1.1.2. Drug Discovery

1. **Phenotypic Drug Discovery:** One conventional approach to drug discovery is phenotypic drug discovery, sometimes referred to as forward pharmacology or classical pharmacology. It identifies compounds with advantageous therapeutic effects by applying the technique of phenotypic screening to sets of artificial small molecules, natural products, or extracts within chemical libraries. This approach involves target identification after determining the in vivo or in vitro functional activity of medications (such as extract drugs or natural products). Phenotypic discovery seeks to identify pharmacologically active compounds and therapeutics that function via novel drug mechanisms by employing a pragmatic and target-independent methodology to produce first leads. When understanding molecular targets is insufficient for effective intervention, this method enables the exploration of disease phenotypes to find potential treatments for conditions with unknown, complex, or multifactorial origins.

2. **Rational Drug Discovery:** The premise that altering a particular biological target may be beneficial for therapeutic purposes is the foundation of rational drug design, also known as reverse pharmacology. Two key components must be present for a biomolecule to be chosen as a therapeutic target. The first is proof that altering the target will change the course of the illness. This information could originate from studies on disease linkage, for instance, which demonstrate a connection between specific disease states and mutations in the biological target. The target's ability to bind to a small molecule and allow that molecule to control its activity is the second. Following the identification of a viable target, the target is typically produced, purified, and cloned. After that, a screening assay is established using the purified protein. Furthermore, the target's three-dimensional structure can be ascertained.

   To find small molecules that bind to the target, libraries of putative medicinal compounds are screened. The screening assay, which is a wet screen, can be used to accomplish this. Furthermore, if the target's structure is known, a virtual screen of potential medications may be carried out. The ideal candidate drug compounds should have characteristics that are expected to result in sufficient chemical and metabolic stability, minimal toxic effects, and oral bioavailability. This is known as drug-likeness. Drug likeness can be estimated using a variety of techniques, including Lipinski's Rule of Five and several scoring techniques like lipophilic efficiency. Numerous techniques for forecasting drug metabolism have also been put forth in academic journals. Multi-objective optimization techniques are occasionally used in drug design due to the large number of properties that must be optimized simultaneously. Finally, drug design still heavily relies on serendipity and bounded rationality due to the shortcomings in the available techniques for activity prediction.

2.1.2. Computer-Aided Drug Design

Predicting whether and how strongly a particular molecule will bind to a target is the primary objective of drug design. The most common method for determining the strength of the intermolecular interaction between a small molecule and its biological target is molecular mechanics or molecular dynamics. These techniques are also employed to model conformational changes in the target that might take place upon the small molecule's binding, as well as to predict the conformation of the small molecule. Density functional theory, semi-empirical methods, and ab initio quantum chemistry techniques are frequently utilized to estimate the electronic properties (polarizability, electrostatic potential, etc.) and to provide optimized parameters for molecular mechanics calculations. of the potential medication that will affect binding affinity.

A semi-quantitative prediction of the binding affinity can also be obtained through the application of molecular mechanics techniques. Additionally, estimates of binding affinity may be obtained using a knowledge-based scoring function. By fitting experimental affinities to computationally determined interaction energies between the small molecule and the target, these methods derive predictive binding affinity equations through statistical techniques such as neural nets, machine learning, and linear regression.

In theory, only one compound needs to be synthesized, saving a significant amount of time and money, since the computational approach should be able to predict affinity before a compound is synthesized. In actuality, current computational techniques are flawed and only yield qualitatively accurate estimates of affinity at best. In actuality, finding the ideal medication often takes multiple design, synthesis, and testing iterations. By lowering the number of iterations needed, computational methods have sped up discovery and frequently produced novel structures (Figure 2.1).

Computer-aided drug design may be used at any of the following stages of drug discovery:

1. hit identification using virtual screening (structure- or ligand-based design)
2. hit-to-lead optimization of affinity and selectivity (structure-based design, QSAR, etc.)
3. lead optimization of other pharmaceutical properties while maintaining affinity

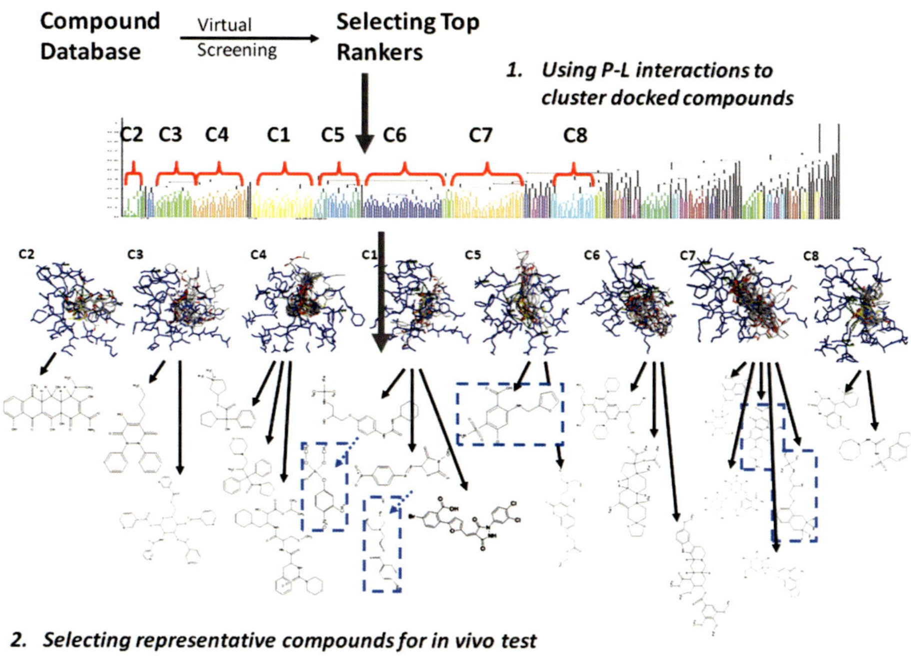

Figure 2.1. *Flowchart of a Usual Clustering Analysis for Structure-Based Drug Design.*

Source: https://upload.wikimedia.org/wikipedia/commons/thumb/5/54/Wiki_Clustering.png/800px-Wiki_Clustering.png.

The protein-ligand interaction and compound 3D structure data are used for analysis to get around the recent scoring functions' inadequate prediction of binding affinity. For structure-based drug design, several post-screening analyzes focusing on protein-ligand interaction have been developed for improving enrichment and effectively mining potential candidates:

1. Consensus scoring
i. Selecting candidates by voting of multiple scoring functions
ii. May lose the relationship between protein-ligand structural information and scoring criterion
2. Cluster analysis
i. Represent and cluster candidates according to protein-ligand 3D information
ii.. Needs meaningful representation of protein-ligand interactions.

2.1.3. Types of Drug Design

There are two major types of drug design. The first is referred to as ligand-based drug design and the second, is structure-based drug design (Figure 2.2).

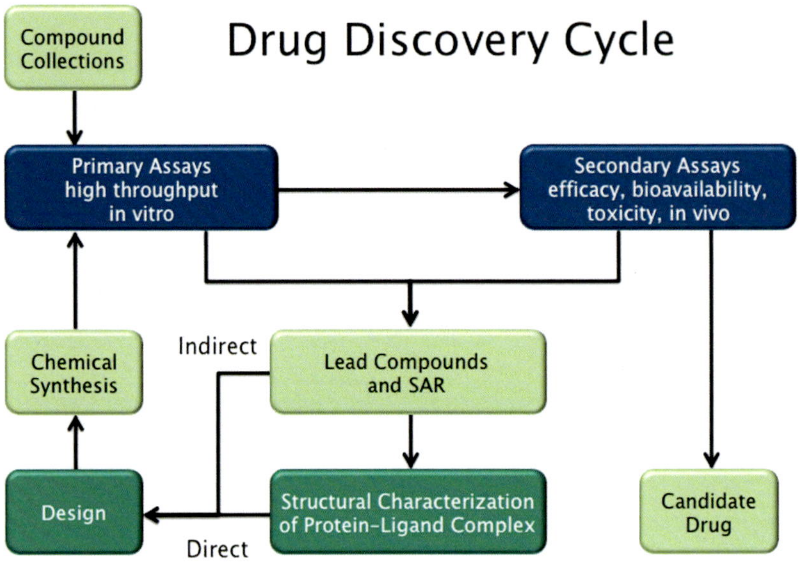

Figure 2.2. *Drug discovery cycle highlighting both ligand-based (indirect) and structure-based (direct) drug design strategies.*

Source: https://upload.wikimedia.org/wikipedia/commons/f/f9/Drug_discovery_cycle_2.png.

2.1.3.1. Ligand-based

Drug design based on ligands, also known as indirect drug design, is dependent on understanding other molecules that attach to the target biological target. A pharmacophore model, which specifies the minimal structural attributes a molecule must have to bind to the target, can be derived from these additional molecules. Based on what binds to the biological target, a model of the target can be constructed. New molecular entities that interact with the target can then be designed using the model. An alternative is to derive a quantitative structure-activity relationship (QSAR), which is a relationship between the properties of molecules that are calculated and their biological activity that is determined through experimentation. The activity of novel analogs may then be predicted using these QSAR relationships.

2.1.3.2. Structure-based

The knowledge of the three-dimensional structure of the biological target, acquired by techniques like X-ray crystallography or NMR spectroscopy, is the foundation of structure-based drug design, also known as direct drug design. If a target's experimental structure is unavailable, a homology model of the target might be constructed using the experimental structure of a related protein. A medicinal chemist's intuition combined with interactive graphics can be used to design candidate drugs that are predicted to bind to the biological target with high affinity and selectivity based on its structure. As an alternative, different automated computational techniques could be employed to propose novel drug candidates.

Three broad categories can be used to roughly categorize the current approaches to structure-based drug design. The first technique involves finding new ligands for a given receptor by utilizing quick approximation docking programs to search through vast databases of small molecule 3D structures to find those that fit the receptor's binding pocket. We call this process "virtual screening". The de novo design of novel ligands falls into a second category. By gradually assembling tiny parts, ligand molecules are constructed using this technique inside the confines of the binding pocket. These fragments may be single atoms or broken molecules. The main benefit of this approach is that new structures that aren't found in any database can be proposed. A third technique involves assessing suggested analogs inside the binding cavity to optimize known ligands.

2.1.3.3. Binding site identification

The initial stage of structure-based design is the identification of binding sites. The ligand should be visible in the structure if the target's or a sufficiently similar homolog's structure is identified when the ligand is bound, in which case the binding site's location is obvious. On the other hand, unoccupied allosteric binding sites might be useful. Additionally, it's possible that the only structures that exist are for apoproteins, or proteins without ligands, and it's difficult to reliably identify empty spaces that could bind ligands with great affinity. To put it briefly, locating concave surfaces on a protein that can hold drug-sized molecules and have the right hot spots (hydrophobic surfaces, hydrogen bonding sites, etc.) is typically necessary for identifying binding sites, which promote ligand binding.

2.1.3.4. Scoring functions

Structure-based drug design applies the concepts of molecular recognition to the structure of proteins to create new ligands. In general, selective high-affinity binding to the target is preferred because it produces medications that are more effective and have fewer side effects. Predicting a ligand's binding affinity to its target and any known anti-targets is crucial for designing or obtaining potential new ligands. This predicted affinity can then be used as a selection criterion. Böhm created one of the first widely used empirical scoring functions to characterize the binding energy of ligands to receptors. This empirical scoring function took the form:

$$\Delta G_{\text{bind}} = \Delta G_0 + \Delta G_{\text{hb}} \Sigma_{h-bonds} + \Delta G_{\text{ionic}} \Sigma_{ionic-int} + \Delta G_{\text{lipophilic}} |A| + \Delta G_{\text{rot}} NROT$$

Where:

- ΔG_0 – empirically derived offset that in part corresponds to the overall loss of translational and rotational entropy of the ligand upon binding.
- ΔG_{hb} – contribution from hydrogen bonding
- ΔG_{ionic} – contribution from ionic interactions
- ΔG_{lip} – contribution from lipophilic interactions where $|A_{lipo}|$ is the surface area of lipophilic contact between the ligand and receptor
- ΔG_{rot} – entropy penalty due to freezing a rotatable in the ligand bond upon binding

A more general thermodynamic "master" equation is as follows:

$$\Delta G_{\text{bind}} = -RT \ln K_{\text{d}}$$

$$K_{\text{d}} = \frac{[\text{Ligand}][\text{Receptor}]}{[\text{Complex}]}$$

$$\Delta G_{\text{bind}} = \Delta G_{\text{desolvation}} + \Delta G_{\text{motion}} + \Delta G_{\text{configuration}} + \Delta G_{\text{interaction}}$$

Where:

- desolvation – enthalpic penalty for removing the ligand from solvent
- motion – entropic penalty for reducing the degrees of freedom when a ligand binds to its receptor
- configuration – conformational strain energy required to put the ligand in its "active" conformation
- interaction – enthalpic gain for "resolvating" the ligand with its receptor

The main concept is that the total binding free energy can be broken down into individual components that play a crucial role in the binding process. Each component represents a specific type of free energy change that occurs during the binding of a ligand to its target receptor. The Master Equation is a sum of these components. By using the Gibbs free energy equation, a relationship was established between the dissociation equilibrium constant, K_d, and the different components of free energy.

Each element of the master equation is estimated using a different computational technique. To estimate the desolvation energy, for instance, one can use the change in polar surface area upon ligand binding. The motion term is proportional to the number of rotatable bonds that are frozen upon ligand binding. Calculations based on molecular mechanics can be used to estimate the configurational or strain energy. Lastly, techniques like the number of hydrogen bonds formed, statistically derived mean force potentials, and changes in the non-polar surface can all be used to estimate the interaction energy. In actuality, multiple linear regression is used to fit the master equation's components to experimental data. This can be achieved with a more limited set of ligands and receptors to produce a more accurate but less general local model, or with a diverse training set including many types of ligands and receptors to produce a less accurate but more general global model.

2.1.3.5. Drug screening

Phenotypic, high-throughput, and virtual screening are among the different types of drug screening. The process of screening medications using cellular or animal disease models to find compounds that change the phenotype and have positive effects on the disease is known as phenotypic screening. New developments in high-throughput screening significantly reduce the needed detection volume and speed up processing. Virtual screening is carried out by a computer, allowing for quick and inexpensive screening of a large number of molecules. Through the use of various computational techniques, virtual screening enables chemists to condense large virtual libraries into more manageable sizes.

2.2. Principles of Drug Design

The process of creating drugs is intricate and multidimensional, incorporating ideas from different scientific fields to create compounds that have therapeutic effects. Fundamentally, the goal of drug design is to develop compounds that interact with particular biological targets to maximize desired pharmacological effects and minimize side effects. A thorough understanding of the molecular causes of disease, structure-activity relationship (SAR) of drug molecules, ligand-receptor interactions, pharmacokinetics, selectivity and specificity, optimization of physicochemical properties, and safety profiling are all included in the principles of drug design. Validating and identifying targets is a basic component of drug design. This involves determining the molecules or biological pathways that are involved in the processes that lead to disease and confirming their suitability as targets for treatment. The identification and characterization of novel drug targets have been made easier by developments in genomics, proteomics, and bioinformatics, opening up new avenues for intervention.

The analysis of structure-activity relationships, or SARs, is essential to logical drug design. In SAR investigations, lead compound chemical structures are methodically changed, and their biological activity is assessed. By clarifying the connection between a molecule's structure and pharmacological characteristics, scientists can pinpoint crucial structural elements necessary for medication effectiveness. The optimization of lead compounds to improve their potency, selectivity, and pharmacokinetic qualities is guided by this iterative process.

The knowledge of ligand-receptor interactions is essential for the development of successful pharmaceuticals. Drug molecules, also known as ligands, attach to particular molecular targets like proteins, enzymes, receptors, or nucleic acids to produce their pharmacological effects. Predicting and analyzing these interactions is done computationally using methods like molecular docking and molecular dynamics simulations. Researchers can design new compounds with better therapeutic profiles by predicting the binding affinity and specificity of drug-target complexes and by elucidating their three-dimensional structure. When determining a drug's pharmacological activity and how it behaves in the body, pharmacokinetics is a key factor. The goal of drug design is to maximize a compound's absorption, distribution, metabolism, and excretion (ADME) characteristics. Through the process of chemical structure modification, researchers can maximize a compound's bioavailability and metabolic stability while lowering the possibility of unfavorable side effects.

To guarantee that medications interact selectively with their intended targets while minimizing off-target effects, selectivity and specificity are crucial factors in drug design. The goal of rational drug design strategies is to maximize a compound's selectivity and specificity by modifying its structure and using targeted delivery methods. This method improves the therapeutic index of medications while lowering the possibility of adverse reactions. To guarantee the pharmaceutical qualities of treatment candidates, physicochemical property optimization is crucial. The absorption, distribution, and bioavailability of a drug are greatly influenced by properties like solubility, lipophilicity, and molecular size. To improve the drug's safety and efficacy profiles, these characteristics must be optimized during the drug design process.

Last but not least, safety profiling is essential for assessing the possible toxicity of medication candidates. Computational modeling aids in predicting and evaluating the safety profile of compounds when paired with preclinical research and experimental assays. Prioritizing the creation of safer and more effective medication candidates allows researchers to identify and mitigate potentially harmful effects early in the drug development process. The field of drug design is multifaceted and dynamic, incorporating concepts from computational modeling, pharmacology, biology, and chemistry. Researchers can systematically design and optimize drug candidates with the potential to address unmet medical needs and enhance patient outcomes by following these principles.

2.2.1. Structure-Activity Relationships (SAR)

A key idea in medicinal chemistry and drug design, Structure-Activity Relationships (SAR) analysis directs the logical creation of therapeutic compounds. To clarify the structural elements necessary for biological efficacy, structural molecular recognition (SAR) investigates the connection between a molecule's pharmacological activity and its chemical structure. Through the methodical alteration of lead compound structures and subsequent assessment of their efficacy, scientists can identify trends that guide the development and refinement of new pharmaceuticals. Fundamentally, the goal of SAR analysis is to locate important structural components in a molecule that influence how it interacts with biological targets, such as enzymes, proteins, receptors, or nucleic acids. The molecule's binding affinity and specificity to its target are determined by these structural characteristics, also known as pharmacophores, which ultimately determine the pharmacological effect of the molecule.

Synthesizing several lead compound analogs or derivatives, each with unique structural modifications, is a common step in the SAR analysis process. These modifications could be substitutions of atoms or groups, adjustments to functional groups, adjustments to stereochemistry, or modifications to molecular scaffolds. The potency, selectivity, and other pharmacological characteristics of each analog are then evaluated employing in vitro or in vivo assays.

Through a methodical correlation between modifications in chemical structure and shifts in pharmacological activity, structural affinity retrieval (SAR) analysis helps scientists pinpoint the essential structural factors that impact a compound's effectiveness. For instance, certain structural characteristics may influence the compound's selectivity or metabolic stability, while other functional groups may be found to be necessary for binding to a target protein. SAR analysis can also shed light on a drug's mode of action and aid in the prediction of both positive and negative side effects. Through an understanding of the effects of structural alterations on a compound's interaction with biological targets, scientists can create molecules that are more effective, less toxic, and have better pharmacokinetic qualities.

Quantitative structure-activity relationship (QSAR) modeling and other computational approaches, which offer predictive tools to direct compound design and optimization, are essential to SAR analysis. Molecular docking and molecular dynamics simulations are two examples of molecular modeling techniques that help scientists rationally design new compounds by enabling them to see and examine the binding interactions between molecules and their targets. On the other hand, QSAR models make use of statistical analyzes to link a compound's structural characteristics with its biological activity, which makes it easier to predict the activity of new analogs. SAR analysis is essential to medicinal chemistry and drug design because it makes therapeutic compounds logically optimized. SAR analysis enables researchers to design molecules with improved efficacy, selectivity, and safety profiles, ultimately advancing the development of novel treatments for a variety of diseases. This is accomplished by clarifying the relationship between chemical structure and pharmacological activity.

From lead optimization to primary screening, many facets of drug discovery depend on structure-activity relationships (SAR). When working with SAR, the first step is determining whether a SAR is present in a group of molecules and the activities that go along with it. Next, one attempts to clarify the specifics of one or more SARs and uses the information to modify their structures to optimize a property or activity. Chemical space is basically infinite in the absence of "sign posts," and it can be rationally explored with a basic understanding of the SAR for a given set of molecules. Developing a chemical series always entails simultaneously optimizing several physical-chemical and biological properties. For instance, the majority of lead optimization initiatives will aim to increase potency, lower toxicity, and guarantee adequate bioavailability, among other characteristics. Even though a medicinal chemist's intuition and experience are invaluable to these efforts, a single chemist may not be able to handle the volume of data produced by contemporary high-throughput experimental techniques. For instance, one might encounter hundreds of chemical series in a primary HTS. In these situations, rapid and effective characterization of SARs is made possible by in silico methods; however, how can the most promising series among them be quickly identified? Using these techniques, one can construct a range of models to identify and encrypt one or more SARs, which can subsequently be utilized to forecast the behaviors of novel compounds. When combined with in silico structural modifications, it is simple to rank large screening decks or even create new compounds from scratch and determine whether or not they are related to the SAR under study. Remember that computational techniques do not take the place of domain knowledge in medicinal chemistry. Instead, through the integration and summarization of copious amounts of pre-existing data, they can serve as a useful guide for the seasoned user, suggesting structural modifications.

While it is true that computational methods can be useful in determining, elucidating, and forecasting structure-activity relationships (SAR), they can also produce misleading results if used carelessly or improperly. SAR models are fundamentally just that—models. That is, a condensed or simplified picture of reality that is full of presumptions and restrictions. These techniques range widely in terms of their utility and complexity. This provides an overview of the various SAR modeling techniques and, more especially, how they help with the process of searching chemical space to clarify and improve structure-activity relationships in a drug discovery context Databases as a source of SAR data will be covered and how they can help to inform and improve the investigation of SAR trends, in addition to modeling algorithms.

2.2.1.1. Capturing SAR

There have been numerous approaches to recording structure-activity relationships over the past sixty years. They can be roughly categorized into two groups: those that are based on data mining or statistical techniques (e.g., regression models) as well as those derived from physical methods (e.g., models of pharmacophores). Readers are directed to literature in the field for an in-depth analysis of QSAR techniques. It is crucial to understand that the modeling technique selected can affect the scope and level of detail that can be explored using a SAR. For instance, crucial components of a SAR that depend on chirality may be missed by statistical QSAR methods based on 2D descriptors that neglect stereochemistry. The nature of the ligand-receptor interactions that underpin an observed SAR can be directly understood using 3D approaches, which are, on the other hand, typically more explicitly informative. Different 3D approaches have different levels of explicitness; docking versus CoMFA is one example. Still, when a crystal structure is available and a few chemical series are being investigated, 3D approaches are generally preferred (Figure 2.3).

Traditional QSAR relies heavily on statistical models that relate biological activities to chemical structure, which is described by numerical descriptors. While some situations are "model-free," others involve the model making distributional assumptions (linear regression).

Either way, a model is created using a training set of molecules. The activity of novel molecules can then be predicted using the model. There is no reason to assume that the structure-activity relationship is linear a priori, even though a large portion of QSAR has concentrated on different types of linear regression (from ordinary least squares to more reliable techniques like PLS or ridge regression). Because of all the intricate processes that take place in vivo, it is unrealistic to expect linear relationships in most biological systems. As a result, contemporary non-linear techniques with high accuracy, like support vector machines and neural networks, have found widespread application.

Making a prediction model, though, is only the first step. The model can be applied to some situations, like virtual screening, and the results are just numerical activity predictions. This article, however, focuses on the application of these predictive models to SAR exploration. The ability to interpret the model and comprehend precisely how it links activity to particular structural features is essential for this kind of investigation. A model should be comprehensible for interpretive purposes, both about the underlying model and the descriptors employed.

The model's predictive power is not its main focus, though statistical models should obviously have statistically significant results. Random forests and linear regression are two examples. When using this kind of usage, one is curious about what the model can reveal about how particular structural elements affect the activity that is being observed. Therefore, it is essential that this data can be extracted from the model. Obviously, interpretability is much more explicit for more physical methods like docking and pharmacophore modeling. Clearly, dissectable models are useful for SAR exploration.

Examples of these interpretive applications for both conventional black box models and simpler models have been documented. It is also true, though, that purely predictive models have their uses, particularly when attempting to distinguish more or less active molecules from a large collection. In this case, users could use a predictive model to generate a preliminary ranking, which would enable them to concentrate on a smaller subset and apply more interpretive techniques.

Visualizing the SAR trends embedded in a model is closely associated with analytical interpretations of QSAR models. One example of a direct visualization of a predictive model in terms of the actual chemical structure is the "glowing molecule" representation that was created. The user can directly comprehend how structural changes made at particular points will impact the property or activity being optimized with this kind of visualization.

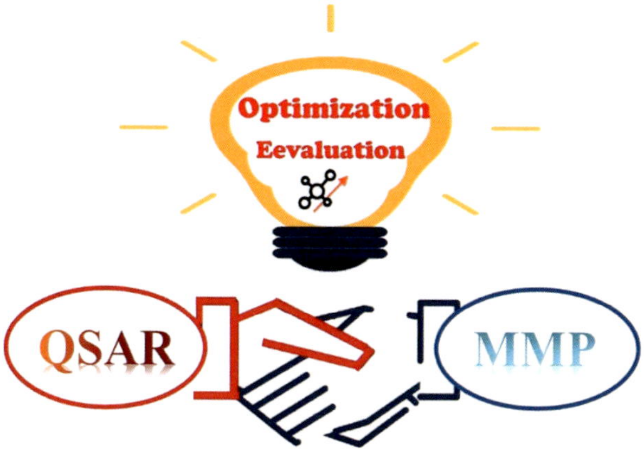

Figure 2.3. *QSAR modeling.*

Source: Yang, ZY., Fu, L., Lu, AP. et al. Semi-utomated workflow for molecular pair analysis and QSAR-assisted transformation space expansion. J Cheminform 13, 86 (2021). https://doi.org/10.1186/s13321-021-00564-6.

It is helpful to incorporate SAR trends into a predictive model so that new properties can be predicted, but there is another way to go about it. In other words, find structures that correspond with a certain activity or activity profile. Rather than focusing on the structure directly, the majority of formulations of this approach seek to derive a set of descriptor values. Finding legitimate structures from a set of descriptor values is the difficult part. The inverse QSAR problem has been worked on by several people. The inverse QSAR analysis of 121 HIV protease inhibitors was conducted using the signature molecular descriptors, and the QSARs of peptides that inhibit ICAM-1 were investigated using the same descriptors. Recently, to address inverse QSAR, a unique descriptor was created. This was then coupled with a kernel method to enable explicit mapping between points in the high-dimensional kernel space (i.e., candidate structures) back to the initial space of descriptors and subsequently to a collection of potential molecules.

- **Is the Model Reliable?:** While any statistical method or machine learning algorithm can be utilized to analyze SAR data and make predictions for new molecules, the reliability of these predictions may vary. These approaches to QSAR modeling rely on the assumption that new molecules being predicted share some structural similarities with the training set. If a new molecule is significantly different, the prediction may not be accurate. Therefore, it is important to establish the "domain of applicability" (DA) of a model to indicate when its predictions can be trusted. This is especially valuable in situations where a model is used over time, as it helps determine when the model needs to be updated due to changes in the molecules being predicted.

Diverse techniques have been devised to delineate areas of relevance. Finding the similarity between a new molecule and the model's training set is the most straightforward method. This method focuses on two factors: the number of closest neighbors in the training set (determined by a user-defined similarity cutoff) and the similarity between the molecule to be predicted and its nearest neighbor in the training set. According to their findings, both of these methods produce a strong indicator of prediction reliability. The training set allows them to measure a molecule's similarity to the entire set by utilizing a new distance metric called the "dimension related distance". Other metrics for measuring distance have also been used, such as the Manhattan and Mahalanobis distances.

There have also been several methods based on descriptor values put forth. The easiest method is to figure out the range of descriptor values in the training set. If the new molecule's values fall outside of this range, the model will have to extrapolate, which will make the prediction inaccurate. Although this method is straightforward conceptually, non-uniformly distributed descriptor values can easily lead to confusion. Reliable predictions can be obtained within the ranges of the principal components that result from PCA, according to alternative methods.

2.2.1.2. Exploring SAR Landscapes

While predictions from QSAR models are a helpful tool for lead optimization, other perspectives on SAR data may also be beneficial. The landscape paradigm of SAR data has drawn attention in recent years and enables us to investigate several facets of structure-activity relationships. This work is an extension of Lajiness's work, which used a 3D representation of chemical structure (represented by the X-Y plane) and bioactivity (represented by the Z-axis) to view the two simultaneously. This directly means that a SAR dataset can be thought of as a landscape with different "topography". Similar molecules in terms of structure and activity are represented by smooth regions, while jagged (i.e., discontinuous) areas are associated with structures that share similarities but display radically different activities (also known as activity cliffs). Indeed, it has been proposed that the later landscape regions are the most intriguing portions of a SAR because they offer the opportunity to make minor structural adjustments that can drastically alter activities. However, these discontinuities can also be problematic because they can cause many QSAR modeling techniques (mainly machine learning or statistical model-based techniques) to perform poorly. Consequently, numerous techniques have been created to mine and characterize SAR landscapes.

This displays the structure similarity against the activity similarity in a pairwise plot. One can identify molecules characteristic of one of four possible behaviors by dividing the resulting plot into four quadrants: smooth regions of the SAR space, (rough) activity cliffs, non-descript (i.e., scaffold hops, which have low structural similarity but high activity similarity, and low structural similarity. Numerous extensions of SAS maps that consider multiple descriptor representations (2D and 3D) have been released recently. Apart from SAS maps, various pairwise metrics like SALI and SARI have been created to describe and illustrate SAR landscapes.

Novel developments in the exploration of SAR data have also resulted from the visualization of landscapes through network diagrams. Compounds are used as nodes in both network representations, and edges are drawn between them according to a metric (SALI for SALI networks, and SARI for NSG's) that describes the pair of nodes in relation to the landscape. After that, the networks can be examined to pinpoint particular SAR patterns. Outlined a method for locating "SAR pathways," or routes in an NSG that link areas with low and high SAR discontinuity. These SAR pathways stand for a group of compounds that, in the right order, display an ongoing sequence of SAR alterations. Although network-based landscape analyzes have seen a lot of activity, another visualization technique abstracted the concept of the SALI metric and expanded it to encompass the receptor.

R-groups have also been subjected to the idea of activity cliffs and the landscape paradigm; an "R-cliff" is when two compounds in a single R-group differ from one another. This clearly places this kind of analysis in the context of analog series derived via R-group decompositions, as it is a specialization of the activity cliff concept.

2.2.1.3. Canned SAR

Many sizable chemical structure databases have become accessible during the past few years. Crucially, in addition to compound structures, many of these databases offer comprehensive details on compound activities. Some notable instances are GVK GOSTAR, PubChem, and ChEMBL. While GOSTAR is a paid service, the first two are freely accessible resources. These databases offer structure-activity information, but the types of data they offer are different. For instance, PubChem offers a bioassay database that houses assay results for different compound sets that have been deposited by the Molecular Libraries Initiative, as well as a compound and substance database where records are individual structures. Because the two databases are connected, it is simple to determine which assays a compound has been tested in or, in the other direction, which structures have been tested in an assay. Assay types include primary screens, secondary screens, confirmatory screens, and both single point and dose-response formats. Assay datasets range in size from two or three compounds to over 300,000 compounds. The assay data may be noisy because PubChem data is not curated, which is given for primary screening data. This is an important point to note. The SAR databases ChEMBL and GOSTAR are both carefully curated, meaning that the structures and activities within them have been hand-picked from the literature and standardized for storage. Furthermore, numerous annotations have been included, including species, assay target, and more. These databases are easily analyzed because they essentially contain "canned" structure-activity relationships.

The GDB-13 database, which is a comprehensive list of small molecule structures with up to 13 heavy atoms (limited to C, H, N, O, S, P, and Cl), is relatively unique. The database can be used as a source of structures for virtual screening even though it lacks activity information related to the structures. It is comparable to databases like ZINC in this regard; the main distinction is that the latter are all commercially available, while the former are essentially entirely virtual. Generally speaking, the main applications for this class of databases are virtual screening techniques, where the objective is to find candidates for further investigation rather than clearly identifying SAR patterns.

2.2.1.4. Alternatives to QSAR

Several other approaches are possible, although QSAR approaches (in all its forms) are by far the most popular ways to capture and investigate SAR trends. They can, despite not being quantitative. Serve as helpful "idea generators".

2.2.1.4.1. Characterizing SAR in Series

One strategy is to use fragments as the starting point for SAR research. There is precedent for this because models based on substructure have been created that are helpful for interpretation as well as prediction. Creating "R-group QSAR" models is one method of utilizing fragments to investigate SAR. These models seek to ascertain whether or not a SAR exists, and if so, how various R-groups impact it. We carry out an R-group decomposition on a set of molecules, producing a number of scaffolds and related substituents. Given a scaffold, we can create an R-group matrix, with observations (i.e., molecules containing the scaffold) in the rows and the R-groups, R_1, R_2, ..., R_n, in the columns. Element (i, j) of the matrix is set to 1 if the i'th molecule contains the j'th substituent. Given this R-group incidence matrix, along with the observed activities for the molecules, one can develop a predictive model. Given that most such R-group matrices will be small, some form of linear regression is likely most suitable. Figure 2.4 shows a schematic diagram summarizing this technique. However, it is obvious that this approach has a number of limitations. Firstly, the number of observations for many scaffolds will be very small (< 10) and hence a reliable model can't be generated. Second, most R-group matrices will be sparse since all substitution points will not be uniformly filled. Also, a binary incidence matrix may not be the most appropriate input for a linear regression model. One way to address this is to replace each of n columns with $n \times d$ columns, where d represents a d-dimensional real-valued descriptor vector derived from the structure of the corresponding R-group. For a scaffold with three or more substitution points, this can lead to an R-group matrix with more columns than rows. Such a matrix will typically have a large number of features, even in cases where this isn't the case (depending on how many descriptors are employed).

Despite these issues, a linear regression model can be created for scaffolds with a sufficient number of observations and comparatively few substitution points. In these situations, the model's predictive accuracy is not the primary concern. Our focus is on the statistical significance of the model, as we believe it to be a true representation of the relationship between the substitutions and the observed activities. Therefore, this might enable us to rank each series separately.

Obviously, for a diverse set of structures, this approach is not very useful.

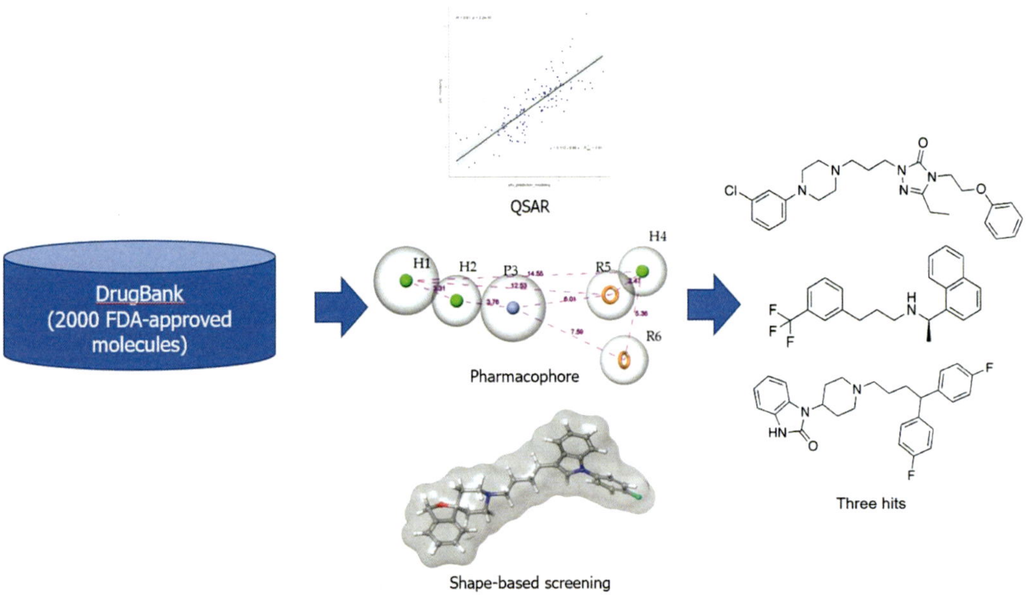

Figure 2.4. *A schematic diagram of R-group QSAR workflow that can be used to rank scaffolds (i.e., chemical series) in terms of whether they exhibit a SAR or not.*

Source: *Yu Y, Dong H, Peng Y, Welsh WJ. QSAR-Based Computational Approaches to Accelerate the Discovery of Sigma-2 Receptor (S2R) Ligands as Therapeutic Drugs. Molecules. 2021; 26(17):5270. https://doi.org/10.3390/molecules26175270.*

2.2.1.4.2. Exploring SAR Via Fragments

Exploring SAR with fragments can also be accomplished by using SAR databases like ChEMBL. The fundamental driving force is the possibility that some segments are connected to high (or low) activity levels, or that they exhibit activity that is biased toward a particular target or target family. We can take an external set of compounds, fragment them, and examine the activity data connected to them in ChEMBL by precompute the fragments for a database such as ChEMBL and storing the fragment-compound associations. Although it's a fairly easy task, there are a few steps involved. With the help of observed activity data and a compound collection, it is possible to create fragments from ChEMBL and determine the activity profiles linked to those fragments, ultimately identifying the specific ChEMBL compounds that are connected to the fragment of interest. As an alternative, one can summarize the selectivity of compound series by characterizing scaffolds according to their activities against various targets (Figure 2.5).

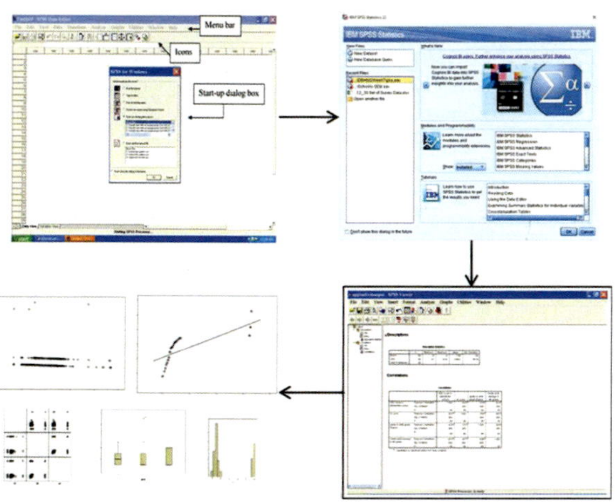

Figure 2.5. *SPSS package in pharmaceutical data analytic.*

Source: Lo, Y.-C., Gui, R., Honda, H., & Torres, J. Z. (2016). Quantitative Methods in System-Based Drug Discovery. InTech. doi: 10.5772/65833.

2.2.2. Quantitative Structure-Activity Relationships (QSAR)

Establishing quantitative relationships between a molecule's chemical structure and biological activity is the goal of Quantitative Structure-Activity Relationships (QSAR) analysis, a potent computational technique in medicinal chemistry and drug design. With the use of QSAR models, scientists can systematically examine and forecast a compound's pharmacological characteristics by taking into account its molecular characteristics. QSAR analysis speeds up the drug discovery process by combining concepts from statistics, biology, and chemistry to enable the logical design and optimization of drug candidates. The fundamental idea of QSAR analysis is that a molecule's physicochemical and structural characteristics can be quantitatively correlated with its biological activity. The process of creating QSAR models involves systematically analyzing a dataset that includes several structurally different compounds with well-established biological activities. For every compound in the dataset, molecular descriptors—information about the chemical structure and characteristics of molecules—are computed. Parameters like molecular size, lipophilicity, electronic characteristics, and topological indices are examples of these descriptors.

Statistical techniques are utilized to establish a correlation between the computed molecular descriptors and the observed biological activities of the compounds. Regression analysis is commonly used in the construction of QSAR models, yielding mathematical equations that predict the quantitative relationship between molecular descriptors and biological activity. The activity of novel compounds that were excluded from the initial dataset can be estimated using these equations, which function as predictive models.

The capacity of QSAR analysis to shed light on the structure-activity relationships of compounds and clarify the molecular characteristics that are essential for their pharmacological effects is one of its main advantages. QSAR analysis directs the logical design of novel compounds with optimal therapeutic properties by pinpointing the structural determinants of a compound's activity. For instance, certain functional groups or molecular motifs that increase binding affinity to a target protein or selectivity against off-targets may be revealed by QSAR models. Moreover, QSAR analysis expedites the drug discovery process by helping to prioritize lead compounds for additional experimental assessment. Researchers can identify promising candidates with low toxicity and high efficacy by using QSAR models to predict the activity of virtual compound libraries.

This reduces the time and resources needed for experimental screening. Apart from drug design, QSAR analysis finds use in chemical risk assessment, environmental toxicology, and material science, among other fields. QSAR models are used to evaluate the safety of chemical compounds, forecast the biological effects of environmental pollutants, and optimize material properties for particular uses.

Notwithstanding its usefulness, QSAR analysis has a number of drawbacks and difficulties. The quality of the input data, the selection of molecular descriptors, and the robustness of the statistical techniques used all affect how accurate and reliable QSAR models are. Furthermore, because biological systems are inherently complex, QSAR models may not fully account for all the variables influencing molecular interactions and pharmacological responses. With its systematic and quantitative approach to elucidating structure-activity relationships and predicting the biological activity of compounds, QSAR analysis is a useful tool in medicinal chemistry and drug design. Through the integration of statistical and computational techniques, QSAR analysis expedites the process of finding and refining new drug candidates, thereby contributing to the advancement of therapeutics for a range of illnesses.

2.3. Molecular Modeling

All theoretical and computational techniques used to simulate or model molecular behavior are collectively referred to as molecular modeling. The techniques are applied to the study of molecular systems, from small chemical systems to large biological molecules and material assemblies, in the domains of computational chemistry, drug design, computational biology, and materials science. Even though the most basic computations can be completed by hand, molecular modeling of any system of a reasonable size ultimately requires computers. The atomistic level description of the molecular systems is a common characteristic of molecular modeling techniques. This could involve modeling protons and neutrons explicitly with their quarks, anti-quarks, and gluons, and electrons with their photons (a quantum chemistry approach) or treating atoms as the smallest individual unit (a molecular mechanics approach).

2.3.1. Molecular Mechanics

One component of molecular modeling is molecular mechanics, which describes the physical foundation of the models using classical mechanics (Newtonian mechanics). Atoms, or the nucleus and electrons together, are usually described in molecular models as point charges with corresponding masses. Van der Waals forces and spring-like interactions—which stand in for chemical bonds—define the interactions between nearby atoms. The latter is often referred to as the Lennard-Jones potential.

On the basis of Coulomb's law, the electrostatic interactions are calculated. In dynamical simulations, atoms can also be given velocities in addition to coordinates in internal or Cartesian space. The macroscopic system temperature is correlated with the atomic velocities. The system internal energy (U), a thermodynamic quantity equal to the sum of the kinetic and potential energies, is connected to the collective mathematical expression known as a potential function. Energy minimization techniques are those that reduce potential energy (e.g., steepest descent and conjugate gradient), whereas molecular dynamics refers to techniques that simulate how a system would behave as time passes.

$$E = E_{\text{bonds}} + E_{\text{angle}} + E_{\text{dihedral}} + E_{\text{non-bonded}}$$

$$E_{\text{non-bonded}} = E_{\text{electrostatic}} + E_{\text{van der Waals}}$$

The molecular potential energy is calculated by this function, also known as a potential function, which adds terms for non-bonded atom pairs that describe van der Waals and electrostatic interactions to the energy terms that describe the deviation of bond lengths, bond angles, and torsion angles from equilibrium values. A force field is the collection of parameters that includes equilibrium bond lengths, bond angles, partial charge values, force constants, and van der Waals parameters. Different mathematical expressions and potential function parameters are used in different molecular mechanics implementations. High-level quantum computations, chemical theory, and experimental reference data were used to develop the common force fields that are used today. The process, known as energy minimization, identifies a local energy minimum, or locations of zero gradient for every atom. Because they are more stable and play a part in chemical and biological processes, lower energy states are frequently studied. In contrast, a molecular dynamics simulation calculates a system's behavior as a function of time. It entails figuring out Newton's laws of motion, especially F=ma, the second law. Atomic trajectories in space and time are obtained by integrating Newton's laws of motion using various integration algorithms. The negative gradient of the potential energy function is the definition of the force acting on an atom. When comparing states of similar systems, the energy minimization method helps obtain a static image, but molecular dynamics offers information about dynamic processes that naturally include temperature effects.

2.3.1.1. Variables

It is possible to model molecules in both vacuum and in the presence of a solvent, like water. Gas-phase simulations are systems that are simulated in a vacuum; explicit solvent simulations are those that include solvent molecules in the simulation. Implicit solvation simulations are a different kind of simulation in which the solvent effect is calculated through an empirical mathematical expression.

2.3.1.2. Coordinate representations

The most practical expression for these Cartesian coordinates is dependent on distance for the majority of force fields. Yet, an internal coordinate system is the most sensible representation due to the relatively rigid nature of bonds that arise between particular atoms and, in essence, define what is meant by the designation molecule. Certain fields refer to the IC representation—which includes the bond's twist angle, length, and angle between bonds as depicted in the figure—as the Z-matrix or torsion angle representation. Sadly, working with force fields in the internal coordinate representation is often difficult when dealing with continuous motions in Cartesian space, which frequently call for discontinuous angular branches in internal coordinates. On the other hand, a straightforward atom displacement in Cartesian space might not follow a straight line trajectory because of the interconnected bonds' prohibitions. As a result, during their iterations, computational optimization programs frequently switch between representations. This can cause cumulative numerical inaccuracy in long-chain molecules and significantly increase the calculation time. Although every conversion algorithm yields mathematically identical results, their speed and numerical accuracy vary. Currently, the Natural Extension Reference Frame (NERF) method is the fastest and most accurate way to convert torsion to Cartesian.

2.3.1.3. Applications

The structure, dynamics, surface characteristics, and thermodynamics of inorganic, biological, and polymeric systems are frequently studied using molecular modeling techniques. These days, a vast array of force field molecular models is easily accessible in databases. Protein folding, enzyme catalysis, protein stability, conformational changes linked to biomolecular function, and molecular recognition of proteins, DNA, and membrane complexes are among the biological activities that have been studied through molecular modeling (Figure 2.6).

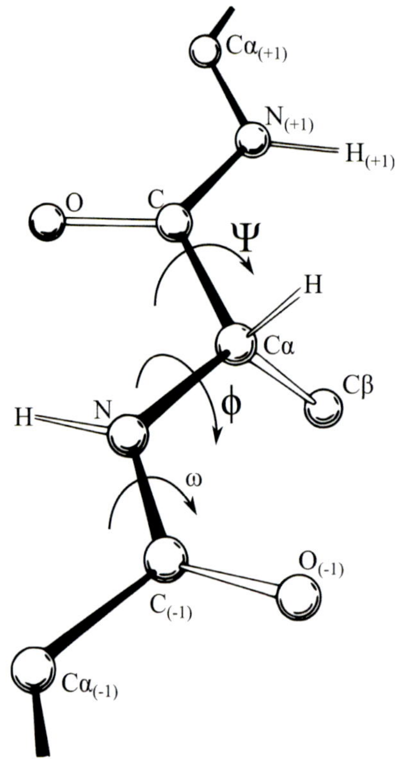

Figure 2.6. *The backbone dihedral angles are included in the molecular model of a protein.*

Source: https://upload.wikimedia.org/wikipedia/commons/thumb/9/97/Protein_backbone_PhiPsiOmega_drawing.svg/315px-Protein_backbone_PhiPsiOmega_drawing.svg.png.

2.4. Molecular Modeling Techniques

A wide range of computational techniques are incorporated into molecular modeling approaches to investigate the atomic-level structure, dynamics, and interactions of molecules. These methods are essential to the fields of molecular biology, materials science, and drug discovery because they enable the logical design of new compounds and offer insightful knowledge about the behavior of molecules. Here, we go over some important molecular modeling methods and how they are used in science studies.

2.4.1. Molecular Docking

A computational method called "molecular docking" is used to anticipate a ligand's (small molecule's) preferred conformation and orientation within a target protein's binding site. Docking algorithms determine possible binding poses and calculate the ligand's binding affinity for the target by modeling the interactions between the ligand and protein. Throughout the drug discovery process, molecular docking is frequently utilized to screen compound libraries, forecast ligand-protein interactions, and create new drug candidates with increased potency and selectivity.

Using a variety of scoring functions to select the best pose produced by each molecule to a rank-order, molecular docking is an in silico technique that identifies the correct binding pose of a protein-ligand complex and assesses its strength. By combining and optimizing factors like hydrophobic, steric, and electrostatic complementarily and estimating their binding free energy, docking techniques try to fit a ligand into the binding site of a target protein. High-resolution X-ray crystallographic structures, NMR structures, or homology-modeled structures with a known binding site are necessary for accurate docking.

The Protein Data Bank (PDB) contains thousands of experimentally determined protein 3D structures. Scientists can experimentally solve the intricate three-dimensional (3D) structures of molecules in their interaction forms thanks to X-ray and NMR equipment. This is a crucial technique for identifying critical residues, assessing the energetics of the interaction forces, and comprehending how molecular structures fit together. Owing to the limitations of current experimental methods, certain proteins' three-dimensional structures are frequently challenging to ascertain and, as a result, are typically not included in the protein data bank (PDB). However, the development of advanced bioinformatics methods has made it possible to use homology modeling servers to model the 3-dimensional structure of a target protein that is not available in the protein data bank (Figure 2.7). The tertiary structure of the target is predicted using homology modeling, which is based on a template with a similar residue. This is supported theoretically by the observation that proteins with similar residues also share similar structures and ancestries. One of the most popular web-based tools for homology modeling is the Swiss Model Server. The exceptionally accurate Alpha fold homology modeling system from DeepMind has further advanced the field of computational structural biology. Jumper and the other brilliant minds at DeepMinds used artificial intelligence (AI) and other potent machine learning tools to design a model that achieved more than 92 % accuracy with 3D-structural protein prediction. This ground-breaking discovery resolved 50 years of major challenges in protein structure prediction. AlphaFold is the most robust webserver/tool available and was rated as the best model/software for homology modeling after being published in Nature. It's interesting to note that RoseTTAFold, a different model that was released on the same day as AlphaFold, also outperformed Deepminds' model in terms of confidence scores and achieved good accuracy in protein prediction. But RoseTTAFold from Baker's lab has an advantage over AlphaFold: it can predict intricate biological assemblies like protein-protein structures. These newly designed models are believed to revolutionize in silico drug discovery in this 21st century.

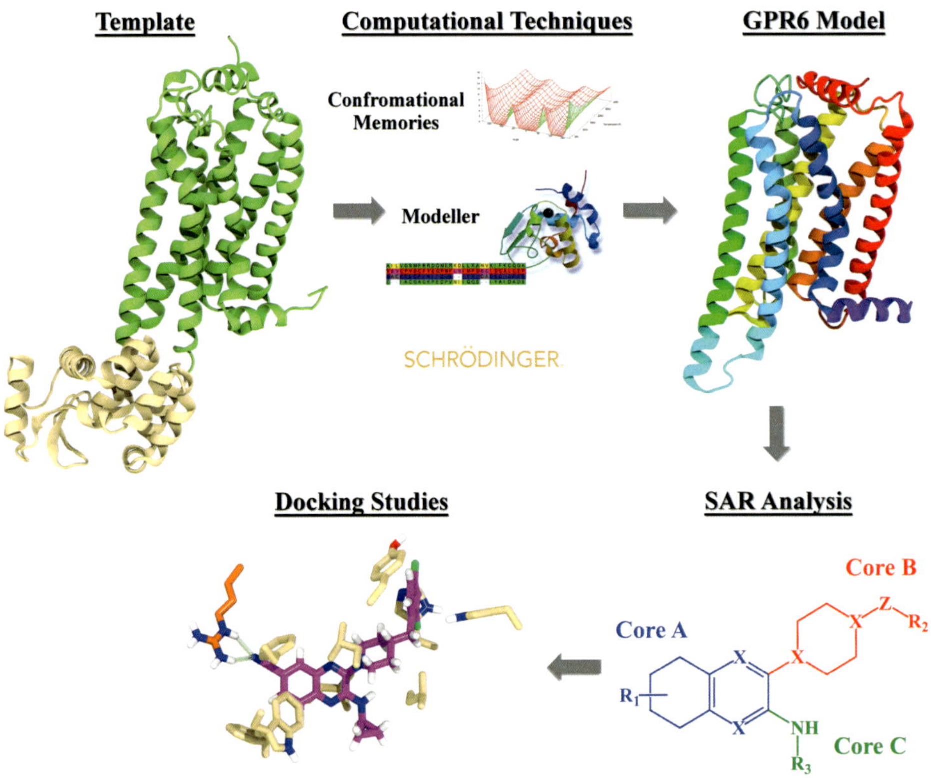

Figure 2.7. *Depicts the homology modeling of proteins.*

Source: Isawi IH, Morales P, Sotudeh N, Hurst DP, Lynch DL, Reggio PH. GPR6 Structural Insights: Homology Model Construction and Docking Studies. Molecules. 2020; 25(3):725. https://doi.org/10.3390/molecules25030725.

Pose prediction, binding affinity estimation, and virtual screening are the three main goals of molecular docking. The ability to distinguish binding sites from non-binding sites and their molecular interactions is a prerequisite for a trustworthy docking method. Furthermore, it is anticipated that the approach utilized will need to effectively separate binding molecules from non-binding molecules and rank the binding molecules among the top compounds in the database when working with big compound libraries. The degree and quality of structural data available about the target protein and the ligand being docked determines how well virtual screening works. Examining the target for the presence of pertinent binding sites is the first step. This is typically accomplished by identifying novel binding pockets using in silico techniques or by analyzing known protein-ligand co-crystal structures (Figure 2.8). Similar pockets are found using techniques such as the catalytic site Atlas, AFT, SURFACE, POCKET SURFER, and PATCH-SURFER. Other in silico methods, like POCKET, work by rolling a spherical probe—a pre-computer representation of an idealized ligand—over the grid surface of the target protein's active pocket to identify the binding site of the protein. Docking-based virtual screening works best and is most useful when the target biomolecule's binding site is known. Therefore, it would be possible to dock a library of ligands with inhibitory potential against the target protein. However, blind docking techniques are typically used when a target protein lacks a known binding site (Figure 2.8 shows the blind docking technique in action). Blind docking may also be used in certain situations to investigate the interaction between the structure of a receptor or protein and the mechanism of action of a possible drug or ligand. This may reveal the agonistic or inhibitory properties of the ligand binding to either the receptor's active or inhibitory site. While blind docking techniques are a feature of most docking programs, they have certain drawbacks, such as being more time-consuming and having a lower success rate than docking into a known binding pocket.

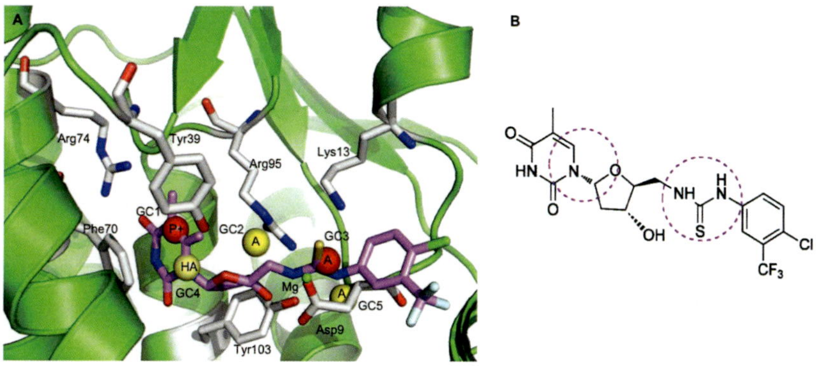

Figure 2.8. *Site-specific docking) and analysis of the docked complex.*

Source: Andrade CH, Pasqualoto KFM, Ferreira EI, Hopfinger AJ. 4D-QSAR: Perspectives in Drug Design. Molecules. 2010; 15(5):3281–3294. https://doi.org/10.3390/molecules15053281.

2.4.1.1. Docking Algorithm

2.4.1.1.1. Search Function

Creating the ideal number of protein-ligand geometries, including the binding pose as determined by experimentation, is the goal of a search algorithm. Following the creation of these binding poses, they are typically evaluated using a scoring algorithm that distinguishes between the experimentally determined binding pose and the other binding mode that the search algorithm predicted. Regarding the approach taken to investigate ligand flexibility, docking programs that utilize a search function can be divided into three primary categories: stochastic, systemic, and deterministic searches. According to the flexibility of the ligand and the protein, docking methods use three main techniques: (1) the protein is considered partially or completely flexible, and all of the ligand's torsional degrees of freedom (TORSDOF) are investigated; (2) the protein is considered rigid, and the ligand's torsional degrees of freedom (TORSDOF) are investigated; (3) the protein is viewed as a rigid entity with no torsional degree of freedom of ligands (conformational, translational, and rotational).

2.4.1.1.2. Ligand Flexibility

Based on the flexibility of the ligand, the search algorithm can be classified into four categories: shape matching, systematic method, stochastic or random method, and simulation method. The principle of 3D-complementarity, which stipulates that the protein-ligand binding surface must complement each other, is used in the shape matching method to insert the ligand into the protein's active site. The search algorithm permits the ligand to have structural degrees of freedom, allowing it to produce different conformations in the protein's binding site. Therefore, ensuring good shape complementarity between the ligand and the protein binding site is the main goal of the shape-matching method. The following docking programs use the shape matching algorithm: EUDOC, ZDOCK, FRED, FLOG, surflex, and ligand fit. Finding every potential structural degree of freedom in a molecule is the goal of a systematic algorithm, which ultimately results in the combinatorial explosion problem. Because of this, it's critical to separate the ligands before gradually docking them into the target protein's active site. Notably, DOCK and FLEX are two programs that use this strategy.

Because it affects the binding interactions between a ligand (small molecule drug candidate) and its target protein, ligand flexibility is an important factor to take into account in drug design and molecular modeling. Both proteins and ligands in biological systems have some degree of conformational flexibility that enables them to adjust for optimal molecular recognition and binding. Accurately predicting binding affinities and creating potent and selective drug candidates require an understanding of and consideration for ligand flexibility.

The ability of a ligand to take on various conformations or geometries in solution or when bound to a target protein is one facet of ligand flexibility. To maximize advantageous interactions like hydrogen bonding, hydrophobic contacts, and electrostatic interactions, ligands may undergo conformational changes to accommodate the protein's binding site. Because of its flexibility, ligands can explore a wider range of binding poses and conformations, which increases the possibility that they will find a binding mode that is energetically favorable.

For precise predictions of binding modes and affinity in molecular modeling and structure-based drug design, ligand flexibility must be taken into consideration. Inaccurate binding predictions may result from traditional docking methods' inability to fully capture the range of ligand conformations and interactions, which typically assume a rigid ligand. By enabling the ligand to sample various conformations within the binding site, sophisticated docking algorithms and molecular dynamics simulations overcome this constraint. These techniques increase the precision of binding affinity predictions and offer more realistic representations of ligand binding by examining the conformational space of the ligand and protein complex.

Furthermore, in fragment-based drug design, where tiny molecular fragments are utilized as building blocks to create larger drug-like compounds, ligand flexibility is also crucial. Finding low molecular weight fragments that bind to the target protein with a high degree of affinity is the foundation of fragment screening. But unlike larger molecules, fragments frequently show more flexibility and conformational variability, making it difficult to predict their binding modes and interactions with accuracy. To explore the conformational space of fragment hits and direct the optimization process to create larger, more potent compounds, advanced computational techniques are utilized, such as conformational sampling and fragment-based docking. Apart from ligand flexibility, molecular recognition and ligand binding are also significantly influenced by protein flexibility. When a ligand binds to a protein, conformational changes may occur, causing the binding site to structurally rearrange to accommodate the ligand. These effects are known as induced-fit effects. For precise molecular interaction modeling and binding affinity prediction, it is imperative to take into account the flexibility of both ligands and proteins.

To precisely predict binding modes, optimize drug candidates, and create potent and selective therapeutics, ligand flexibility must be taken into account in drug design and molecular modeling. Through the integration of sophisticated computational techniques that consider ligand flexibility, scientists can enhance the precision of binding forecasts and expedite the drug discovery procedure.

2.4.1.1.3. Protein Flexibility

Since proteins have dynamic, flexible structures, one of the main objectives of molecular docking is to treat the protein as such throughout the docking procedure. Induced-fit and conformational selection are two molecular recognition models that can be applied to the flexibility of proteins. The induced-fit model states that a protein frequently undergoes a conformational rearrangement upon ligand-protein binding. The protein-ligand complex that results from these molecular modifications in protein conformation has a stronger binding. Based on the observation that proteins exist as an ensemble of conformations in solution and molecular dynamics, and that these structures can be experimentally generated using NMR, the conformational selection model was developed. The relaxed complex scheme, which generates different protein conformations for docking, is an illustration of this preparation. According to the conformational selection model, small molecules choose the protein conformation that they bind to the strongest from the ensemble of conformations.

The protein-ligand docking methods have been implemented using these two models. The conformational complexity of proteins has been described by the induced-fit, which also explains how complementarity is attained through conformational selection. Therefore, it is important to highlight that conformational selection and induced-fit do not conflict with one another; rather, they each focus on a different facet of the intermolecular recognition process. The induced fit model is typically cited in selective docking methods that support local flexibility, while the conformational selection model can be directly linked to ensemble docking methods that rely on a collection of rigid protein conformations. Schrodinger's Glide induced-fit docking (IFD) is an example of a program that has been used for the induced-fit model, whereas OE-Docking v 3.0. 0 has been utilized to address the ensemble of protein conformational models through the use of its HYBRID program.

2.4.1.1.4. Scoring Function

An algorithm called scoring functions is used to determine how well a protein-ligand complex binds. The scoring function predicts the binding pose that best captures the real structure of the protein-ligand complex when a ligand attaches to its target receptor. In contrast, the scoring function should be able to rank one ligand concerning another in addition to identifying the actual configuration and orientation if certain sets of ligands need to be computed. Therefore, the scoring function must be created in a way that allows it to rank different protein-ligand complex poses.

A scoring function can be used to evaluate the binding energy of a protein-ligand complex by making several assumptions and simplifications to get as close to the true binding energy as possible in the shortest amount of time. Force-field, empirical, and knowledge-based scoring functions are currently the three types of scoring functions in use.

Physical interactions such as van der Waals interactions, electrostatic interactions, and bond length, bond angle, and bond torsions have all been taken into consideration when developing the force field scoring functions. Typically, ab initio quantum mechanical calculations and experiments are used to determine all of these parameters. The way solvents are handled during ligand binding presents a problem for the force-field function. Different force-field parameters serve as the basis for different force-field scoring functions. For instance, the Autodock force-field parameter uses AMBER, and the G-score force-field parameter uses Tripos. One popular program that uses the force-field scoring function algorithm to calculate protein-ligand interactions is called DOCK. The fact that charged groups prefer aqueous environments while non-polar groups prefer to remain in non-aqueous environments—a phenomenon known as the de-solvation effect—is one of the main problems with the force-field function. More difficult than the de-solvation effect, accurately predicting the entropic effect is another issue with the force-field scoring function. Because columbic interactions favor ligands with the highest charges only, these difficulties may actually restrict the resulting interactions of the protein-ligand docking system. One must consider the effect of water on the complex both before and after complex formation, as well as the mechanism by which the complex is mediated by the effect of water, to have a meaningful docking interaction.

Using solvent models to indirectly examine the impact of solvent on protein-ligand interactions, certain scientific teams analyzed and improved the current function. The electrostatic interactions, a precomputed receptor potential, and the ligand desolvation penalties were determined and computed using DelPhi and HYDREN, respectively. The van Der Waals interactions and the protein's electrostatic potentials were modeled using the Poisson-Boltzmann method and the Lennard-Jones potential, respectively.

In empirical scoring functions, the binding energy score of a protein-ligand complex is evaluated by adding up a set of weighted empirical energy terms which induce VDW energy, hydrogen bonding energy, electrostatic energy, entropy term, desolvation term, hydrophobicity term, etc.

$$\Delta G = \Sigma i W i \cdot \Delta G i$$

where "ΔGi" stands for individual empirical energy terms, and the corresponding coefficients "Wi" are computed by generating the binding affinity data of a training set of protein-ligand complexes with identified three-dimensional structures with the use of least square fittings. In comparison with other scoring functions, the empirical scoring functions are usually much more computationally productive due to their simple energy terms. A number of empirical scoring functions have been developed, such as SCORE2, Chem Score, Rank Score, Lig Score, Glide Score, HINT, etc.

Protein-ligand complex structural data obtained through experimental methods is used to generate knowledge-based scoring functions. The potential mean force (PMF) principle, which states that the energy of a complex is the total of all the interaction terms between protein and ligand atom pairs, forms the basis of the scoring functions. Introducing a suitable reference state for an optimal description of the residue-residue or atom-atom pairs in the non-interaction state is a crucial part of knowledge-based scoring functions. Many knowledge-based scoring functions have the important benefit of being computationally simple, which makes screening huge compound databases more effective. The fact that their derivation is essentially predicated on data implicitly encoded in certain subsets of the target-ligand complex is a disadvantage. Some common knowledge-based functions include DrugScore, PMF, MScore, SMoG, BLEEP and ITScore/SE

2.4.1.2. Molecular Dynamics Simulation

By simulating the motion of atoms and molecules over time, a computational technique known as molecular dynamics (MD) simulation enables scientists to examine the dynamic behavior of biomolecular systems at the atomic level. Proteins, nucleic acids, and other macromolecules in solution or in complex with ligands can be predicted by MD simulations based on the solutions to Newton's equations of motion. This includes changes in conformation, flexibility, and interactions. Protein engineering, drug discovery, and an understanding of biological processes are all aided by the insights that MD simulations offer into protein folding, ligand binding, and biomolecular function.

2.4.2. Pharmacophore Modeling and Quantitative Structure-Activity Relationships (QSAR)

Quantitative Structure-Activity Relationships (QSAR) and pharmacophore modeling are two potent computational approaches used in drug discovery and design that provide distinct insights into the connection between chemical structure and biological activity. In contrast to pharmacophore modeling, which aims to pinpoint the critical structural elements required for ligand binding and activity, QSAR analysis quantitatively links a molecule's chemical structure to its biological activity or other characteristics. Both strategies guide the optimization of drug candidates and hasten the discovery of novel therapeutics, and they complement one another in the process of rational drug design.

The first step in pharmacophore modeling is to identify biologically active substances that have been shown to have specific actions against a target. These substances function as a training set for the pharmacophore model, which is a representation of the fundamental characteristics needed for ligand recognition and target-protein interaction. Hydrophobic regions, aromatic rings, hydrogen bond donors and acceptors, and other structural components essential for binding are typical pharmacophore features. Pharmacophore models can be created using two methods: structure-based approaches, which use the target protein's three-dimensional structure to identify important interactions, or ligand-based approaches, in which the alignment of training set compounds reveals common pharmacophoric features. Pharmacophore models are useful tools for virtual screening because they let scientists prioritize compounds for additional experimental testing and find possible drug candidates from compound libraries with similar pharmacophoric features.

2.4.2.1. Pharmacophore Modeling

To determine the essential structural and chemical characteristics required for a molecule to interact with a biological target and produce a particular pharmacological effect, pharmacophore modeling is a computational technique used in drug design. The idea behind pharmacophore modeling is the following: regardless of their overall chemical structures, molecules with similar pharmacophoric features are likely to exhibit similar biological activities. Pharmacophore models are three-dimensional depictions of these fundamental characteristics that direct drug candidate design and optimization.

The first step in the pharmacophore modeling process is usually to identify a group of physiologically active compounds that have been shown to have specific activities against a target. These substances—referred to as the training set—are utilized to create a pharmacophore model that identifies the shared structural components in charge of their activity. Different computational techniques, such as ligand-based approaches, structure-based approaches, or a combination of both, can be used to generate pharmacophore models.

The training set compounds in ligand-based pharmacophore modeling are aligned according to their shared pharmacophoric characteristics, such as hydrophobic regions, aromatic rings, and hydrogen bond donors and acceptors. The spatial arrangement of these features is then determined by computational algorithms, which produce a pharmacophore hypothesis that depicts the crucial interaction pattern needed for activity. Ligand-based pharmacophore models are especially helpful in situations where it is difficult or impossible to determine the target protein's three-dimensional structure.

On the other hand, structure-based pharmacophore modeling obtains the pharmacophore model by using the target protein's three-dimensional structure. Identification of important interactions between the protein and ligand is done computationally using techniques like molecular docking or molecular dynamics simulations. Based on the spatial arrangement of these interactions within the binding site, pharmacophore features are then obtained. Designing ligands with enhanced binding affinity and selectivity is possible through the application of structure-based pharmacophore modeling, which also sheds light on the precise protein-ligand interactions that underpin activity.

When a pharmacophore model is created, compound libraries can be virtually screened to find possible drug candidates with comparable pharmacophoric characteristics. Finding molecules that match the pharmacophore hypothesis entails virtual screening, which involves matching the pharmacophore model to the structures of potential compounds. To expedite the drug discovery process, compounds that match the pharmacophore model are then given priority for additional experimental testing.

There are many uses for pharmacophore modeling in drug design and discovery. It can be applied to lead optimization, clarify structure-activity relationships, and create new compounds with enhanced potency and selectivity. Furthermore, fragment-based drug discovery, in which smaller molecule fragments are methodically put together to create larger drug-like compounds, can make use of pharmacophore models. All things considered, pharmacophore modeling is a useful computational tool that helps with the thoughtful design of therapeutic agents and speeds up the creation of new medications to treat a variety of illnesses.

2.4.2.2. Quantitative Structure-Activity Relationship (QSAR) Modeling

A statistical method for relating a molecule's chemical structure to its biological activity or other characteristics is called QSAR modeling. Molecular descriptors, which encode details about the physicochemical characteristics and structural elements of molecules, are used to construct QSAR models. QSAR models predict the activity of novel compounds by comparing their structural similarity to the training set, which is derived from an analysis of a dataset containing compounds with known activities. Drug design, environmental toxicology, and chemical risk assessment all make extensive use of QSAR modeling to rank lead compounds, maximize molecular characteristics, and forecast biological effects.

A Closer Look

Drug Discovery

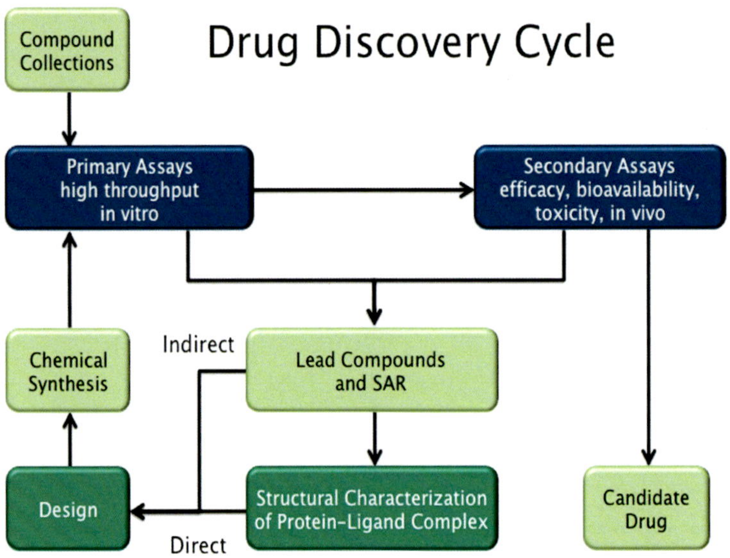

The methodical and complex process of drug discovery seeks to find and create new therapeutic agents to fight illnesses. It happens in a number of interrelated steps, each of which is essential to the final success of releasing a novel medication onto the market. Target identification and validation is the first step in the process, in which particular molecular targets linked to disease pathways are identified and their potential for use as therapeutic intervention sites is validated. This phase typically entails a blend of genetic investigations, biochemical tests, and computer simulations to pinpoint targets that are both druggable and biologically significant. The procedure moves on to hit identification and lead generation after target validation. This stage involves finding compounds, or hits, that interact with the target and show some biological activity by screening compound libraries or using computational techniques. Following optimization, lead compounds with potential therapeutic efficacy are produced by enhancing the potency, selectivity, and pharmacokinetic characteristics of the hits.

Lead optimization is the next step, in which medicinal chemists alter lead compounds to maximize their drug-like qualities and reduce their toxicity. Preclinical testing is the next step, in which the safety, effectiveness, and pharmacokinetics of lead compounds are thoroughly examined in cellular and animal models. The most promising applicants move on to clinical trials, which are a series of closely monitored human experiments intended to assess the safety and efficacy of the medication in patients.

Successful drug discovery ultimately leads to regulatory approval and commercialization, allowing the novel therapy to be made available to patients who require it. However, the process of finding new drugs is difficult and time-consuming; it frequently takes years and involves large sums of money. Notwithstanding these difficulties, drug discovery is still an essential activity that spurs innovation and enhances patient outcomes in the medical field.

Summary

- Molecular modeling plays a crucial role throughout the drug design process by providing detailed insights into molecular interactions, dynamics, and energetics.
- Drug design, often referred to as rational drug design or simply rational design, is the inventive process of finding new medications based on the knowledge of a biological target.
- Rational drug design begins with a hypothesis that modulation of a specific biological target may have therapeutic value.
- Ligand-based drug design relies on knowledge of other molecules that bind to the biological target of interest. These other molecules may be used to derive a pharmacophore model that defines the minimum necessary structural characteristics a molecule must possess to bind to the target.
- Drug design is a complex and multifaceted process that integrates principles from various scientific disciplines to develop therapeutically effective compounds.
- Quantitative Structure-Activity Relationships (QSAR) analysis is a powerful computational approach in drug design and medicinal chemistry that aims to establish quantitative relationships between the chemical structure of molecules and their biological activity.
- Molecular modeling encompasses all methods, theoretical and computational, used to model or mimic the behavior of molecules.
- Molecular modeling techniques encompass a diverse array of computational methods used to study the structure, dynamics, and interactions of molecules at the atomic level.
- Molecular docking is a computational technique used to predict the preferred orientation and conformation of a ligand (small molecule) within the binding site of a target protein.

References

1. Agrafiotis, D. K., Wiener, J. M., Skalkin, A., & Kolpak, J. (2011). Single R-group polymorphisms (SRPs) and R-cliffs: An intuitive framework for analyzing and visualizing activity cliffs in a single analog series. *Journal of Chemical Information and Modeling, 51*(5), 1122–1131.
2. Austin, C. P., Brady, L. S., Insel, T. R., & Collins, F. S. (2004). NIH molecular libraries initiative. *Science, 306*, 1138–1139.
3. Banerjee, A., Schepmann, D., Köhler, J., Würthwein, E. -U., & Wünsch, B. (2010). Synthesis and SAR studies of chiral non-racemic dexoxadrol analogues as uncompetitive NMDA receptor antagonists. *Bioorganic & Medicinal Chemistry, 18*(22), 7855–7867.
4. Blum, L. C., & Reymond, J. -L. (2009). 970 million druglike small molecules for virtual screening in the chemical universe database GDB-13. *Journal of the American Chemical Society, 131*(25), 8732–8733.
5. Blum, L. C., van Deursen, R., Bertrand, S., Mayer, M., Bürgi, J. J., Bertrand, D., & Reymond, J. -L. (2011). Discovery of α7-nicotinic receptor ligands by virtual screening of the chemical universe database GDB-13. *Journal of Chemical Information and Modeling, 51*(12), 3105–3112.
6. Bohacek, R. S., McMartin, C., & Guida, W. C. (1996). The art and practice of structure-based drug design: A molecular modeling perspective. *Medicinal Research Reviews, 16*(1), 3–50.

7. Breiman, L. (2001). Statistical modeling: Two cultures. *Statistical Science, 16*, 199–231.

8. Brown, N., & Lewis, R. A. (2006). Exploiting QSAR methods in lead optimization. *Current Opinion in Drug Discovery & Development, 9*(4), 419–424.

9. Chatterjee, S., & Hadi, A. S. (1986). Influential observations, high leverage points, and outliers in linear regression. *Statistical Science, 1*(3), 379–416.

10. Chen, B., & Wild, D. J. (2010). PubChem BioAssays as a data source for predictive models. *Journal of Molecular Graphics and Modelling, 28*(5), 420–426.

11. Churchwell, C. J., Rintoul, M. D., Martin, S., Visco Jr, D. P., Kotu, A., Larson, R. S., Sillerud, L. O., Brown, D. C., & Faulon, J. -L. (2004). The signature molecular descriptor. 3. Inverse-quantitative structure-activity relationship of ICAM-1 inhibitory peptides. *Journal of Molecular Graphics and Modelling, 22*(4), 263–273.

12. Cook, R. D. (1977). Detecting influential observations in linear regression. *Technometrics, 19*, 15–18.

13. Cruz-Monteagudo, M., Borges, F., & Cordeiro, D. S. (2008). Desirability-based multiobjective optimization for global QSAR studies: Application to the design of novel NSAIDs with improved analgesic, anti-inflammatory, and ulcerogenic profiles. *Journal of Computational Chemistry, 29*(14), 2445–2459.

14. Dudek, A. Z., Arodz, T., & Gálvez, J. (2006). Computational methods in developing quantitative structure-activity relationships (QSAR): A review. *Combinatorial Chemistry & High Throughput Screening, 9*(3), 213–228.

15. Eriksson, L., Jaworska, J., Worth, A. P., Cronin, M. T. D., McDowell, R. M., & Gramatica, P. (2003). Methods for reliability and uncertainty assessment and for applicability evaluations of classification- and regression-based QSARs. *Environmental Health Perspectives, 111*(10), 1361–1375.

16. Faulon, J. -L., Visco, D. P., & Pophale, R. S. (2003). The signature molecular descriptor. 1. Using extended valence sequences in QSAR and QSPR studies. *Journal of Chemical Information and Computer Sciences, 43*, 707–720.

17. Guha, R. (2008). On the interpretation and interpretability of QSAR models. *Journal of Computer-Aided Molecular Design, 22*(12), 857–871.

18. Guha, R., & Jurs, P. C. (2004). The development of QSAR models to predict and interpret the biological activity of artemisinin analogues. *Journal of Chemical Information and Computer Sciences, 44*, 1440–1449.

19. Guha, R., & Van Drie, J. H. (2008). The structure-activity landscape index: Identifying and quantifying activity-cliffs. *Journal of Chemical Information and Modeling, 48*(3), 646–658.

20. Guha, R., Stanton, D. T., & Jurs, P. C. (2005). Interpreting computational neural network QSAR models: A detailed interpretation of the weights and biases. *Journal of Chemical Information and Modeling, 45*, 1109–1121.

21. Irwin, J. J., & Shoichet, B. K. (2005). ZINC - a free database of commercially available compounds for virtual screening. *Journal of Chemical Information and Modeling, 45*(1), 177–182.

22. Jaworska, J., Nikolova-Jeliazkova, N., & Aldenberg, T. (2005). QSAR applicability domain estimation by projection of the training set in descriptor space: A review. *Alternatives to Laboratory Animals, 33*, 445–459.

23. Lajiness, M. S. (1991). Evaluation of the performance of dissimilarity selection methodology. In *QSAR: Rational Approaches to the Design of Bioactive Compounds* (pp. 201–204). Leiden, Netherlands: Escom.

24. Maggiora, G. M. (2006). On outliers and activity cliffs–why QSAR often disappoints. *Journal of Chemical Information and Modeling, 46*(4), 1535.

25. Medina-Franco, J. L., Martínez-Mayorga, K., Bender, A., Marín, R. M., Giulianotti, M. A., Pinilla, C., & Houghten, R. A. (2009). Characterization of activity landscapes using 2D and 3D similarity methods: Consensus activity cliffs. *Journal of Chemical Information and Modeling, 49*(2), 477–491.

26. Nicolotti, O., Giangreco, I., Miscioscia, T. F., & Carotti, A. (2009). Improving quantitative structure-activity relationships through multiobjective optimization. *Journal of Chemical Information and Modeling, 49*(10), 2290–2302.

27. Nicolotti, O., Gillet, V. J., Fleming, P. J., & Green, D. V. S. (2002). Multiobjective optimization in quantitative structure-activity relationships: Deriving accurate and interpretable QSARs. *Journal of Medicinal Chemistry, 23*, 5069–5080.

28. Nikolova-Jeliazkova, N., & Jaworska, J. (2005). An approach to determining AD for QSAR group contribution models: An analysis of SRC KOWWIN. *Alternatives to Laboratory Animals, 33*, 461–470.

29. Novotarskyi, S., Sushko, I., Körner, R., Pandey, A. K., & Tetko, I. V. (2011). A comparison of different QSAR approaches to modeling CYP450 1A2 inhibition. *Journal of Chemical Information and Modeling, 51*(6), 1271–1280.

30. Papa, E., Villa, F., & Gramatica, P. (2005). Statistically validated QSARs, based on theoretical descriptors, for modeling aquatic toxicity of organic chemicals in *Pimephales promelas* (fathead minnow). *Journal of Chemical Information and Modeling, 45*(5), 1256–1266.

31. Peltason, L., & Bajorath, J. (2007). SAR index: Quantifying the nature of structure-activity relationships. *Journal of Medicinal Chemistry, 50*(23), 5571–5578.

32. Roberts, D. W., Patlewicz, G., Kern, P. S., Gerberick, F., Kimber, I., Dearman, R. J., Ryan, C. A., Basketter, D. A., & Aptula, A. O. (2007). Mechanistic applicability domain classification of a local lymph node assay dataset for skin sensitization. *Chemical Research in Toxicology, 20*(7), 1019–1030.

33. Schultz, T. W., Hewitt, M., Netzeva, T. I., & Cronin, M. T. D. (2007). Assessing applicability domains of toxicological QSARs: Definition, confidence in predicted values, and the role of mechanisms of action. *QSAR & Combinatorial Science, 26*, 238–254.

34. Seebeck, B., Wagener, M., & Rarey, M. (2011). From activity cliffs to target-specific scoring models and pharmacophore hypotheses. *ChemMedChem. 2011 Sep 5;6(9):1630-9, 1533.*

35. Segall, M., Champness, E., Obrezanova, O., & Leeding, C. (2009). Beyond profiling: Using ADMET models to guide decisions. *Chemistry & Biodiversity, 6*(11), 2144–2151.

36. Shen, M. -Y., Su, B. -H., Esposito, E. X., Hopfinger, A. J., & Tseng, Y. J. (2011). A comprehensive support vector machine binary hERG classification model based on extensive but biased end point hERG data sets. *Chemical Research in Toxicology, 24*(6), 934–947.

37. Sheridan, R. P., Feuston, B. P., Maiorov, V. N., & Kearsley, S. K. (2004). Similarity to molecules in the training set is a good discriminator for prediction accuracy in QSAR. *Journal of Chemical Information and Computer Sciences, 44*(6), 1912–1928.

38. Sisay, M. T., Peltason, L., & Bajorath, J. (2009). Structural interpretation of activity cliffs revealed by systematic analysis of structure-activity relationships in analog series. *Journal of Chemical Information and Modeling, 49*(10), 2179–2189.

39. Stanforth, R. W., Kolossov, E., & Mirkin, B. (2007). A measure of domain of applicability for QSAR modeling based on intelligent k-means clustering. *QSAR & Combinatorial Science, 26*(7), 837–844.

40. Stanton, D. T. (2003). On the physical interpretation of QSAR models. *Journal of Chemical Information and Computer Sciences, 43*(5), 1423–1433.

41. Tetko, I. V., Bruneau, P., Mewes, H. W., Rohrer, D. C., & Poda, G. I. (2006). Can we estimate the accuracy of ADME-Tox predictions? *Drug Discovery Today, 11*(15, 16), 700–707.

42. Tropsha, A., Gramatica, P., & Gombar, V. K. (2003). The importance of being earnest: Validation is the absolute essential for successful application and interpretation of QSPR models. *QSAR & Combinatorial Science, 22*, 69–77.

43. von Korff, M., & Sander, T. (2006). Toxicity-indicating structural patterns. *Journal of Chemical Information and Modeling, 46*, 536–544.

44. Wawer, M., Peltason, L., & Bajorath, J. (2009). Elucidation of structure-activity relationship pathways in biological screening data. *Journal of Chemical Information and Modeling, 52*(4), 1075–1080.

45. Wawer, M., Peltason, L., Weskamp, N., Teckentrup, A., & Bajorath, J. (2008). Structure-activity relationship anatomy by network-like similarity graphs and local structure-activity relationship indices. *Journal of Medicinal Chemistry, 51*(19), 6075–6084.

46. Weaver, S., & Gleeson, M. P. (2008). The importance of the domain of applicability in QSAR modeling. *Journal of Molecular Graphics and Modelling, 26*(8), 1315–1326.

47. Winkler, D. A. (2002). The role of quantitative structure–activity relationships (QSAR) in biomolecular discovery. *Briefings in Bioinformatics, 3*(1), 73–86.

48. Wong, W. W., & Burkowski, F. J. (2009). A constructive approach for discovering new drug leads: Using a kernel methodology for the inverse-QSAR problem. *Journal of Cheminformatics, 1*, 4.

49. Xu, Y. J., & Gao, H. (2003). Dimension related distance and its application in QSAR/QSPR model error estimation. *QSAR & Combinatorial Science, 22*, 422–429.

50. Yongye, A. B., Byler, K., Santos, R., Martínez-Mayorga, K., Maggiora, G. M., & Medina-Franco, J. L. (2011). Consensus models of activity landscapes with multiple chemical, conformer, and property representations. *Journal of Chemical Information and Modeling, 51*(6), 1259–1270.

51. Zvinavashe, E., Albertinka, J. M., & Rietjens, I. M. C. M. (2008). Promises and pitfalls of quantitative structure-activity relationship approaches for predicting metabolism and toxicity. *Chemical Research in Toxicology, 21*(12), 2229–2236.

Chapter 3

DRUG DELIVERY SYSTEMS

Contents

Introduction

Drug delivery involves the administration of drugs or pharmaceuticals to humans or animals to achieve a therapeutic outcome. Different technologies are used to ensure that the drugs have their intended effect while minimizing any negative side effects, affecting how the drug is absorbed, distributed, metabolized, and eliminated from the body.

Numerous novel drug candidates have been developed as a result of developments in biotechnology and medicine, but many of them are unsuccessful in pre-clinical testing because of their low solubility, low stability, and limited bioavailability. To enhance the pharmacokinetics and pharmacodynamics of therapeutic agents and facilitate their delivery at the intended site in the desired dose at the right time and rate, drug delivery systems (DDS) have been extensively studied and developed. Novel drug delivery systems (DDS) are being developed to address advanced therapeutic needs, such as targeted delivery, controlled release, improved solubility, on-demand activation, and novel routes of administration (nasal, ocular, and transdermal). Examples of these DDS include transdermal patches, antibody-drug conjugates, nano- and microparticles, inhalers, and drug reservoir implants. The drug's characteristics, intended release rate, preferred site of action, and mode of administration all influence the choice of DDS.

Drug formulations with nanoparticles (NP) that are targeted, safe, and effective are now possible thanks to significant advancements in nanotechnology. Systems for delivering drugs via nanotechnology have shown great promise in increasing the solubility of hydrophobic drugs, optimizing pharmacokinetics and biodistribution, and facilitating preferential accumulation at the target site.

Drugs can be conjugated or absorbed onto the particle surface, encapsulated in the core, or dissolved within the particle matrix of nanodelivery systems. By adding targeting moieties to the surface of the particle, drug-loaded nanoparticles can be more precisely directed to a particular disease site. Drug delivery formulations have made use of a variety of nanocarriers, including liposomes, polymer micelles, dendrimers, polymer-drug conjugates, inorganic nanoparticles, and carbon-based nanomaterials. The most popular and thoroughly studied nanocarriers are liposomes, but polymer nanoparticles have become one of the most cutting-edge methods for drug delivery. Polymeric drug delivery nanoparticles can be made from synthetic or natural polymers that are biocompatible (Figure 3.1).

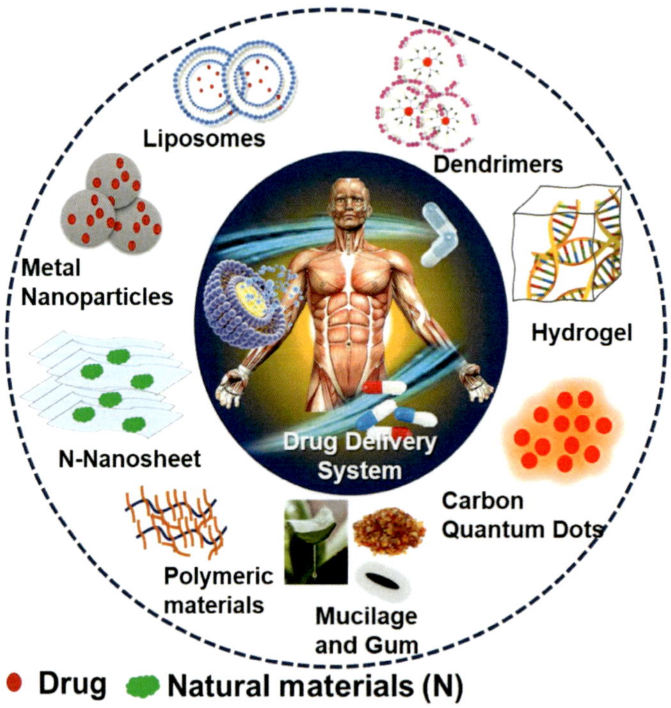

Figure 3.1. *Drug delivery.*

Source: Veerapandian M, Ramasundaram S, Jerome P, Chellasamy G, Govindaraju S, Yun K, Oh TH. Drug delivery application of functional nanomaterials synthesized using natural sources. Journal of Functional Biomaterials. 2023; 14(8):426. https://doi.org/10.3390/jfb14080426.

Orientation and Directional Terms

Term	Definition	**Illustration**
Drug delivery	Drug delivery refers to approaches, formulations, manufacturing techniques, storage systems, and technologies involved in transporting a pharmaceutical compound to its target site to achieve a desired therapeutic effect.	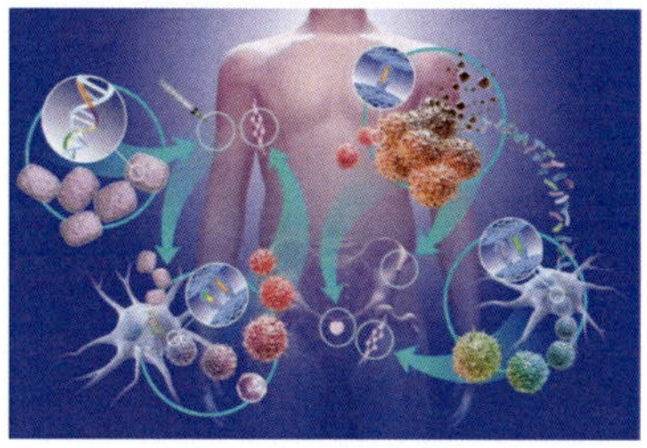
Transmucosal routes	The transmucosal route includes oral, nasal, vaginal, and urethral and presents a challenge in the field of novel drug delivery technology.	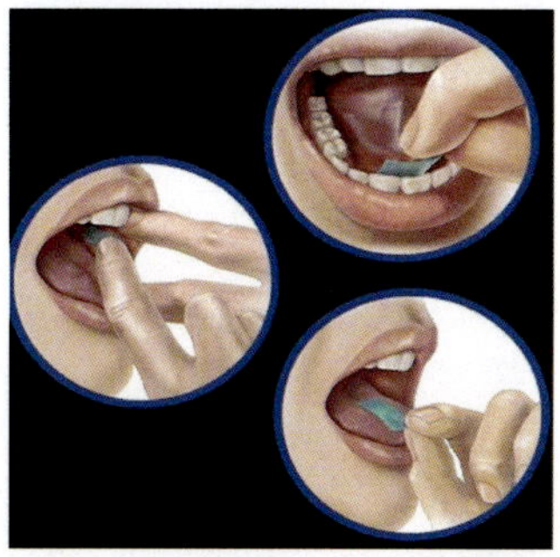
Oral route	The oral route is the most common route for drug administration. It is the most preferred route, due to its advantages, such as non-invasiveness, patient compliance and convenience of drug administration.	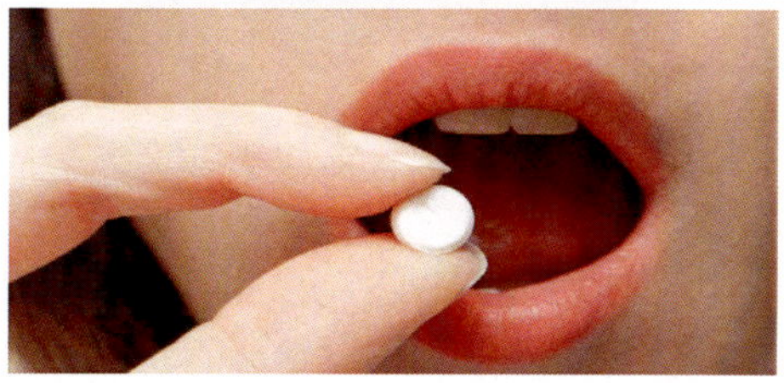
Drug transport	Drug transport is the process by which a drug enters or leaves a cell or organelle.	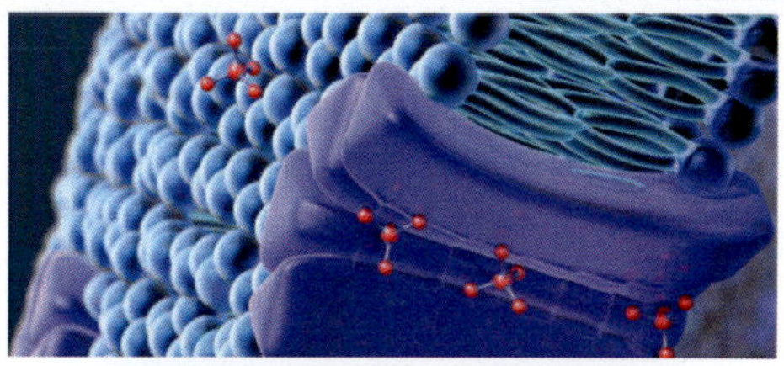
Drug administration	Drug administration means an act in which a single dose of a prescribed drug or biological is given to a resident by an authorized person in accordance with this Part.	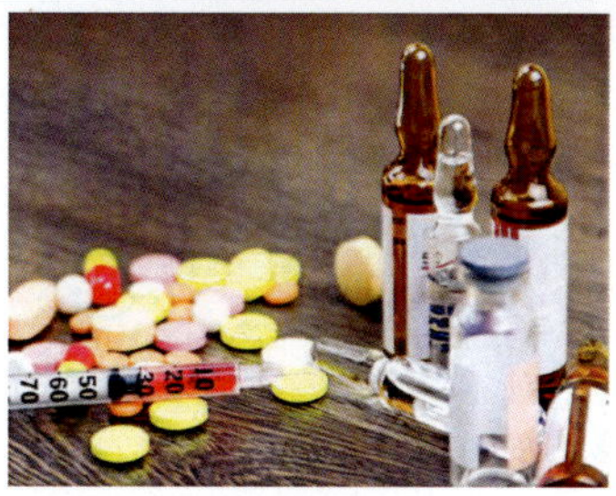

3.1. Drug Delivery Routes

The human body can absorb drugs through a variety of anatomical pathways. They might target specific organs and diseases, or they might be designed to have systemic effects. The illness, the desired outcome, and the product that is available all influence the route of administration selection. Medication can be given systemically with a target organ infection or directly to the diseased organ (Figure 3.2).

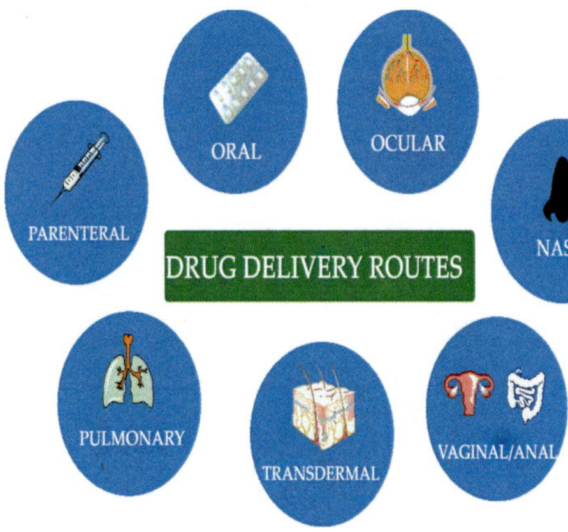

Figure 3.2. *A classification of various anatomical routes for systemic drug delivery.*

Source: Kurczewska J. Recent reports on polysaccharide-based materials for drug delivery. Polymers. 2022; 14(19):4189. https://doi.org/10.3390/polym14194189.

3.1.1. Oral Drug Delivery

Oral drug administration has historically been the most popular method for delivering both traditional and cutting-edge medications. This preference is clearly supported by the patients' widespread acceptance of it and the ease of administration. Major limitations of oral route of drug administration are:

- Drugs taken orally for systemic effects have variable absorption rate and variable serum concentrations which may be unpredictable. This has led to the development of sustained-release and controlled-release systems.
- The high acid content and ubiquitous digestive enzymes of the digestive tract can degrade some drugs well before they reach the site of absorption into the bloodstream. This is a particular problem for ingested proteins. Therefore, this route has limitations for the administration of biotechnology products.
- Many macromolecules and polar compounds cannot effectively traverse the cells of the epithelial membrane in the small intestines to reach the bloodstream. Their use is limited to local effect in the gastrointestinal tract.
- Many drugs become insoluble at the low pH levels encountered in the digestive tract. Since only the soluble form of the drug can be absorbed into the bloodstream, the transition of the drug to the insoluble form can significantly reduce bioavailability.
- The drug may be inactivated in the liver on its way to the systemic circulation. An example of this is the inactivation of glyceryl trinitrate by hepatic monooxygenase enzymes during the first-pass metabolism.
- Some drugs irritate the gastrointestinal tract, and this is partially counteracted by coating.
- The oral route may not be suitable for drugs targeted to specific organs.
- Despite its disadvantages, the oral route remains the preferred route of drug delivery. Several improvements

have taken place in the formulation of drugs for oral delivery to improve the action.

3.1.2. Parenteral Drug Delivery

Parenteral refers, technically, to the injection of drugs via subcutaneous, intramuscular, intravenous, and intra-arterial routes; in actuality, the term refers to the introduction of substances into the body by routes other than the gastrointestinal tract. The administration of drugs through injections into particular body organs will be covered under the different therapeutic areas.

Parenteral drug administration is the most widely used invasive method of drug delivery and is now a standard part of medical practice. The parenteral form is the only way to obtain many significant medications. Typical disposable syringes are made of plastic or glass and contain needles. Retractable needles or autodestruct syringes that lock after injection are included with nonreusable syringes and needles. The advantages of parenteral administration are:

- Rapid onset of action
- Predictable and almost complete bioavailability
- Avoidance of the gastrointestinal tract with problems of oral drug administration
- Provides a reliable route for drug administration in very ill and comatose patients, who are not able to ingest anything orally Major drawbacks of parenteral administration are:
- Injection is not an ideal method of delivery because of the pain involved and patient compliance becomes a major problem.
- Injections have limitations for the delivery of protein products particularly those that require sustained levels.

Comments on various types of injections are given in the following text.

- **Subcutaneous:** This entails using a hypodermic needle to inject the medication into a layer of subcutaneous fatty tissue. Patients can administer subcutaneous injections to large areas of the body, such as when administering insulin for diabetes. Various factors that influence drug delivery by subcutaneous route are:
  - Size of the molecules as the larger molecules have slower penetration rates than smaller ones.
  - Viscosity may impede the diffusion of drugs into body fluids.
  - The anatomical characteristics of the site of injection such as vascularity and amount of fatty tissue influence the rate of absorption of the drug.

Compared to intramuscular or intravenous injections, subcutaneous injections typically have a slower rate of absorption and a delayed onset of action. Hyaluronidase infiltration has the potential to speed up the absorption rate. Disadvantages of subcutaneous injection are:

- The rate of absorption is difficult to control from the subcutaneous deposit.
- Local complications include irritation and pain at the site of injection.
- Injection sites have to be changed frequently to

avoid accumulation of the unabsorbed drug which may cause tissue damage.

There are numerous options for self-administration subcutaneous injection systems, such as autoinjectors, pen pumps, pre-filled glass syringes, conventional syringes, and needleless injectors. The subcutaneous route of delivery for peptides and macromolecules is still dependable and manageable.

- **Intramuscular Injections:** These are injected deeply into the skeletal muscles, typically the gluteal or deltoids. Compared to subcutaneous injection, intramuscular injection has a quicker start of action, but it takes longer than intravenous injection to take effect. Although the drug's absorption is diffusion-controlled, the high vascularity of the muscle tissue causes it to happen more quickly. The physicochemical characteristics of the solution injected as well as physiological factors like muscle blood flow and activity level influence the rate of absorption. Disadvantages of the intramuscular route for drug delivery are:
  - Pain at the injection site.
  - Limitation of the amount injected according to the mass of the muscle available.
  - Degradation of peptides at the site of injection.
  - Complications include peripheral nerve injury and the formation of hematoma and abscess at the site of injection.
  - Inadvertent puncture of a blood vessel during injection may introduce the drug directly into the blood circulation.

The majority of injectables are administered intramuscularly. For this route, a variety of dosage forms are available, including reconstituted powders, colloidal suspensions, and oil-in-water emulsions. When a drug is in a product form where it is not completely dissolved, the absorption process is typically slower and the effects take longer to manifest. Drugs injected intramuscularly usually create a depot in the muscle mass, from which the drug is absorbed gradually. Peak drug concentrations are usually seen from 1 to 2 h. Factors which affect the rate of release of the drug from such a depot include the following:

- Compactness of the depot as the release is faster from a less compact and more diffuse depot
- The concentration and particle size of the drug in the vehicle
- Nature of solvent in the injection
- Physical form of the product
- The flow characteristics of the product
- Volume of the injection

- **Intravenous Administration:** This entails either a continuous infusion through a catheter or needle inserted into a deep or superficial vein, or an injection of an aqueous into a superficial vein. For some drugs, this is the only way to administer them, and because of how quickly the injection takes effect, it is the preferred option in emergency scenarios. Less medication is needed than with other routes of administration, so theoretically none of the medication is lost. One can regulate the infusion rate to enable continuous and extended administration. There are devices available for intravenous catheter-based timed administration of intermittent doses. Depending on the size of the particles, the intravenous solution's particles are distributed to different organs. Smaller particles accumulate in the bone marrow, while those larger than 7 μm are trapped in the lungs. The spleen and liver absorb those whose diameter falls between 0 and 7 μm. When targeting different organs with a drug, this information is helpful. Disadvantages of the intravenous route are:

- Immune reactions may occur following injections of proteins and peptides.
- Trauma to veins can lead to thrombophlebitis.
- Extravasation of the drug solution into the extravascular space may lead to irritation and tissue necrosis.
- Infections may occur at the site of catheter introduction.
- Air embolism may occur due to air sucked in via the intravenous line.

By utilizing nanovesicles like liposomes, the kinetics of drug distribution and metabolic profile can now be altered for intravenous administration.

- **Intra-arterial:** Administering therapeutic drugs through direct injection into the arteries is not a common practice. For angiography, arterial puncture and contrast material injection have been performed. The majority of arterial perfusions through catheters inserted into arteries or intra-arterial injections are used for localized chemotherapy of specific organs and limbs. Brain cancerous tumors have been treated with intra-arterial chemotherapy.

3.1.3. Transdermal Drug Delivery

Transdermal drug delivery is a method that replaces oral, intravascular, subcutaneous, and transmucosal routes for the therapeutic administration of drugs through the skin. A special report on this subject provides a thorough description of the technologies and business aspects of development.

It includes the following categories of drug administration:

- Local application formulations, e.g., transdermal gels
- Penetration enhancers
- Drug carriers, e.g., liposomes and nanoparticles
- Transdermal patches
- Transdermal electrotransport
- Use of physical modalities to facilitate transdermal drug transport
- Minimally invasive methods of transdermal drug delivery, e.g., needle-free injections

Transdermal drug delivery is seeing an increase in the use of microneedles and iontophoresis. An easy, one-step method for delivering biomacromolecules transdermally under control has been reported, utilizing hydrogel-forming microneedle arrays and electrophoresis. It increases the variety of medications that can be applied topically.

3.1.4. Transmucosal Drug Delivery

All of the body's internal passageways and orifices are covered in mucous membranes, and different anatomical locations can accommodate the introduction of drugs. Here, we will limit our discussion to a few generalizations that apply to all mucous membranes; the specifics will be covered location-specific, such as buccal, nasal, and rectal.

Diffusion is the method by which penetrants pass through mucous membranes. The amount of a substance that crosses the tissue in a unit of time is constant at steady state, and neither the direction of nonelectrolyte transfer nor the concentration of the solutions affects the permeability coefficients. The routes of penetration through the epithelial barriers are intercellular rather than intracellular, as is the case with the skin's epidermis. The use of surfactants, such as sodium lauryl sulfate, a cationic surfactant, can increase the permeability. In vitro, the oleic acid unsaturated fatty acid can enhance the diffusion of propranolol through the porcine buccal mucosa by acting as a vehicle consisting of propylene glycol. Delivery of biopharmaceuticals across mucosal surfaces may offer several advantages over injection techniques which include the following:

- Avoidance of an injection
- Increase of therapeutic efficiency
- Possibility of administering peptides
- Rapid absorption as compared to oral administration
- Bypassing first-pass metabolism by the liver
- Higher patient acceptance as compared to injectables
- Lower cost than injections

By preventing the drug from becoming diluted in bodily fluids, enabling targeted and localized delivery of the medication at a particular location, and preserving the drug concentration between toxic and effective levels, mucoadhesive controlled-release devices can increase the efficacy of transmucosal delivery. Hydrogels based on acrylic have found widespread application as mucoadhesive systems. Their flexibility and nonabrasive properties in the partially swollen state make them ideal for bioadhesion because they lessen the attrition that damages the tissues in contact. Devices made of cross-linked polymerics may stick to the mucosa. For instance, tethering long, flexible poly(ethylene glycol) chains can increase the hydrogels' adhesive properties. The resultant hydrogels have improved the anchoring of the chains with the mucosa, exhibiting mucoadhesive properties.

- **Buccal and Sublingual Routes:** The lipid solubility of the non-ionized drug, salivary pH, and the partition coefficient—an indicator of the drug's relative affinity for the vehicle in relation to the epithelial barrier—all affect buccal absorption. A high partition coefficient value suggests that the drug has poor affinity for the vehicle. A high interaction between the drug and the vehicle, which decreases the drug's release from the vehicle, is indicated by a small partition coefficient value. The drug's minimally soluble vehicle is the optimal one. Buccal drug administration has the following attractive features:

- Quick absorption into the systemic circulation with rapid onset of effect due to absorption from the rich mucosal network of systemic veins and lymphatics.
- The tablet can be removed in case of an undesirable effect.
- Oral mucosal absorption avoids the first-pass hepatic metabolism.
- A tablet can remain for a prolonged period in the buccal cavity which enables development of formulations with sustained release effect.
- This route can be used in patients with swallowing difficulties. Limitations to the use of buccal route are:
- The tablet must be kept in place and not chewed or swallowed.
- Excessive salivary flow may cause too rapid dissolution and absorption of the tablet or wash it away.
- A bad-tasting tablet will have a low patient acceptability.
- Some of these disadvantages have been overcome by the use of a patch containing the drug which is applied to the buccal mucosa or the using the drug as a spray.

3.1.5. Nasal Drug Delivery

For years, medications have been applied topically to produce both systemic and topical effects. Agents for the treatment of sinusitis, rhinitis, nasal congestion, and associated allergic and other chronic conditions are included in topical administration. Corticosteroids, antihistamines, anticholinergics, and vasoconstrictors are a few examples of different medications. The drug of choice can be administered via the nasal route, which is appealing because it can circumvent issues with oral administration, such as drug degradation in the gastrointestinal tract and high first-pass metabolism. Although direct drug delivery to the brain is also possible, the nasal route has received more attention in recent years for systemic drug delivery.

- **Surface Epithelium of the Nasal Cavity:** A squamous and transitional epithelium covers the anterior one-third of the nasal cavity, an olfactory epithelium covers the upper part of the cavity, and a typical airway epithelium—ciliated, pseudostratified, and columnar—covers the remaining portion of the cavity. The columnar cells are connected to adjacent cells by both interdigitations of the cell membrane and tight junctions at the apices. The cilia play a crucial role in introducing mucus into the throat. Mucous clearance is hampered by the drug's toxic effects on the cilia. The safety of nasal delivery drugs has been investigated through in vitro effects on mucous layer physical properties and ciliary beating reversibility.
- **Intranasal Drug Delivery:** Intranasal administration is a viable option for medications that are not effective when taken orally, are used regularly, need small dosages, and are intended to enter the bloodstream quickly. Compound physicochemical properties affect the rate of diffusion of the compounds through nasal mucous membranes, as they do through

other biological membranes. However, the physicochemical characteristics of the medication have little effect on the in vivo nasal absorption of compounds with a molecular weight of less than 300. More significant than lipophilicity and ionization state are variables like molecule size and the compound's capacity to form hydrogen bonds with membrane constituents. The aqueous channels in the membrane are most likely the route by which medications are absorbed from the nasal mucosa. Therefore, the drug will be absorbed quickly through the membrane's aqueous path as long as it is in solution and has a small molecular size. As the molecular size increases, the absorption from the nasal cavity decreases. Factors which affect the rate and extent of absorption of drugs via the nasal route are:

- The rate of nasal secretion. The greater the rate of secretion, the smaller the bioavailability of the drug.
- Ciliary movement. The faster the ciliary movement, the smaller the bioavailability of the drug.
- Vascularity of the nose. An increase in blood flow leads to faster drug absorption and vice versa.
- Metabolism of drugs in the nasal cavity. Although enzymes are found in the nasal tissues, they do not significantly affect the absorption of most compounds except peptides which can be degraded by aminopeptidases. This may be due to low levels of enzymes and short exposure time of the drug to the enzyme.
- Diseases affecting nasal mucous membrane. The effect of the common cold on nasal drug absorption is also an important consideration.
- A major limitation of nasal delivery is rapid mucociliary clearance resulting in low absorption and hence poor bioavailability of the drug. In situ nasal gelling drug delivery systems have been explored to overcome this and provide sustained delivery via the nasal route.

3.1.5.1. Enhancement of Nasal Drug Delivery

Reducing drug metabolism, extending the duration of drug residence in the nasal cavity, and boosting absorption are three ways to improve nasal drug delivery.

Prodrugs, parent molecule chemical modification, and physical permeability enhancement techniques can all be used to achieve nasal drug absorption. As a special excipient comes into contact with the nasal mucosa during nasal preparations, it may have some effect on facilitating drug transport. Compared to the pores in the epidermis, the mucosal pores are simpler to open. The following characteristics should be considered in choosing an absorption enhancer:

- The enhancer should be pharmacologically inert.
- It should be non-irritating, nontoxic, and nonallergic.

- Its effect on the nasal mucosa should be reversible.
- It should be compatible with the drug.
- It should be able to remain in contact with the nasal mucosa long enough to achieve maximal effects.
- It should not have any offensive odor or taste.
- It should be relatively inexpensive and readily available.

It is necessary to test how nasal absorption enhancers affect ciliary beating because any negative impact on mucociliary clearance will reduce the patient's willingness to accept the nasal formulation. An enhancer of absorption is chitosan, a naturally occurring polysaccharide that is extracted from the shells of crustaceans. Because chitosan is bioadhesive, it binds to the mucosal membrane and extends the formulation's retention period on the nasal mucosa. Chitosan may also speed up absorption by encouraging paracellular transport or by using other strategies. Chitosan nasal technology can be utilized in the form of solution, dry powder, or microsphere formulations to enhance the efficiency of the compound delivery system. Significant enhancements in bioavailability have been attained with various substances. When compared to oral or subcutaneous administration, nasal chitosan technology can offer a fast peak concentration for compounds that need a quick start of action.

- ***Advantages of Nasal Drug Delivery***
  - High permeability of the nasal mucosa compared to the epidermis or the gastrointestinal mucosa
  - Highly vascularized subepithelial tissue
  - Rapid absorption, usually within half an hour
  - Avoidance of first-pass effect that occurs after absorption of drugs from the gastrointestinal tract
  - Avoidance of the effects of gastric stasis and vomiting, for example, in migraine patients
  - Ease of administration by the patients who are usually familiar with nasal drops and sprays
  - Higher bioavailability of the drugs than in case of gastrointestinal route or pulmonary route
  - Most feasible route for the delivery of peptides
- ***Disadvantages of Nasal Drug Delivery***
  - Diseases conditions of the nose may result in impaired absorption.
  - The dose is limited due to the relatively small area available for absorption.
  - Time available for absorption is limited.
  - Little is known of the effect of the common cold on transnasal drug delivery, and it is likely that instilling a drug into a blocked nose or a nose with a surplus of watery rhinorrhea may expel the medication from the nose.
  - The nasal route of delivery is not applicable to all drugs. Polar drugs and some macromolecules are not absorbed in sufficient concentration due to poor membrane permeability, rapid

clearance, and enzymatic degradation into the nasal cavity.

Alternative methods are presently being developed to help get past these nasal barriers. Phospholipids and surfactants are examples of absorption enhancers that are frequently used, but their concentration must be used carefully. To improve the bioavailability of medications administered intranasally, researchers are looking into a variety of drug delivery methods, such as liposomes, cyclodextrins, and micro- and nanoparticles.

After weighing the benefits and drawbacks, nasal drug delivery emerges as a viable delivery method that rivals pulmonary drug delivery, which is also displaying a lot of promise. The nearly total bioavailability and dosage accuracy are two crucial factors.

3.1.1.2. Nasal Drug Delivery to the CNS

The prevailing belief is that medications cross the blood–brain barrier (BBB) and enter the central nervous system (CNS) through the olfactory epithelium in the nasal cavity. Since the olfactory nerve is the only location in the human body where the CNS is directly expressed on the nasal mucosal surface, it is the target when direct absorption into the brain is the aim.

3.1.6. Colorectal Drug Delivery

Even though humans have been administering drugs directly to their rectums since 1500 BC, most pharmaceutical users are reluctant to do so. On the other hand, medications intended to act systematically or that are directed toward the large intestine can be safely and gradually absorbed in the colon. Ingested materials stay in the colon for a significantly longer period of time even though the colon has a lower capacity for absorption than the small intestine. Food stays in the colon for two to three days after passing through the small intestine in a matter of hours. The basic requirements of drug delivery to the colorectal area are:

- The drug should be delivered to the colon either in a slow release or targeted form ingested orally or introduced directly by an enema or rectal suppository.
- The drug must overcome the physical barrier of the colonic mucous.
- Drugs must survive metabolic transformation by numerous bacterial species resident in the colon which are mainly anaerobes and possess a wide range of enzymatic activities.

1. Factors Which Influence Drug Delivery to Colorectal Area

- The rate of absorption of drugs from the colon is influenced by the rate of blood flow to and from the absorptive epithelium.
- Dietary components such as complex carbohydrates trap molecules within polysaccharide chains.
- Lipid-soluble molecules are readily absorbed by passive diffusion.
- The rate of gastric emptying and small bowel transit time.
- Motility patterns of the colon determine the rate of transit through the colon and hence the residence time of a drug and its absorption.
- Drug absorption varies according to whether the drug is targeted to the upper colon, the lower colon, or the rectum.

2. Advantages of the Rectal Route for Drug Administration
- A relatively large amount of the drug can be administered.
- Oral delivery of drugs that are destroyed by the stomach acid and/or metabolized by pancreatic enzymes.
- This route is safe and convenient, particularly for the infants and the elderly.
- This route is useful in the treatment of emergencies in infants such as seizures when the intravenous route is not available.
- The rate of drug absorption from the rectum is not influenced by ingestion of food or rate of gastric emptying.
- The effect of various adjuvants is generally more effective in the rectum than in the upper part of the gastrointestinal tract.
- Drugs absorbed from the lower part of the rectum bypass the liver.
- Degradation of the drugs in the rectal lumen is much less than in the upper gastrointestinal tract.

3. Disadvantages of the Rectal Route for Drug Administration
- Some hydrophilic drugs such as antibiotics and peptide drugs are not easily absorbed from the rectum, and absorption enhancers are required.
- Drugs may cause rectal irritation and sometimes proctitis with ulceration and bleeding.

Oral administration is another option for medications intended to act in the colon. Colon targeting is known to offer a number of therapeutic benefits, including the oral delivery of medications that are broken down by stomach acid and/or processed by pancreatic enzymes. Drugs that are released gradually from the colon can help treat arthritis, angina, and nocturnal asthma. Drugs delivered locally to the affected area are more effective in treating colonic pathologies, including Crohn's disease, ulcerative colitis, and colorectal cancer. When an oral anticancer medication is administered specifically to the colon to treat colorectal cancer, its concentration is increased at the target site, lowering the dosage and lowering the risk of side effects. Similarly, lower dosages are needed for colonic delivery of vermicides and colonic diagnostic agents.

3.1.7. Pulmonary Drug Delivery

Although different types of aerosols have been used since the middle of the 20th century to treat respiratory disorders, there has recently been interest in using the pulmonary route for systemic drug delivery. The lung's demonstrated potential as a portal for peptide entry and the viability of gene therapy for cystic fibrosis has stoked interest in this strategy even more. To use this route effectively, one must comprehend the mechanism of macromolecule absorption by the lungs.

3.1.7.1. Mechanisms of Macromolecule Absorption by the Lungs

Inhaled air is distributed by the lung deep within the tissue to a vast surface area known as the alveolar epithelium, which covers about 100 m^2 in adults. There are roughly 500 million tiny air sacs on this enormous surface called alveoli, which are surrounded by an equally massive capillary network. The airways, which begin with a single trachea and branch multiple times to reach the grape-like clusters of tiny alveoli, aid in the delivery of inhaled air to the alveoli. Compared to the airway volume of 400 ml, the alveolar volume ranges from 4,000 to 6,000 ml, offering a larger area for absorption of the substances inhaled. Large molecule medications, like peptides and proteins, are difficult to pass through the surface of the airway because it is almost completely impermeable due to a thick layer of ciliated mucus-covered cells. In contrast, the alveoli possess a thin layer of a single cell that allows for absorption into the bloodstream. Some barriers to the absorption of substances in the alveoli are:

- Surfactant, a thin layer at the air/water interface and may trap the large molecules.
- A molecule must traverse the surface lining fluid which is a reservoir for the surfactant and contains many components of the plasma as well as mucous.
- The single layer of epithelial cells is the most significant barrier.
- The extracellular space inside the tissues and the basement membrane to which the epithelial cells are attached.
- The vascular endothelium which is the final barrier to systemic absorption is more permeable to macromolecules than the pulmonary epithelium.

Although the mechanism of absorption of macromolecules by the lungs is still poorly understood, the following mechanisms are considered to play a part:

1. **Transcytosis (Passage Through the Cells):** This may occur and may be receptor-mediated, but it is not very significant for macromolecules >40 kDa.
2. Paracellular Absorption. This is usually thought to occur through the junctional complex between two cells. The evidence for this route of absorption is not very convincing in the case of the lungs. Molecules smaller than 40 kDa may enter via the junctional pores.
3. Drug transporter proteins of the lung epithelium play a role in pulmonary drug delivery, e.g., transporter-dependent absorption of β2-agonists in respiratory epithelial cells.

The entry of macromolecules into the blood is more predictable once they cross the epithelial barrier. The main route for absorption is provided by lymph vessels and venules. It is also possible for direct absorption to happen across the capillary endothelium's tight junctions.

3.1.7.2. Pharmacokinetics of Inhaled Therapeutics for Systemic Delivery

It is a difficult experimental task to accurately estimate the pharmacokinetics of inhaled therapeutics for systemic delivery. Numerous models have been reported for the investigation of lung absorption and disposition for inhaled therapeutic molecules in vivo, in vitro, and ex vivo settings. Because they enable the direct acquisition of pharmacokinetic data through repeatable dosing and control of regional distribution in the lungs through the use of various administration techniques, in vivo methods in small rodents remain the cornerstone of assessment. Lung epithelial cell lines cultured in vitro offer a means of delving deeper into the kinetics and mechanisms of transepithelial drug transport. Some of the drawbacks of in vivo and in vitro models are addressed by the ex vivo model of the isolated perfused lung. The preparation, in conjunction with a novel kinetic modeling analysis, allows for the independent determination of kinetic descriptors for lung absorption and nonabsorptive clearances, i.e., while controlling lung regional distributions. Before moving forward with clinical trials for future inhaled therapeutic entities for systemic delivery, scientists must carefully consider the pros and cons of each model at each stage of the research and development program.

- **Advantages of Pulmonary Drug Delivery**
  - Large surface area is available for absorption.
  - Close proximity to blood flow.
  - Avoidance of first-pass hepatic metabolism.
  - Smaller doses are required than the oral route to achieve equivalent therapeutic effects.
- **Disadvantages of Pulmonary Drug Delivery**
  - The lungs have an efficient aerodynamic filter which must be overcome for effective drug deposition to occur.
  - The mucous lining the pulmonary airways clears the deposited particles toward the throat.
  - Only 10–40% of the drug leaving an inhalation device is usually deposited in the lungs by using conventional devices.

3.1.7.3. Techniques of Systemic Drug Delivery via the Lungs

The focus here is on using the lungs for systemic drug delivery, though drugs may be given to the lungs for local treatment of pulmonary conditions. Inhalation anesthesia has historically been administered using straightforward inhalation apparatuses and aerosols containing a variety of medications. The use of dry powder formulations for deposition in the deep lung, which necessitates placement within the tracheal bronchial tree rather than simple aerosol inhalation, has arisen due to the current interest in peptide and protein delivery via this route. Various technologies that are in development for the systemic delivery of drugs by the pulmonary route are:

- **Dry Powders:** Dry powders often contain more active ingredients than liquid forms for many drugs. Dry powder aerosol particles can contain up to 50–95 % pure drug, compared to only 1–2 percent in aqueous aerosols, where the remaining portion is water. This implies that the majority of medications can be administered therapeutically in one to three puffs as a dry powder aerosol. Metered-dose inhaler (MDI) systems can carry about five times as much drug in a single breath as dry powder aerosols, and currently marketed liquid or nebulizer systems cannot carry nearly as much. When compared to nebulizers, a dry powder system might shorten the dosing duration for medications that need larger dosages, like insulin or α1-antitrypsin. Nebulizer delivery of insulin, for instance, necessitates many more puffs per dose, e.g., as much as 50–80 per dosage in one diabetic study. The last justification for emphasizing dry powders is the possibility of microbial development in the formulation. Liquids carry a higher risk of microbial growth than solids, which can result in life-threatening lung infections.

- **Inhalers:** Liquid medicine formulations can be delivered by a variety of aerosols. The aerosol is produced and delivered straight to the patient by inserting the liquid units into the apparatus. By doing this, any issues arising from turning proteins into powders are avoided. This technique can be used to deliver insulin and morphine.
- **Nanoparticle Formulations for Pulmonary Drug Delivery:** Both the bioavailability and drug delivery to the deep lung are greatly enhanced by nanoparticulate formulations. Spray-drying a nanoemulsion yields nanoparticles (less than 100 nm) that can be evenly distributed throughout the propellant to create a pressurized metered-dose inhaler formulation that is incredibly stable. Techniques for creating and characterizing drug-loaded polymeric nanoparticles made from charged, biodegradable, branched polyesters; employing a vibrating mesh nebulizer to aerosolize the nanosuspensions; and assessing the pharmacokinetics of the nanoscale drug delivery vehicles in the lungs.
- **Controlled-release pulmonary drug delivery:** his is appropriate for pharmaceuticals meant to be inhaled, either for systemic absorption or for local action in the lungs. Potential applications for the controlled release of drugs delivered through the lungs are:
  - It enables the reduction of dosing frequency for drugs given several times per day.
  - It increases the half-life of drugs which are absorbed very rapidly into the blood circulation and are rapidly cleared from the blood.
  - An inhaled formulation may lead to the development of products that might otherwise be abandoned because of unfavorable pharmacokinetics.
  - Pulmonary controlled release could decrease development cycles for drug molecules by obviating the need for chemical modification.

2.1.7.4. Conclusions and Future Prospects of Pulmonary Drug Delivery

Now that the pulmonary route of drug administration has been established, drugs can be delivered systemically. This method can be used to deliver a variety of medications, but the delivery of proteins and peptides is particularly appealing. Peptide and protein therapeutic products are becoming more and more common, so biotechnology companies will be investing in this field. Developments in the manufacturing of dry powder formulations will be just as crucial as the creation of apparatus for administering medications to the lungs. It is possible to create effervescent carrier particles with a sufficiently small particle size for deep lung deposition. This makes it possible to investigate this technology in the future to deliver a wide range of substances to the lungs with potentially better release than with traditional carrier particles.

As large molecules become more potent and sensitive and small particles become more chemically and physically robust, issues pertaining to microparticle formation for lung delivery will become increasingly important. Notwithstanding these drawbacks, the goal of pulmonary delivery of biopharmaceuticals is worthwhile and doable. Prospective findings are being obtained in the investigation of nanoparticles for pulmonary drug delivery. A large number of the safety concerns have been resolved.

Medications that are either on the market or in development to lessen influenza symptoms, minimize nausea and vomiting after chemotherapy for cancer, and administer vaccinations are among the non-biotherapeutic drugs being developed for inhalation. Inhalable antibiotics may be used in the future to treat lung conditions like tuberculosis locally and in large doses. Alternatively, drugs that are known to upset the stomach, like erythromycin, antidepressants, or migraine painkillers, might be packaged for inhalation. Drugs that are inhaled have the potential to eliminate common side effects associated with oral dosages, such as low solubility, food interactions, and low bioavailability. Fast-acting therapies, such as inhalables for pain, spasms, anaphylaxis, and seizures, may be beneficial for a variety of medical conditions because they enter the bloodstream more quickly than pills and some injections.

Anticipate a medicine cabinet filled with inhalable medications that will take the place of injectables, which are dreaded, and oral medications that have a host of adverse effects. Delivering biotherapeutics and other medications to the lungs is a broad challenge that will benefit from new approaches.

3.1.8. Cardiovascular Drug Delivery

Because the vascular system supplies blood and nutrients to all of the body's organs, its anatomy and physiology make it different from other systems when it comes to drug delivery. Medication can be administered via the vascular system to affect the entire body or specifically target an organ by way of the local blood supply. Devices are employed in addition to standard drug formulations like controlled release. Devices are used in a significant portion of cardiovascular therapeutics, especially for major and serious disorders. While some of these can be inserted surgically, others can be inserted using minimally invasive techniques like catheterization. Device placement necessitates the use of sophisticated cardiovascular imaging systems. Drug delivery to the cardiovascular system involves more than just putting medications in a controlled-release formulation; it also involves giving the heart cutting-edge treatments.

Methods for local administration of drugs to the cardiovascular system include the following:

- Drug delivery into the myocardium: direct intramyocardial injection, drug-eluting implanted devices
- Drug delivery via the coronary venous system
- Injection into coronary arteries via a cardiac catheter
- Intrapericardial drug delivery
- Release of drugs into arterial lumen from drug-eluting stents

3.1.9. Drug Delivery to the Central Nervous System

One of the challenges in treating disorders of the central nervous system (CNS) is getting medication into the brain. The blood-brain barrier (BBB), which restricts drug access to brain tissue, is the main barrier to CNS drug delivery. In the past, medications that were given systemically were primarily used to treat CNS diseases. This pattern keeps happening. The majority of research on CNS disorders focuses on finding medications and formulations for controlled release; the process by which these medications are delivered to the brain has received less attention. Figure 3.3 lists different ways to deliver medications to the central nervous system.

3.1.9.1. Drug Delivery across the BBB

Drug delivery to the central nervous system is still hampered by the BBB. Strategies for bridging the BBB based on nanotechnology have significantly advanced this field. This book includes a chapter on the creation of BBB model systems to locate, evaluate, and identify new nanoparticles that can be used for in vitro brain delivery. The authors of this work outline a procedure for screening nanoparticles with different sizes and levels of surface functionalization to identify the physicochemical properties that underlie the creation of nanoparticles that can effectively cross the blood-brain barrier.

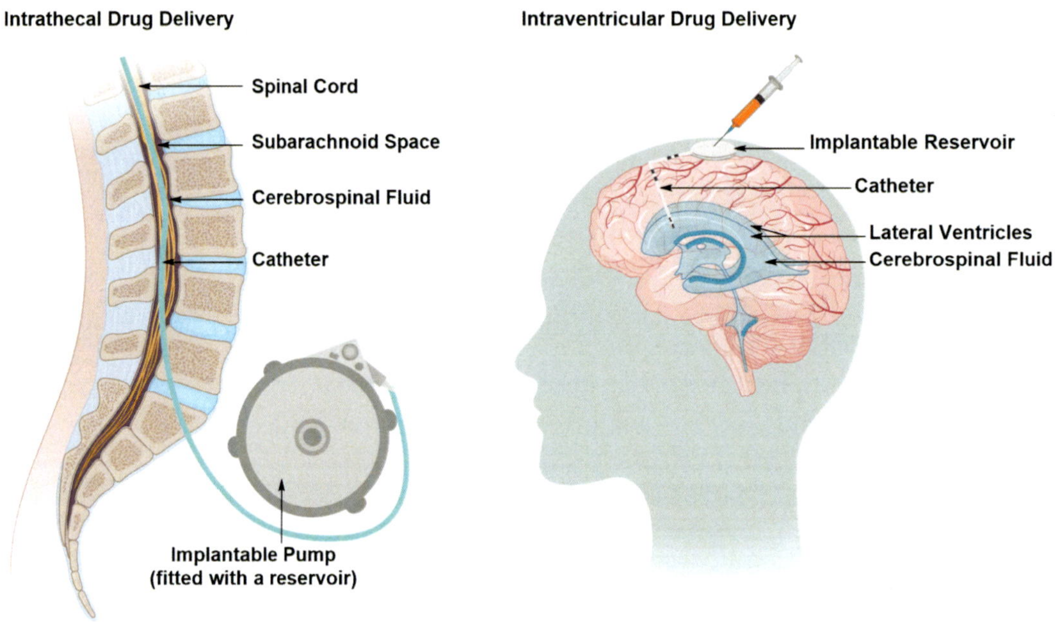

Figure 3.3. *Various methods of drug delivery to the central nervous system.*

Source: Abdul Razzak R, Florence GJ, Gunn-Moore FJ. Approaches to CNS drug delivery with a focus on transporter-mediated transcytosis. International Journal of Molecular Sciences. 2019; 20(12):3108. https://doi.org/10.3390/ijms20123108.

3.2. Drug Formulations

Delivery methods are always evolving; this includes new device discoveries as well as adjustments to established techniques. This section will cover some of the drug modifications and administration techniques. Figure 3.4 provides a classification of technologies that impact drug availability and release.

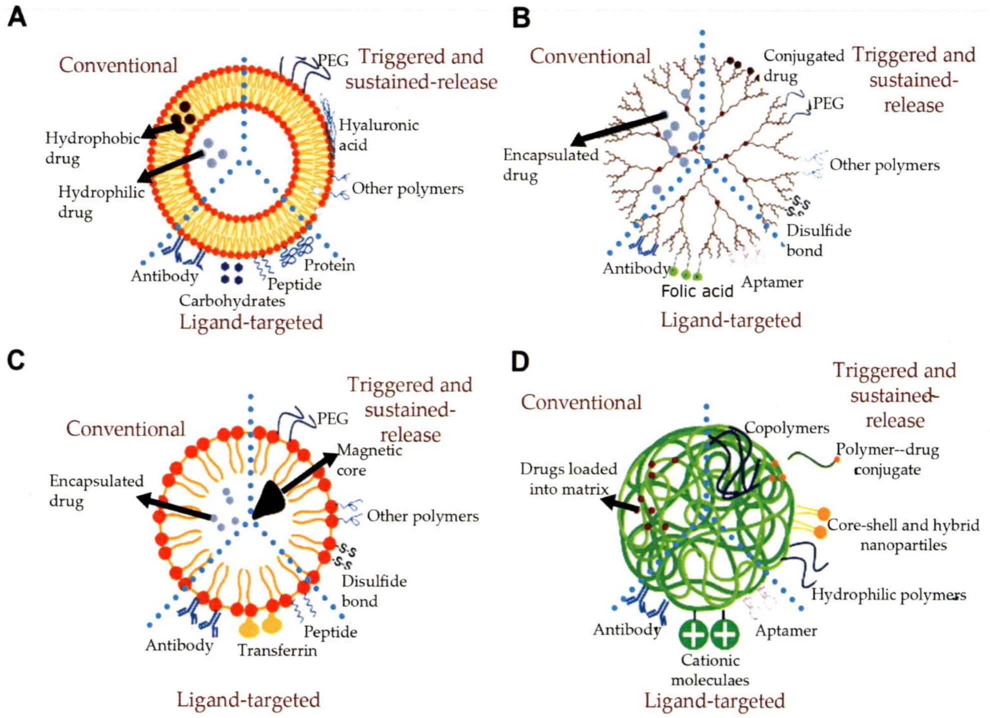

Figure 3.4. *Sustained drug release.*

Source: Bai X, Smith ZL, Wang Y, Butterworth S, Tirella A. Sustained drug release from smart nanoparticles in cancer therapy: a comprehensive review. Micromachines. 2022; 13(10):1623. https://doi.org/10.3390/mi13101623.

3.2.1. Sustained Release

Although sustained-release (SR) preparations are not new, there are a few new changes that are being implemented. When compared to "rapid" or "conventional" release preparations, they are also known as "long-acting" or "delayed-release.". There are instances where this phrase is used synonymously with "controlled release," which denotes more intricate control over release that is not limited to the temporal dimension. Although controlled release suggests consistency, drug release in SR preparations might not be reliable. The rationales of developing SR are:

- To extend the duration of action of the drug
- To reduce the frequency of dosing
- To minimize the fluctuations in the plasma level
- To improve drug utilization
- To lessen adverse effects

Limitations of SR products are:

- Increase in drug cost.

- Variation in the drug-level profile with food intake and from one subject to another.
- The optimal release form is not always defined, and the multiplicity of SR forms may confuse the physician as well as the patient.
- SR is achieved by either chemical modification of the drug or modifying the delivery system, e.g., the use of a special coating to delay the diffusion of the drug from the system. Chemical modification of drugs may alter such properties as distribution, pharmacokinetics, solubility, or antigenicity. One example of this is the attachment of polymers to the drugs to lengthen their lifetime by preventing cells and enzymes from attacking the drug.

3.2.2. Controlled Release

Controlled release refers to the administration of a medication, usually through a device. The control's goal is to deliver the medication, regardless of the surrounding conditions, at a given rate for a predetermined amount of time. Delivery times can range from days to years and are typically far longer than in SR cases. Controlled release may also include techniques to help the drug localize at an active site. This kind of control is described by the terms "targeted delivery systems" and "site-specific delivery systems.".

3.2.3. Programming the Release at a Defined Time

Chemical processes like enzymatic degradation or physical mechanisms like swelling with bursting can be employed to achieve programmed or pulsatile release. It is possible to design capsules that will rupture in an aqueous environment after a set amount of time. The osmotic pressure of the contents, the wall's thickness, elasticity, and the sphere's radius are all physical parameters that can be changed. The Port system, a semipermeable capsule with an osmotic charge and an insoluble plug, and the Chronset system, an osmotically active compartment in a semipermeable cap, are two examples of pulsatile-release oral drug delivery techniques.

3.2.4. Prodrugs

A prodrug is an active drug that is pharmacologically inert and needs to be converted to the parent compound in vivo through an enzymatic or chemical reaction to have any therapeutic effect.

The following are required for a prodrug to be useful for site-specific delivery:

- Prodrugs must have adequate access to their pharmacological receptors.
- The enzyme or chemical responsible for activating the drug should be active only at the target site.
- The enzyme should be in adequate supply to produce the required level of the drug to manifest its pharmacological effects.
- The active drug produce at the target site should be retained there and not diffuse into the systemic circulation.

L-dopa, the precursor of dopamine, is an example of a prodrug since it is distributed systemically after oral administration. The brain's corpus striatum converts it to dopamine, which has the intended therapeutic effects.

3.2.5. Novel Carriers and Formulations for Drug Delivery

Since the first injections and the straightforward administration of pills and capsules, numerous innovative delivery techniques have been developed. Figure 3.5 displays implants that are biodegradable.

3.2.6. Antibody Targeted Systems

Immunoglobulins can be used as the macromolecule in drug delivery systems that employ macromolecular attachment for delivery. This system's ability to be directed towards the site of antibody specificity is undoubtedly advantageous. The benefits include a significant decrease in side effects and a lower dosage requirement.

Antibodies are used to target liposomes when drugs are covalently or noncovalently bound to them or encapsulated in vesicles like microspheres or liposomes. Covalent attachments reduce the antigen-binding capacity and are typically ineffective. One way to raise the drug/antibody ratio during conjugation is to use an intermediate carrier molecule. These intermediaries consist of poly-L-glutamic acid or dextran.

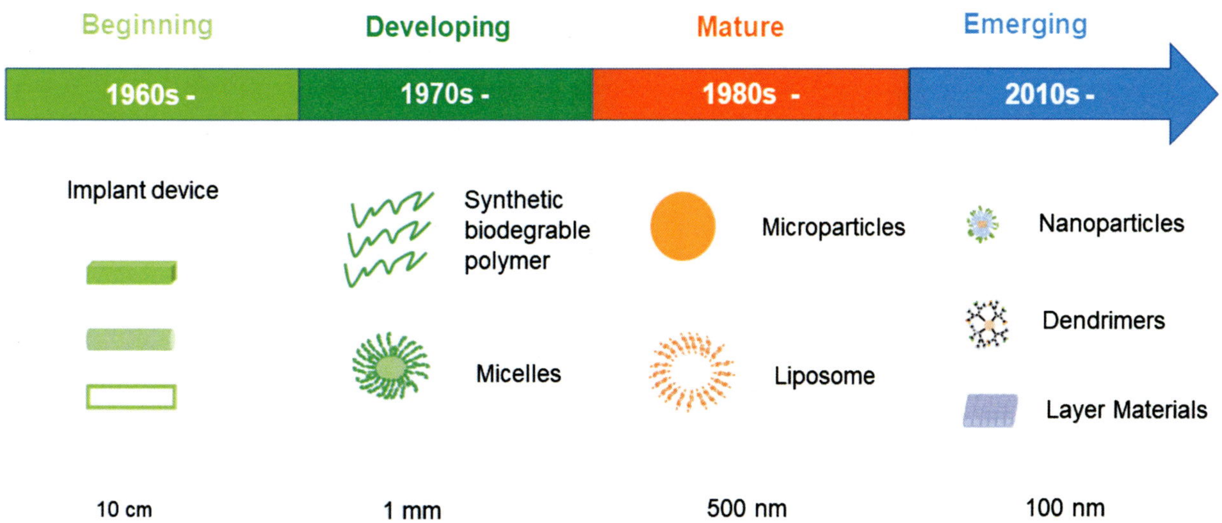

Figure 3.5. *Biodegradable drug delivery systems.*

Source: Zhu M, Whittaker AK, Han FY, Smith MT. Journey to the market: The evolution of biodegradable drug delivery systems. Applied Sciences. 2022; 12(2):935. https://doi.org/10.3390/app12020935.

Anticancer medications are one type of medication that has been conjugated to antibodies or their fragments. Many antibody–liposome combinations have been studied for the delivery of genes and medications. Liposomes containing drug cargo that have had their surfaces conjugated to antibodies are referred to as immunoliposomes. The primary benefit of an antibody-targeted system is the potential to mitigate the side effects of anticancer medications through the utilization of monoclonal antibodies that selectively recognize tumor antigens.

In clinical practice, radiolabeled antibodies are employed for imaging and therapeutic applications in addition to research. They offer a chance to combine medication administration with diagnosis. Radiolabeled monoclonal antibodies are used as direct therapeutic agents for cancer radioimmunotherapy due to their specific targeting of tumor antigens.

3.2.7. Gene Therapy as a Drug Delivery Method

Gene therapy is generally understood to be the process of introducing specific genetic material to patient target cells with the ultimate goal of preventing or treating a given disease state. Gene therapy is an effective means of delivering therapeutics; alternative delivery modalities are employed for genes.

Through a process known as "bactofection," certain bacteria that naturally select specific tumors have been employed as gene vectors to deliver genes or gene products to the tumor environment. In one chapter, methods for investigating this phenomenon in vivo and in vitro for invasive and noninvasive bacteria are covered. These bacteria can be used as tumor-specific therapeutic delivery vehicles in rodent models to transfer plasmid DNA to mammalian cells. Figure 3.6, which lists the different technologies used in gene therapy, provides an overview of the wide range of applications. Targeted and regulated gene therapy shows promise.

3.2.7.1. Delivery of siRNAs

Effective delivery of siRNAs is necessary for the successful silencing of genes. Numerous techniques have been employed for the delivery of siRNA, such as lipid-based technologies for targeted delivery. One chapter describes a novel microfluidic-based manufacturing process for the rapid manufacture of siRNA–lipid nanoparticles (siRNA–LNP), along with protocols for characterizing the size, polydispersity, RNA encapsulation efficiency, RNA concentration, and total lipid concentration of the resulting nanoparticles. SiRNA–LNPs have the potential to be used in therapeutic applications.

3.2.8. Cells as Vehicles for Drug Delivery

Drugs are delivered by means of cells. Examples of these include drugs encapsulated in red blood cells (RBC), gene therapy delivered through cells, and encapsulated cells that secrete therapeutic proteins that are implanted.

3.2.8.1. Cell-Mediated Gene Therapy

Because cells can act as biological pumps for the release of therapeutic substances, transplanting cells with specific functions is a recognized procedure for the treatment of human diseases. Cells are genetically modified, amplified in vitro, and then injected into target tissues as part of a process known as cell-mediated gene therapy. Cell-mediated gene therapy has been applied to a variety of cell types.

By genetically modifying stem cells to secrete desired gene products, it may be possible to use stem cells' capacity to home to areas of acute injury as a method of local drug delivery. It has been demonstrated that mesenchymal stem cells (MSCs) can migrate toward and engraft into tumor sites. This suggests that MSCs may be used as carriers for cancer gene therapy through nonviral transfection.

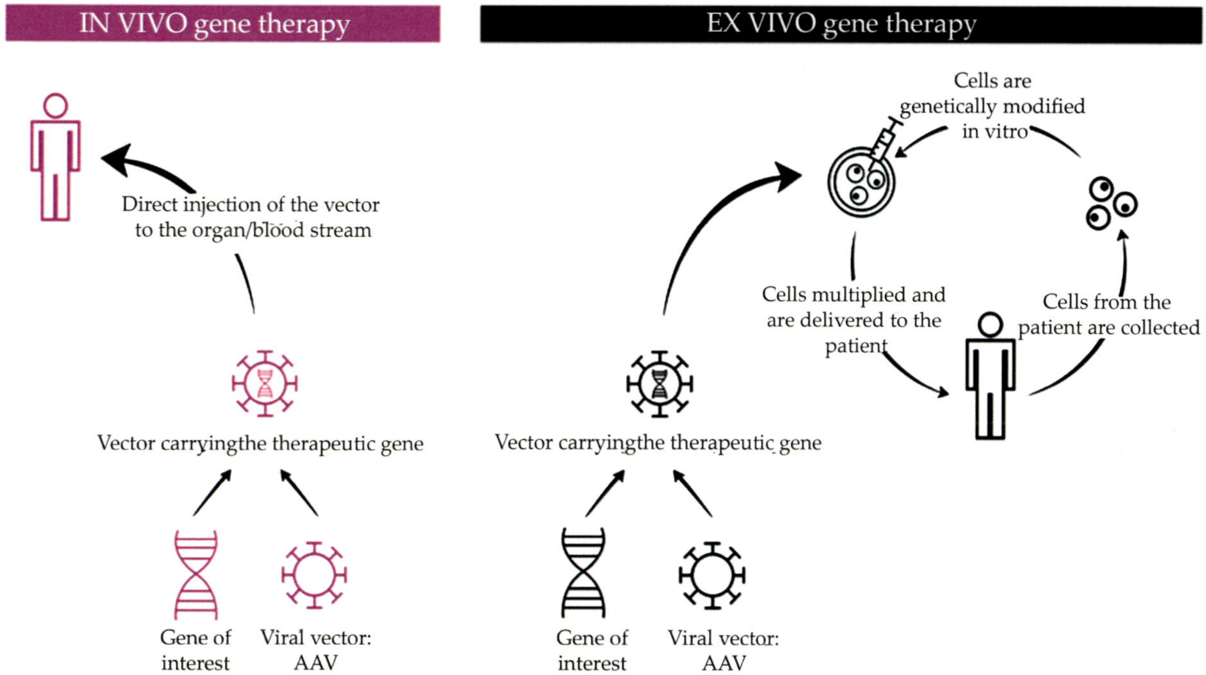

Figure 3.6. *Gene therapy.*

Source: de Castro MJ, del Toro M, Giugliani R, Couce ML. Gene therapy for Neuronopathic mucopolysaccharidoses: State of the Art. International Journal of Molecular Sciences. 2021; 22(17):9200. https://doi.org/10.3390/ijms22179200.

3.2.8.2. RBCs as Drug Delivery Vehicles

Red blood cells (RBCs) are naturally occurring drug delivery vehicles because of their exceptional bloodstream longevity, biocompatibility, and secure physiological metabolism. Many patient infusion protocols for medications encapsulated in red blood cells are being investigated. RBC carriage may be advantageous for drug delivery, especially for medications that target phagocytic cells and those that must act within the vascular lumen. RBC drug delivery can be achieved through two methods: (1) coupling of drugs to the surface of RBCs, and (2) encapsulation into isolated RBCs ex vivo followed by infusion in compatible recipients. Those controlling the immune response. Without the need for ex vivo modification or RBC infusion, safe anchoring of cargoes to circulating RBC is made possible by RBC drug delivery via injection of therapeutics conjugated with fragments of antibodies (Figure 3.7).

RBCs swell with membrane rupture and pore formation when they are placed in a hypotonic medium. This makes it possible to encapsulate 25% of the medication or enzyme in a solution.

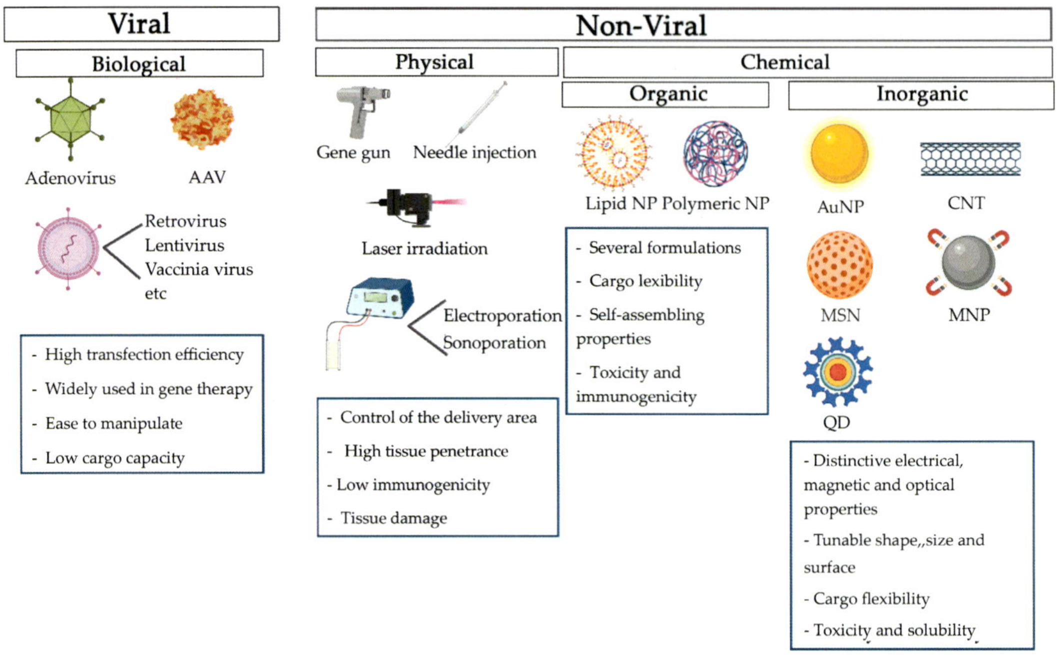

Figure 3.7. *Delivery of cells for therapeutic purposes.*

Source: Mirón-Barroso, S., Domènech, E. B., & Trigueros, S. Nanotechnology-based strategies to overcome current barriers in gene delivery. International Journal of Molecular Sciences. 2021; 22(16), 8537. https://doi.org/10.3390/ijms22168537.

The membrane is resealed by restoring the tonicity of the solution. Potential uses of loaded RBCs as drug delivery systems are:

- They are biodegradable and non-immunogenic.
- They can be modified to change their resident circulation time; depending on their surface, cells with little surface damage can circulate for a longer time.
- The entrapped drug is shielded from immunological detection and external enzymatic degradation.
- The system is relatively independent of the physicochemical properties of the drug.

The drawbacks of using RBCs are that the damaged RBCs are sequestered in the spleen and the storage life is limited to about 2 weeks.

3.2.8.2. Drug Delivery Systems for Cell Therapy

Drug delivery systems are necessary for both gene and cell therapies, even though cells may also deliver therapeutics similar to how gene therapy vectors do. Transporting materials to encourage cell growth is a key goal in cell therapy for regenerative medicine. The creation of a self-assembling peptide hydrogel and its possible application in a rodent model of myocardial infarction as a means of delivering cells and growth factors to the infarcted heart.

3.2.9. Ideal Properties of Material for Drug Delivery

The properties of an ideal macromolecular drug delivery or biomedical vector are:

- Structural control over size and shape of drug or imaging agent cargo space
- Biocompatible, nontoxic polymer/ pendant functionality
- Precise, nanoscale container and/ or scaffolding properties with high drug or imaging-agent capacity features
- Well-defined scaffolding and/or surface-modifiable functionality for cell-specific targeting moieties
- Lack of immunogenicity
- Appropriate cellular adhesion, endocytosis, and intracellular trafficking to allow therapeutic delivery or imaging in the cytoplasm or nucleus
- Acceptable bio-elimination or biodegradation
- Controlled or triggerable drug release
- Molecular level isolation and protection of the drug against inactivation during transit to target cells
- Minimal nonspecific cellular and blood-protein binding properties
- Ease of consistent, reproducible, clinical-grade synthesis

3.2.10. Innovations for Improving Oral Drug Delivery

The oral route is still the most popular way to administer medication. There is continuous work to improve the speed and efficiency of this route.

3.2.10.1. Fast-Dissolving Tablets

Fast-disintegration technology is used for manufacturing these tablets. The advantages of fast-dissolving tablets are:

- Convenient to take without the use of water
- Easier to take by patients who cannot swallow
- Rapid onset of action due to faster absorption
- Less gastric upset because the drug is dissolved before it reaches the stomach
- Improved patient compliance

3.2.10.1. Softgel Formulations

Drugs passing through the upper gastrointestinal tract to be absorbed later have been shielded by capsules and other protective coatings. Additionally, the coatings lessen gastrointestinal discomfort. The softgel offers the benefits of a solid dosage form while delivering medication in solution. Hydrophobic drugs, which have low bioavailability due to their inability to dissolve easily in water or digestive juices, are especially well-suited for softgel capsules. When hydrophobic medications are combined into solid dosage forms, there may be a slow rate of dissolution, variable absorption, and insufficient bioavailability. Fatty acids, such as those found in food, enhance bioavailability. g. diglycerides or mono-cerides. Drugs that are hydrophobic, like griseofulvin, isotretinoin, and hydrochlorothiazide, can be quickly absorbed in the gut by solubilizing them with fatty acids. Hydrophobic drugs are dissolved in a hydrophilic solvent and then enclosed. The medication is instantly released in the gastric juice and is absorbed from the gastrointestinal tract into the bloodstream when softgels are crushed or chewed. The intended therapeutic effects therefore start to take effect quickly. Advantages of softgels over tablets are:

- The development time for softgel is shorter due to lower bioavailability concerns, and such solutions can be marketed at a fraction of the cost.
- Softgel formulations, e.g., that of ibuprofen, have a shorter time to peak plasma concentration and greater peak plasma concentration compared to a marketed tablet formulation. Cyclosporin can give therapeutic blood levels which are not achievable in tablet form. Similarly, oral hypoglycemic glipizide in softgel is also known to have better bioavailability results compared with tablet form.
- Softgel delivery systems can also incorporate phospholipids or polymers or natural gums to entrap the drug active in the gelatin layer with an outer coating to give desired delayed-/ controlled-release effects. The advantages of softgel capsules over other hard-shell capsules are:
- Sealed tightly in an automatic manner.
- Easy to swallow.
- Allow product identification, using colors and several shapes.
- Better stability than other oral delivery systems.
- Good availability and rapid absorption.
- Offer protection against contamination, light, and oxidation.
- Unpleasant flavors are avoided due to content encapsulation.

3.2.10.1. Improving Drug-Release Mechanisms of Oral Preparations

Depending on the preparation method and nature, the drug-release rates of orally administered products typically decrease from the matrix system over time. Geometric configurations are used in a number of ways to address issues related to drug-release mechanisms and release rates, such as the cylindrical rod and cylindrical donut methods. The three-dimensional printing (3DP) provides the following advantages:

- • Zero-order drug delivery
- • Patterned diffusion gradient by microstructure diffusion barrier technique
- • Cyclic drug release

The 3DP method prints a binder into specific regions of powder layers that have been deposited one after the other using ink-jet printing technology to create a solid object. The active agent may be incorporated into the apparatus as discrete units within the matrix structure or as a dispersion along the polymeric matrix. The choice of polymer and binder materials can be optimized to meet specific needs, such as controlled release, for the drug-release mechanism.

3.2.11. Drug Delivery Devices

Implanting the drug-delivery system into body tissue and using it as a sustained-release medication is one of the most straightforward methods available. Table 3.10 provides a classification of drug delivery devices.

Drug delivery devices are not a new idea; instead, they are utilizing new technologies. Sometimes implantation requires specific injection tools and surgical methods. These implants' materials have to be biocompatible, i.e., the polymers utilized shouldn't irritate the implantation site or encourage the formation of an abscess. Currently, one of the methods used to explore the possibilities of sustained delivery systems is subcutaneous implantation. There are good absorption sites available, and you can take the device out whenever you want.

Numerous other medications, such as insulin, thyroid hormones, cardiovascular agents, and nerve growth factor, have also been inserted subcutaneously. Certain implantable devices are more than just straightforward drug diffusion sources. Certain devices can release insulin in response to variations in osmotic pressure, while pellets can release their drug load encapsulated by magnetism. Many of the drawbacks of the majority of implantable drug delivery systems would be eliminated with such external control of an embedded device.

3.2.11.1. Pumps and Conduits for Drug Delivery

Mechanical pumps are typically tiny devices that deliver medications into the right vessels or other parts of the body. Examples of these devices are percutaneous infusion catheters and implantable infusion pumps. There are numerous commercially available pumps, implantable catheters, and infusion devices. Examples of applications of these devices are:

- Intrathecal morphine infusion for pain control
- Intraventricular drug administration for disorders of the brain
- Hepatic arterial chemotherapy
- Intravenous infusion of heparin in thrombotic disorders
- Intravenous infusion of insulin in diabetes

The advantages of these devices are:

- The rate of drug diffusion can be controlled.
- Relatively large amounts of drugs can be delivered.
- The drug administration can be changed or stopped when required.

3.2.11.2. Controlled-Release Microchip for Drug Delivery

Liquid solutions have been released pulsatile through the use of microchip technology. A microchip made of solid-state silicon with flow channels and micrometer-sized pumps can release one or more chemicals under control when needed. The electrochemical dissolution of thin anode membranes covering microreservoirs containing chemicals in various forms forms the basis for the release mechanism. Chemical substances in solid, liquid, or gel form can be released in different quantities in a pulsatile, continuous, or mixed manner. The entire device can be implanted into the body or mounted on the tip of a tiny probe.

Microchip Technology Inc. uses its technology to create a drug delivery device that is controlled-release iontophoretic transdermal and can use a smaller battery size and lighter battery overall. All that is required for wearable patch-based iontophoresis devices are small footprint microcontrollers. Conventionally, controlled drug release from polymeric materials occurs in reaction to certain stimuli, including light, enzymes, electric and magnetic fields, and ultrasound. In adults with type 1 diabetes, continuous glucose monitoring has been linked to better glycemic control. Microchip Technology, Inc. is creating an implanted, long-term continuous glucose monitor that uses wireless technology to provide convenient, accurate, dependable, and continuous glucose readings that help direct the administration of insulin. Additionally, the device's clinical trial for the delivery of PTH1–34 for the treatment of osteoporosis was successfully completed by the company.

As advances in micro- and nanotechnologies are incorporated, drug delivery based on lab-on-a-chip technology is evolving. The three main lab-on-a-chip drug delivery systems under development are (1) the synthesis of smart particles as drug carriers at the tissue level; (2) the integration of a concentration gradient generator with a cell culture platform at the cellular level; and (3) microneedles and implantable devices with fluid-handling components at the organism level.

The development of an autonomous controlled-release implant, also known as "pharmacy-on-a-chip," or a highly controlled tablet (smart tablet) for drug delivery may be possible in the future with the right choice of biocompatible material. By engineering the chips, the researchers hope to be able to respond to commands transmitted through the skin by altering the medication type or drug-release schedule. Every microchip has many distinct reservoirs from which telemetry can regulate the delivery of doses.

3.2.11.3. Use of Physical Agents for Controlled Release of Therapeutic Substances

Physical agents like heat and ultrasound are used to control the release of therapeutic agents. An example outlined in a chapter of this book is a noninvasive, nonviral method of gene therapy delivery using ultrasound for targeted gene delivery. This innovative technology uses gas-filled, acoustic microspheres for imaging and therapy, potentially aiding in the development of single gene replacement therapy.

3.2.12. Particulate Drug Delivery Systems

The idea of employing particles to transport medications to specific body locations came from their application as radiodiagnostic agents in medical research on the reticuloendothelial system, which includes the liver, spleen, bone marrow, and lymph nodes. Particles with sizes varying from 20 µm to 300 µm have been suggested for use in drug delivery. The particles can be injected directly into the systemic circulation or into a specific body compartment due to their small size. A close mixture of the drug may be present in particulate drug delivery systems, and the drug may either be encapsulated by the carrier material or dispersed as an emulsion in the core material. Factors which influence the release of drugs from particulate carriers are:

- The drug: Its physicochemical properties, position in the particle, and drug–carrier interaction
- Particles: Type, size, and density of the particle
- Environments: Temperature, light, presence of enzymes, ionic strength, and hydrogen ion concentration
- Various particulate drug carrier systems can be grouped into the following classes:
- Microspheres are particles larger than 1 µm but small enough not to sediment when suspended in water (usually 1–100 µm).

- Nanoparticles are colloidal particles ranging in size between 10 and 1,000 nm.
- Glass-like sugar matrices.
- Liposomes.
- Cellular particles such as resealed erythrocytes, leukocytes, and platelets.

3.2.12.1. Microspheres

Cross-linked protein microspheres have been employed as biodegradable medication delivery systems. Small drug molecules are released from protein microspheres at a comparatively quick rate; however, this issue can be solved by using a variety of techniques, such as complexing the drug with macromolecules. Acrylamides (e.g., starch) and a variety of man-made polymers have been employed in the production of microspheres. A barrier membrane encircling a solid or liquid core sets microcapsules apart from microspheres, and this is advantageous for peptides and proteins. Special applications of microspheres and microcapsules are:

- Poly- D,L-lactide- co-glycolide-agarose microspheres can encapsulate proteins and stabilize them for drug delivery.
- Multicomponent, environmentally responsive, hydrogel microspheres, coated with a lipid bilayer can be used to mimic the natural secretory granules for drug delivery.
- Microencapsulation of therapeutic agents to provide local controlled drug release in the central nervous system across the blood–brain barrier.
- Microspheres can be used for the chemoembolization of tumors in which the vasculature is blocked while an anticancer agent is released from the trapped microparticles.
- Microcapsules, produced at the ideal size for inhalation (1–5 μm), can be used in formulating drugs for pulmonary delivery, both for local delivery and for systemic absorption.
- Microspheres can be used as nasal drug delivery systems for systemic absorption of peptides and proteins.
- Poly- D,L-lactide- co-glycolide microspheres can be used as a controlled-release antigen delivery system—parenteral or oral.
- Delivery of antisense oligonucleotides.
- Nano-encapsulation of DNA in bioadhesive particles can be used for gene therapy by oral administration.

3.2.12.2. Glass-Like Sugar Matrices

These are glass-like sugar matrix microparticles. Spray drying is the process of spraying a sugar and insulin solution as a mist into a hot, dry air stream, quickly drying the mist to a powder. The quick change from a liquid to a glassy powder keeps the insulin from becoming denaturated. Sugar microspheres can also be used to preserve medications and vaccines, which typically need to be refrigerated when transported to far-flung locations worldwide. By “propping up” the active structure of the drug molecules, sugar molecules shield them from denaturing when the water molecules are extracted.

3.2.13. Nanotechnology-Based Drug Delivery

Nanotechnology is the manipulation of matter at the nanoscale length scale to create and use materials, devices, and systems, i.e., in terms of molecules, atoms, and supramolecular structures. The phrase is commonly used to describe the creation and application of useful structures that have at least one characteristic dimension measured in nanometers; one nanometer is equivalent to one billionth of a meter (10^{-9} m).

Before nanotechnology was used in drug delivery, there was already a trend toward the miniaturization of carrier particles. Size and porosity are two factors that determine whether or not a nanoparticle is suitable for use in drug delivery. Drugs can be given to patients via a variety of delivery methods with the help of nanoparticles. When a drug is delivered intravenously, it can safely travel through the tiniest blood vessels in the body. When a drug is delivered via inhalation, its surface area is increased and it dissolves more quickly. All of these uses of nanoparticles are crucial. Porosity is crucial for the entrapment of gases in nanoparticles, regulating the rate at which drugs release, and directing drug delivery to particular areas.

Many hydrophobic drugs release too slowly from the nanoparticles used to deliver them, making it difficult to formulate them for sustained release and reducing the effectiveness of the delivery system. While maintaining the intended sustained-release profile of these medications, it is possible to accelerate the release by altering the water uptake into the nanoparticles. By altering the porosity of the nanoparticles during the manufacturing process and selecting from a broad range of materials to include in the shell, water uptake into nanoparticles can be altered.

Nanobiotechnology provides the following solutions to the problems of drug delivery:

- Improving solubilization of the drug.
- Using noninvasive routes of administration eliminates the need for administration of drugs by injection.
- Development of novel nanoparticle formulations with improved stabilities and shelf lives.
- The development of nanoparticle formulations for improved absorption of insoluble compounds and macromolecules enables improved bioavailability and release rates, potentially reducing the amount of dose required and increasing safety through reduced side effects.
- Manufacture of nanoparticle formulations with controlled particle sizes, morphology, and surface properties would be more effective and less expensive than other technologies.
- Nanoparticle formulations that can provide sustained-release profiles up to 24 h can improve patient compliance with drug regimens.
- Direct coupling of drugs to targeting ligand restricts the coupling capacity to a few drug molecules, but coupling of drug carrier nanosystems to ligands allows import of thousands of drug molecules by means of one receptor-

targeted ligand. Nanosystems offer opportunities to achieve drug targeting with newly discovered disease-specific targets.

3.2.13.1. Nanomaterials and Nanobiotechnologies Used for Drug Delivery

Various nanomaterials and nanobiotechnologies used for drug delivery are shown in Table 3.1.

3.2.13.2. Liposomes

Liposomes are tiny vesicles composed of phospholipids and other amphipathic lipids, known for their stability. The properties of liposomes can significantly differ based on factors such as lipid composition, size, surface charge, and preparation method.

Table 3.1. Evolution of Nanoparticles from 1991 to 2022 in Detail Discussed Here

Year	Types of NPs	Drug Delivery Approaches	Diseases	Applications	Characterization
1991	Poly-alkyl-cyanoacrylate nanoparticles	Carrier that delivers drug to target specific site.	Cancer	Cancer chemotherapy and intracellular antibiotherapy.	Scanning electron microscope (SEM)
1992	Calcium hydroxyapatite ceramic (CHC)	Drug gentamicin placed in the porous blocks of calcium hydroxyapatite antibiotics (CHA).	Chronic osteomyelitis (animal model)	The bactericidal activity was retained and drug shows effective results.	No in vivo experiments performed
1993	Nano and micro particles	Micro-particulate system used for the administration of the drug.	Enhance oral immune system (immunization)	In vitro, self-diffusion, liberation due to erosion, pulsed delivery due to oscillating field.	In vitro experiments performed
1994	Acrylic acid copolymer NPs	Acrylic acid, acrylic amide, acrylic-butyl ester, and methacrylic methyl ester used as copolymer in drug delivery.	No	Help opsonin to reach specific target site and also enhance reticuloendothelial system.	Small angle X-ray scattering

1995	Poly-alkyl-cyanoacrylate (PECA) nanoparticles	Ofloxacin (OFX) and perfloxacine entrapped in PECA nanoparticles. OFX system more efficient than PFX system.	Bacterial diseases	The fluoro-quinolone-loaded nanoparticles enhance antimicrobial activity of the drug.	Freeze fracture electron microscopy, physicochemical characterization
1996	Protein and peptides-based NPs	Monoclonal antibodies, recombinant proteins transported to BBB by chimeric peptide approach.	Alzheimer's disease	Avidin conjugate with BBB vector to transport all proteins across BBB. Vasoactive intestinal peptide cures brain diseases.	No characterization of physiologic-based strategy
1997	Nanoparticle	Nanoparticles as carrier to deliver drug to intra-arterial localization system. Cather based delivery	Restenosis (arterial reobstruction)	Easily penetrate into the arterial wall and without causing injury. Biocompatible and effective for restenosis treatment.	No
1998	Diblock copolymer nanoparticles	Micelles and nanosphere carry genes and hydrophobic drugs to target site.	No	Help to sustain drug rate. Solubilize, release, and protect drugs. Enhance retention time in the blood.	No
1999	Chitosan nanoparticles	Potential of chitosan nanoparticles to improve absorption of insulin through nasal cavity.	Diabetes	MicroAB assay used to determine insulin loading and release.	Zeta potential, laser doppler anemometry, photon correlation spectroscopy

2000	Liposome with hyperthermia as nanoparticles	Increased drug delivery to tumor. Hyperthermia helps liposome to work properly.	Ovarian carcinoma	Helpful in human cancer treatment.	Experiments performed
2001	PEGylated poly-cyano-acrylate nanoparticles	Efficient drug carrier to deliver therapeutic molecules in prion disease test.	Prion Diseases	Long retention time in blood as compared to non-PEGylated nanoparticles. Brain and spleen target tissues show uptake higher in scrapie-infected animals.	Experiments performed
2002	Transferrin mediated receptor endocytosis	Transferrin and transferrin receptor in drug and in gene transference via the BBB.	Cancer and Brain diseases	Transferrin receptor interceded iron uptake; regulation of transferrin receptor expression, anticancer drugs site-specific to tumor cells.	No
2003	L-nanoparticles	Intravenous injection of L-particles loaded with green dye shows hepatocellular carcinoma in humans.	I-Hepatitis B II-Hepatocellular carcinoma III-Hemophilia	Hepatitis B virus infects liver hepatocyte cells. L-nanoparticles deliver drugs or genes efficiently and specifically to the targeted hepatocyte cells in a mouse xenograft model.	No

2004	Colloidal gold nanoparticles	Colloidal gold nanoparticles used as vector to carry tumor necrosis factor (TNF) towards specific part of tumor in mice.	MC-38 carcinoma tumor	The designed vector PT-cAu-TNF bound on the surface of the gold NPs. Intravenous injection shows effective results in MC-38 carcinoma tumor.	TEM, dynamic light scatter, and differential centrifugal sedimentation, zeta potential
2005	Liposomes, nanoparticles	Vitamin Folic acid placed inside cationic liposomes and conjugate liposomes to folate ligand act as carrier and chemotherapeutics agents, and DNA attaches to the receptor-bearing cancer cells in vitro.	Cancer (human nasopharyngeal and prostate tumor)	Folate-associated, lipid-based nanoparticles transport DNA with high transfection efficacy and constraining tumor progress with intratumoral shot into human nasopharyngeal and prostate malignancy using an HSV-tk/GCV treatment system.	No
2006	Folate-conjugated starch nanoparticles (StNP's)	Folate changed with PEG coupled to the exterior of starch NPs to attain the FA-PEG/StNPs. Doxorubicin loaded on FA-PEG/StNP.	Liver cancer	In vitro, FA-PEG/StNP targeted on liver cells BEL7404. It reduced DOX toxicity. This combination can be suitable for cancer targeting drug haulers in future.	AFM and zeta potential, UV Spectro-photometer characterize particle size determination

2007	Gold nanoparticles (AuNPs)	Drug and gene delivery approach to deliver drugs and genes by using gold nanoparticles. The transfection efficacy for beta galactosidase with various MMPCs.	Human nasopharyngeal carcinoma	Properties of drug transfer like reduced toxicity, treating acute diseases, uptake and release rate using fluorophore AuNPs provide added insight in future.	Fluorescence and bright-field microscopy
2008	PEGylated gold nanoparticles	Very effective drug transfers with AuNPs' vector for in vivo photodynamic treatment in cancer.	Cancer	The diversity in medicine released in vitro in two-phase solution system. In vivo in cancer-bearing mice shows that the way of drug carriage is enormously well-planned, and submissive targeting prefers the tumor area.	TEM and image analysis, DLS measurement, UV-vis, and fluorescent spectrophotometer
2009	Alginate/ Chitosan (Alg/Chi) nanoparticles	Nanoparticles of alginate/chitosan polymers were arranged by pre-gel preparation method via drop-wise addition of several concentrations of $CaCl_2$ to a definite concentration of sodium alginate.	No	Optimization of Alg/Chi NPs and preparation are areas of this research. Some parameters like ratio of Alg/Chi, ratio of $CaCl_2$/ Alginate and N/P can disturb size and loading ability of these particles.	Zeta potential, photon correlation spectroscopy, scattering particle size analyzer, FTIR analysis, DSC analysis

2010	Mesoporous silica nanoparticles	Targeted carriage of chemotherapeutic mediator methotrexate (MTX) to tumor cells by means of poly (ethylene mine)-functionalized mesoporous silica small units as vectors for drug delivery.	Cancer	(a) Choice of adaptable surface functionalization; (b) High level of cell specificity and effective cellular uptake; (c) A slight grade of early seepage and the measured release of the medicine; (d) Low cytotoxicity of the transporter.	Scanning electron microscope (SEM)
2011	Nano diamond (ND) or diamond nanoparticles	Nano diamonds have ability to transport small interfering RNA into sarcoma (Ewing) cells. Was examined with evaluation of the route of in vivo anticancer nucleic acid drug transfer.	Ewing Sarcoma Cells (Cancer)	Well-organized delivery of oligonucleotide by a cationic nano-diamond nanoparticle: (i) Suitably robust adsorption of the biomolecule on the particle surface across the cell membrane deprived of damage of material; (ii) The severance of the compound on the time-scale of a cell division cycle.	FT-IR confirm the absorption of PAH on nano-diamonds and zeta potential

2012	Silver nanoparticles	This method was to design stable silver NP vector to make larvicides of mosquitos to destroy mosquitos' life with drugs.	Malaria, Dengue fever, Filariasis	The leaf potage of *Annona squamosa* used as an active capping and reducing mediator for the fusion of silver nanoparticles.	Ultraviolet spectrophotometry, X-Ray diffraction, FT-IR, SEM
2013	Silver nanoparticle	Nanoparticles of noble metal show potential as photo-activated vectors for drug delivery. SNPs conjugated with thiol-terminated photo-liable DNA oligonucleotides.	Photo-activated gene silencing	Good consistency to nucleases, hybridization amplified action upon photo release, and effective cellular uptake as associated to commercial transfection vectors.	UV-spectrophotometer, fluorescent confocal microscopy
2014	Silver nanoparticles as drug-loading vector	Silver nanoparticles synthesized from plant *Pongamia pinnata* by green method.	Dengue	Medically active plant and earth eco-friendly. Larvicidal action of silver nanoparticles and leaf extract contrary to *Aedes aegypti* showed positive results.	UV-visible absorption spectrum, TEM, XRD, FTIR
2015	Polyamidoamine nanoparticles	Polyamidoamine nanoparticles work as nanocarrier and deliver anti-malarial drug to the targeted sites. It also works as nanomedicine.	Malaria	Union of doxorubicin and polymers increases drug solubility, enhances its blood half-life, decreases toxicity, and enhances targeting.	Fluorescence-assisted cell sorting, transmission electron microscopy, confocal immunofluorescence

2016	Solid Lipid nanoparticles (SLNP)	Electroporation and nanocarrier used to deliver drugs. In this study, SLNP laden with cyanine type IR-780, flavonoid derivatives, photosensitizer through solvent diffusion method.	Colon cancer	Drug transfer potential of therapeutics compressed with electroporation.	Confocal laser scanning microscopy (CLMS) for the estimation of F-actin AFM and DLS
2017	Filamentous bacteriophage and phage-mimetic nanoparticles	Delivery of drug and gene through phage particles. Phage can be chemically altered or genetically designed to load drugs and transfer foreign genes.	Bacterial and viral diseases	Filamentous bacteriophage used in the making of mark medicine transfer as virus-based delivery system. The bacteriophage uncovered with mark-definite peptides or antibodies can be bound with other carriers (such as liposomes, inorganic NPs) to make a unique transfer scheme.	No
2018	Mesoporous silica nanoparticles (MSNs)	Through electrostatic absorption, MSNs loaded with surface-hyper-branching polymerized poly (ethylene- mine) for loading siRNA.	No	The practice of non-viral vectors can solve most of these problems like short time, noxiousness while inorganic, and non-viral vectors, like MSNs, are also very affordable and vigorous.	Transmission electron microscopy, dynamic light scattering (DLS), and zeta potential involved in particle size determination

2019	Chitosan nanoparticles	Drug loaded on chitosan nanoparticles to deliver to targeting sites. All types of drug delivery sites involved.	No	Ocular drug delivery, vaccine delivery, perioral delivery, vaccine transfer, mucosal and nasal drug transfer, gene carriage, pulmonary drug delivery, buccal medicine distribution, vaccine transfer, and cancer treatment.	No
2020	Mesoporous silica NPs with folic acid (MSN–COOH-Tet-HBP-FA)	This approach is pH subtle drug delivery system built on folic-acid-targeted HBP to re-form/reshape the mesoporous silica nanoparticles.	Cancer	The hyper-branched polymer HBP encapsulates the drug particles in the mesopores as a lid, which progresses the permanency of the carrier material and permits the drug to attain "zero pre-release" within 20 h in a usual physiological atmosphere.	XRD, TEM, HNMR spectra, SEM, UV-analysis, Thermogravimetric analysis (TGA)
2021	Novel silver nanoparticles	In this approach, DNA or messenger RNA (mRNA) sequences are transported to the body to produce proteins, which copy disease antigens to arouse the immune response.	SARS-CoV-2	The nucleic acid vaccines comprise cell-mediated and humoral immunity activation, affluence of strategy, quick malleability to altering pathogen strains, and customizable multi-antigen vaccines. To fight the SARS-CoV-2 epidemic and many other ailments, nucleic acid vaccines seem to be a hopeful way.	No

2021	1-Lipid based nanoparticles 2-Metal and metal oxide NPs 3-Resveratrol-zinc NPs	These nanoparticles have crucial role in the COVID-19 success rate. Metals such as Au, Ag, Zn, Cu have potential in controlling coronavirus due to their discrete features. It is a drug delivered via carrier. It gives immuno-anti-inflammatory viral retort.	COVID-19 SARS-Cov-2 viral disease COVID-19	It helped in the COVID-19 treatment vaccines, such as Doxil and Onpattro, and has a good success rate. Such NPs have been used in prevention like face masks, various immune sensors, and coatings on various things. Resveratrol-zinc nanoparticles possess a chief pharmacokinetic gain for COVID-19.	No COVID-19 mono and adjuvant therapy
2022	1-Iridium oxide NPs 2-Chitosan nanoparticles	A nanoprobe was synthesized for in vivo fluorescence tomography of microRNA and coactive photothermal dealings of lump. It is a biotic macromolecule-based medicine transfer system to advance the curative potential of non-natural neural control networks.	Cancer Nervous breakdown	Nanoprobe helped in vivo in healing studies and continuously killed the lump growth. Theses neuroprotective mediators are merged into the structure of NGCs and delivered into brain via NPs.	No Nanocarriers are biocompatible, biodegradable, non-immunogenic, constant, and hold tunable properties

Source: Afzal O, Altamimi ASA, Nadeem MS, Alzarea SI, Almalki WH, Tariq A, Mubeen B, Murtaza BN, Iftikhar S, Riaz N, et al. Nanoparticles in Drug Delivery: From History to Therapeutic Applications. Nanomaterials. 2022; 12(24):4494. https://doi.org/10.3390/nano12244494.

They are therefore divided into three classes based on their size and number of bilayers:

1. Small unilamellar vesicles are surrounded by a single lipid layer and are 25–50 nm in diameter.

2. Large unilamellar vesicles are a heterogeneous group of vesicles similar to and are surrounded by a single lipid layer.
3. Multilamellar vesicles consist of several lipid layers separated from each other by a layer of aqueous solution.

Liposome lipid bilayers have a structure akin to that of living cell membranes, and they have the same ability to transport lipophilic materials like medications within them. The permeability and fluidity of the lipid bilayer, as well as its composition, determine the pharmaceutical properties of liposomes. Liposome formulations often contain cholesterol, an essential component of many cell membranes that decreases permeability and increases stability of the phospholipid bilayers.

Up until recently, liposomes' toxicity and our limited understanding of their biochemical behavior prevented their use as therapeutic vectors. Liposomes are most commonly used as delivery systems for medications and antibodies intended to specifically target and deliver anticancer agents. Issues with stability, delivery to the appropriate location, and drug release upon arrival at the intended site may restrict the application of liposomes. To lengthen the time that liposomes circulate in the bloodstream, polyethylene glycol (PEG) units can be easily attached to the bilayer of the liposome (creating what are known as stealth liposomes). Moreover, liposomes can be coupled to ligands or antibodies to improve medication therapy that is target-specific.

Innovative drug delivery technologies that require piercing multiple membranes to reach the intended site of action have made use of liposome-based strategies. The novel MITO-Porter system, which is covered in a different chapter of this book, has been designed to deliver a broad range of carrier-encapsulated molecules, irrespective of size or physicochemical characteristics, to mitochondria by means of membrane fusion. This strategy requires the liposomes to fuse with the organelle membrane to deliver cargos to the target organelles.

3.2.13.3. Polymer Nanoparticles

Poly(ethylene glycol) (PEG)-coated poly(lactic acid) (PLA) nanoparticles, chitosan (CS)-coated poly(lactic acid–glycolic acid) (PLGA) nanoparticles, and chitosan (CS) nanoparticles are examples of biodegradable polymer nanoparticles. These nanoparticles have the ability to transport proteins through the intestinal and nasal mucosa in an active form. Furthermore, PEG coating helps the encapsulated protein, tetanus toxoid, pass through the nasal and intestinal mucous membranes and increases the stability of PLA nanoparticles in gastrointestinal fluids. In addition, these nanoparticles produced strong and sustained immune responses when administered intranasally.

Drug delivery that is targeted and controlled can be achieved through the use of thermo-sensitive polymers, which use temperature as a triggering signal. An assessment of the polymers' cytotoxicity, as well as the synthesis and characterization of a thermoresponsive polymer and its use in a drug delivery model using bovine serum albumin.

3.2.13.4. Chitosan Nanoparticles

The naturally occurring biodegradable polymer chitosan (CS) is derived from chitin. the effectiveness of using chitosan nanoparticles of various sizes as drug delivery vehicles for anticancer medications and discovered that chitosan-100 kDa outperformed chitosan-15 and chitosan-200 KD as drug carriers.

A water-soluble derivative of CS, N-(2-hydroxyl) propyl-3-trimethyl ammonium chitosan chloride is produced when glycidyltrimethyl ammonium chloride reacts with CS. The mucoadhesive CS coating of PLGA nanoparticles increases the nasal transport of the encapsulated tetanus toxoid and increases the stability of the particles in the presence of lysozyme. CS-only nanoparticles are stable when incubated with lysozyme. Furthermore, after intranasal administration, these particles are highly effective in enhancing both the systemic and local immune responses to tetanus toxoid and the nasal absorption of insulin. Through intranasal delivery, chitosan–siRNA nanoparticle formulation can be administered directly into the brain.

3.2.13.5. Polymeric Micelles

A potential remedy for the delivery issues related to these substances is the use of micelles, which are biocompatible nanoparticles with sizes ranging from 50 to 200 nm and which can be used to encapsulate poorly soluble medications. By using these micelles to direct the drugs to specific parts of the body, toxicity issues may be resolved. Drug delivery systems that are pH-sensitive can be designed to release their contents or alter their physicochemical characteristics in response to changes in the acidity of their environment.

3.2.13.6. Nanosponge for Drug Delivery

Cyclodextrin polymers are hyper-cross-linked and nanostructured into three-dimensional networks, known as nanosponges. This is achieved by complexing cyclodextrin with a cross-linker, such as carbonyldiimidazole. Another technique for creating a nanosponge is to scrunch a long, linear molecule into a sphere with a diameter of roughly 10 nm by using a lot of internal cross-linking. Using this method, a nanoparticle with many surface sites where drug molecules can be attached is created rather than trying to encapsulate drugs in nanoscale containers. The nanosponge and its cargo can pass through biological barriers and enter particular intracellular compartments thanks to a molecular transporter that is attached to it. Drugs that are poorly soluble have been made more soluble and stable by using nanosponges. Oral drug delivery using β-cyclodextrin nanosponges containing the anticancer agent tamoxifen has been implemented. After 24 and 48 hours of incubation, tamoxifen nanosponge complex, which has particles the size of 400–600 nm, was found to be more cytotoxic than regular tamoxifen.

3.2.13.7. Future Prospects of Nanotechnology- Based Drug Delivery

Smart drug delivery systems that can interact with the human body are a desirable state of affairs in the drug delivery industry. This is a field in which nanotechnology will be very significant. Nanoparticles are even used in time-release tablets, which have a relatively straightforward coating that dissolves in particular places. Pharmaceutical companies are already utilizing nanotechnology to develop smart drug delivery systems. For instance, the drug's or particle's interface with the human body can be programmed to become active when the drug reaches its intended target. For drug-release devices utilizing nanotechnology, autonomous device operation is necessary. For instance, autonomous device operation would require biochemical recognition to generate forces to stimulate various valves and channels in the drug delivery systems, so that it does not require any external control, as opposed to converting a biochemical signal into a mechanical signal and being able to control and communicate with the device.

3.2.14. Receptor-Mediated Targeted Drug Delivery

The process by which extracellular macromolecules and particles enter intracellular environments is known as receptor-mediated endocytosis. Complex transmembrane proteins called cell surface receptors mediate extremely specific interactions between cells and their extracellular environment. Receptor-mediated endocytosis is a process that the cells use for processing, transport, defense, and nutrition. Drugs attached to either a targeting carrier or a targetable polymeric carrier can only be absorbed by cells through receptor-mediated endocytosis. Receptors are expressed differently in different cell types and tissues, so using them as markers could be a useful approach to drug delivery. The targeted delivery of the medication to the target cells that carry receptors can be accomplished through receptor-mediated uptake. Numerous receptors, including those for asialoglycoprotein, low-density lipoprotein, and transferrin, have been employed to deliver medications to particular cell or tissue types.

Recent developments in targeted drug delivery have largely concentrated on controlling the body's natural membrane trafficking system to help deliver medications into target tissues through receptor-mediated endocytosis. Known as molecular motors, vesicle motor proteins (myosin, cytoplasmic dynein, and kinesin) are crucial to membrane trafficking processes. It's critical to comprehend the processes involved in the endocytosis process, which brings extracellular and surface-bound materials into the cell. It's also critical to understand the sorting processes that take place within the endocytic pathways that control the drug's final fate and intracellular destination. No accumulation within the cell is possible if the drug is internalized and then recycled or degraded. Improved drug delivery can result from strategies for controlling such occurrences. Gene delivery in hepatocytes through receptor-mediated endocytosis is one instance.

Factors that influence the efficiency of the receptor-mediated uptake of targeted drug conjugate are:

- Affinity of the targeting moieties
- The affinity and nature of target antigen
- Density of the target antigen
- The type of cell targeted
- The rate of endocytosis
- The route of internalization of the receptor–ligand complex
- The ability of the drug to escape from the vesicular compartment into the cytosol
- The affinity of the carrier to the drug

Receptor-mediated drug delivery is especially useful for gene therapy and cytotoxic cancer therapy.

3.2.15. Targeted Delivery Systems

Numerous carrier systems and homing devices, including glass-like matrices, monoclonal antibodies, resealed erythrocytes, microspheres, and liposomes, are being developed for targeted and controlled delivery. More advanced systems based on gene delivery, nanotechnology, and molecular mechanisms exist.

3.2.15.1. Polymeric Carriers for Drug Delivery

Alternative drug administration techniques are being developed in an attempt to increase the specificity of treatment options due to the limitations of currently available drug therapies, especially for the treatment of diseases localized to specific organs. Using biodegradable polymeric carriers to transport medications to the disease site and deposit them there for prolonged periods of time while minimizing systemic drug distribution is one strategy for achieving this goal. The medication is released into the body, and soon after, the polymeric carrier is broken down and removed. The polymers are divided into three groups:

1. Nondegradable polymers. These are stable in biological systems. These are mostly used as components of implantable devices for drug delivery.
2. Drug-conjugated polymers. In these, the drug is attached to a water-soluble polymer carrier by a cleavable bond. These polymers are less accessible to healthy tissues as compared with the diseased tissues. These conjugates can be used for drug targeting via systemic administration or by implanting them directly at the desired site of action where the drug is released by cleavage of the drug–polymer bond. Examples of such polymers are dextrans, polyacrylamides, and albumin.
3. Biodegradable polymers. These degrade under biological conditions to nontoxic products that are eliminated from the body.

Macromolecular complexes of various polymers can be divided into the following categories according to the nature of molecular interactions:

- Complexes formed by interaction of oppositely charged polyelectrolytes
- Charge transfer complexes
- Hydrogen-bonding complexes
- Stereocomplexes

Polyelectrolyte complexes have various applications such as microcapsules, medical implants, and protein binding for pharmaceutical products. Polyphosphazenes are a novel class of organometallic polymers that have emerged in recent years. Polyphosphazenes are a good material for controlled-release technologies because of their synthetic flexibility. Desirable characteristics of a polymeric system used for drug delivery are:

- Minimal tissue reaction after implantation
- High polymeric purity and reproducibility
- A reliable drug-release profile
- In vivo degradation at a well-defined rate in case of biodegradable implants

There are two types of polymeric delivery systems that are used to implant drugs at specific sites: reservoirs, in which the drug is evenly distributed within a polymer matrix, and matrixes, in which the drug is encapsulated into a polymeric envelope that functions as a diffusional rate-controlled membrane. The majority of biodegradable systems are matrix-based, releasing the medication through a mix of dissolution, erosion, and diffusion. The inability to modify dosage once implanted and the need for surgery to remove the implant to stop therapy are drawbacks of the implants. Repeated implantations are necessary for persistent long-term release. Because injectable biodegradable drug delivery systems are easier to use and offer more localized drug delivery over longer periods of time than traditional ones, this has opened up new possibilities for controlled drug delivery. For this, polymers that are synthetic and natural have both been employed. They solidify at the intended location after being injected in a fluid state. These delivery systems have been extensively studied for the delivery of a wide range of therapeutic agents, including insulin and proteins and peptides as well as antineoplastic agents.

3.2.15.2. Evaluation of Polymers in Vivo

The use of biodegradable polymers in implantable drug delivery systems has garnered significant interest. The challenges of accurately characterizing in vivo, however, create uncertainty when extrapolating in vitro results to in vivo systems, which is a major problem in the development of these systems. To get around this restriction, drug release and polymer degradation have been studied in vitro and in vivo using non-electron paramagnetic resonance (EPR) and magnetic resonance imaging (MRI). With MRI, one can keep an eye on the amount of water present, the shape of the tablet, and the biological system's reaction, including encapsulation and edema. The MRI experiment results provide the first direct in vivo evidence of proposed mechanisms of polymer erosion. EPR spectroscopy can be used to learn more about the microviscosity inside the implant and the mechanism of drug release by using nitroxide radicals as model drug-releasing compounds. The application of these non-invasive techniques to in vivo process monitoring yields novel insights into the mechanisms underlying drug release and polymer degradation.

3.2.15.3. Avidin–Biotin Systems for Targeted Drug Delivery

Both streptavidin, a bacterial analog of avidin from *Streptomyces avidinii*, and avidin, which was first isolated from chicken eggs, have a very high affinity for biotin. This special quality forms the cornerstone of avidin-biotin technology. A review of the current state of avidin-biotin systems and their application to vector targeting and pretargeted drug delivery can be found elsewhere. Some of the useful applications are:

- Targeting antibodies and therapeutic molecules are administered separately leading to a reduction of drug dose in normal tissues compared with conventional (radio) immunotherapies.
- Introducing avidin gene into specific tissues by local gene transfer, which subsequently can sequester and concentrate considerable amounts of therapeutic ligands.
- Enables transductional targeting of gene therapy vectors.

3.2.15.4. Targeted Delivery of Biologicals with Controlled Release

A key component of therapeutics is targeted delivery to the organ, site, or lesion in the body. This is especially crucial for biologicals, where delivery is frequently paired with either intrinsic or extrinsic mechanisms to regulate the drug's or the therapeutic molecule's release. The process for creating a gold nanoparticle-based smart drug delivery system, which releases the bioactive ingredient in response to an intracellular stimulus, i.e., gradient of glutathione concentration.

3.2.16. Methods of Administration of Proteins and Peptides

Various possible routes for administration of proteins and peptides are:

- Parenteral
- Transdermal
- Inhalation
- Transnasal
- Oral
- Rectal
- Implants
- Cell and gene therapies
- Use of special formulations

The most popular way to deliver proteins and peptides is still by injection. Injections without needles or with minimal pain are being used, and parenteral routes of controlled delivery are being improved.

3.2.16.1. Delivery of Peptides by Subcutaneous Injection

The subcutaneous route of delivery for peptides and macromolecules is still dependable and manageable. For prolonged and repeated delivery, however, there is a need for increased convenience and reduced costs. MEDIPAD (Elan Pharmaceutical Technologies) is an example of how subcutaneous delivery has been refined. It combines the idea of a "patch" with a sophisticated, miniature pump that runs on gas generation. The transdermal drug delivery report included a description of it.

3.2.16.2. Depot Formulations and Implants

They must guarantee the stability of proteins and peptides because they are typically given by injection. The sustained release poly(lactide-coglycolide) formulation is one of the ones utilized. Leuprolide is an example of a product that has been approved for sale. In addition to requiring invasive administration, implants also need to guarantee protein/peptide stability. Osmotic pumps-driven implantable titanium systems deliver medication release. Growth hormone is among the other proteins to which this technology has been applied. The first long-acting growth hormone formulation was Nutropin Depot (Genentech/Alkermes), which contains the hormone in biodegradable microspheres that release the hormone gradually after injection. In children with growth hormone deficiency, it lowers the injection frequency from once daily to once a month.

3.2.16.3. Poly(ethylene Glycol) Technology

The water-soluble polymer poly(ethylene glycol), or PEG, is a well-known remedy for constipation. PEG modifies the characteristics of proteins when covalently bound to them, expanding the range of possible applications. PEGylation, the chemical modification of proteins and other bioactive molecules with PEG, is a technique that can be used to modify or add new molecular functions, as well as remove undesirable properties to better suit specific applications. This strategy can be applied to enhance the delivery of peptides and proteins.

3.3. New Concepts in Pharmacology That Influence Design of DDS

Pharmacology has historically impacted drug delivery formulations, especially pharmacokinetics and pharmacodynamics. Some of the newer developments in pharmacology and therapeutics that influence the development of DDSs are:

1. Pharmacogenetics
2. Pharmacogenomics
3. Pharmacoproteomics
4. Pharmacometabolomics
5. Chronopharmacology

3.3.1. Pharmacogenetics

Pharmacogenetics, a term coined in the pregenomic era of pharmacology, is the study of how genetic factors affect a drug's action rather than how genes cause disease. The relationship between a person's genotype and their capacity to metabolize an alien substance is currently being studied. Pharmacodynamics (interaction with the target or the site of action) and pharmacokinetics (absorption, distribution, and metabolism) determine a drug's pharmacological effect. It also discusses how different factors affect these processes. One of the main factors influencing drug clearance and the primary cause of interindividual variations in pharmacokinetics is drug metabolism.

Pharmacological response varies more between members of a population than it does within an individual or between monozygotic twins at different times. Hereditary factors as a determinant of drug response are consistent with the existence of large population differences with small intrapatient variability. Twenty to 95 % of the variation in drug disposition and effects is thought to be hereditary. It has been established that genetic variations in drug-metabolizing enzymes, transporters, receptors, and other drug targets are related. The initial definition has led to a broader scope that now includes overlaps with pharmacogenomics. Genes affect both pharmacokinetics and pharmacodynamics. Pharmacogenetics has a threefold role in the pharmaceutical industry, which is relevant to the development of personalized medicines:

1. For study of the drug metabolism and pharmacological effects
2. For predicting genetically determined adverse reactions
3. Drug discovery and development and as an aid to planning clinical trials

3.3.2. Pharmacogenomics

A separate field within genomics called pharmacogenomics continues the tradition by using the large-scale systemic approaches of genomics to comprehend the fundamental mechanisms and apply them to the development of new drugs. Pharmacogenomics, which connects the domains of medicinal chemistry and genomics, currently aims to investigate how drugs affect cells as shown by gene expression patterns. A number of drug response markers are instances of the interaction between pharmacogenomics and pharmacogenetics, both of which are critical to the creation of customized medications. Although the terms "pharmacogenetics" and "pharmacogenomics" are sometimes used interchangeably, it's important to understand their distinctions.

These intricate multifactorial situations can be analyzed using a variety of technologies to provide genotypic and gene expression data for each individual. These same instruments can be used to investigate the range of drug effects in various populations. By helping to design clinical trials so that nonresponders would be eliminated from the patient population and taking the guesswork out of prescribing medications, pharmacogenomics promises to enable the development of safer and more effective drugs. It will also make sure that the appropriate medication is administered to the appropriate patient right away. To determine which drug regimen best suits a patient's genetic makeup, clinicians could, before prescribing, test the patient for specific single nucleotide polymorphisms (SNPs) known to be associated with nontherapeutic drug effects. The inherited nature of these variations in drug disposition and effects is being clarified by pharmacogenomic studies at a rapid pace. This advances drug discovery and strengthens the scientific foundation for tailoring drug therapy based on the genetic makeup of individual patients.

Pharmacogenomics offers a fresh perspective on time-tested issues, i.e., how to locate and focus on the key element of the disease pathway (s). Drug delivery systems will become more crucial as a result of these modifications, and they must be modified to reflect our evolving understanding of disease. Drug delivery issues must be taken into account at every step of the drug development process, from discovery to clinical application.

3.3.3. Pharmacoproteomics

The word "proteomics" refers to the systematic study of tissue protein profiles and proteins expressed by a genome. Since the life of a cell is a dynamic process and deoxyribonucleic acid (DNA) sequence information only offers a static snapshot of the various ways the cell might use its proteins, there is a growing interest in proteomic technologies. "Pharmacoproteomics" refers to the role of proteomics in drug development. A specific target-based therapy may be matched to a specific marker in a subgroup of patients with the aid of proteomics-based characterization of multifactorial diseases. Leading the way in this area's development is the industrial sector. Differential protein expression could serve as the basis for customized treatment instead of a genetic polymorphism.

3.3.4. Chronopharmacology

The term "chronopharmacology" refers to differences in a drug's effect based on when it is administered during the day. The biological processes of mammals are arranged in accordance with circadian rhythms, which last roughly 24 hours. A biological clock located in the hypothalamic suprachiasmatic nuclei (SCN) regulates them. These rhythms show that they are endogenous because they continue to exist in a constant environment. Disease can change certain rhythms. Treatment can be adjusted over the course of a 24-hour period by taking into account the rhythms of the disease and pharmacology.

Understanding these rhythms seems especially important for treating and/or understanding hypertension and ischemic coronary artery disease. The circadian rhythm of systolic or diastolic blood pressure can be separated from the rest-activity cycle in both rats and humans, indicating that it is regulated by an oscillator that is not dependent on the SCN. This finding may allow for treatment adjustments based on abnormalities in the blood pressure rhythm. The morning peak of myocardial infarction in humans is caused by the combination of multiple risk factors, blood coagulability, blood pressure, oxygen consumption, and myocardial ischemia susceptibility, all of which have a 24-hour cycle. Clinical prerequisites for the chronopharmacology of cardiovascular medications, such as nitrate derivatives, and the existence of these rhythms are necessary for the treatment of heart disease.

It is well known that the circadian phase can affect how sensitive tumor cells are to chemotherapy drugs. Within tissues, there may be variations in the rhythmicity of cells. Certain cells within a tumor may be able to evade the drug's effects if they are not phased in the same way. It could be more effective to synchronize the cells before administering medication to eradicate the tumor. Mice of both the wild type and circadian mutants show pronounced differences in how they react to the anticancer medication cyclophosphamide. The sensitivity of Clock mutant mice to treatment is consistently high, whereas that of wild-type mice varies significantly based on when the drug is administered. These results will serve as justification for not only delaying chemotherapy treatments to make them less toxic, but also serving as a starting point for the hunt for pharmacological drug toxicity modulators that operate through circadian system regulators. This finding may considerably lower the morbidity connected with anticancer treatment and raise the therapeutic index.

Drug formulations that follow a chronopharmacological pattern can deliver the drug's ideal serum levels at the right time of day or night. For instance, drug release is optimized for early mornings when action is desired. In contrast, when using traditional drug administration techniques, the peak of the drug's effects is reached early in the night, and when using controlled release, the patient's level remains high all night long. In addition to increasing treatment efficacy, successful chronopharmacotherapeutics will create new markets. Appropriate drug delivery systems are necessary for this treatment strategy.

3.3.5. Impact of Current Trends in Pharmaceutical Product Development on DDS

Over the past 20 years, the pharmaceutical industry has made significant advancements. Technologies for drug delivery are now a significant component of the biopharmaceutical sector.

3.3.6. Impact of New Biotechnologies on Design of DDS

Over the past ten years, new biotechnologies have had a significant influence on DDS design. Among these, nanobiotechnology is the most important (Figure 3.8 and Table 3.2).

Table 3.2. Some selected Examples of Micro-/Nanosystems for the Treatment of CVDs

Micro-/ Nanosystems	Applications	Advantages/Benefits
Liposomes containing vascular endothelial growth factor (VEGF)	To treat MI and improve cardiac function	High enhancement in fractional shortening and improvement in systolic function; excellent improvements in cardiac function and vascular structure
Polylactic co-glycolic acid NPs containing VEGF	To repair the heart after MI	Enhancement in the angiogenic and therapeutic potency of VEGF for treating ischemic heart disease.
Polymeric NPs	For the targeted delivery of nitric oxide (NO); treatment of portal hypertension	Non-toxicity; these NPs could alleviate the hemodynamic disorders in bile duct-ligated-induced portal hypertension, evidenced by reducing portal pressure and unchanging mean arterial pressure.
Niosomes	For the delivery of lacidipine; the management of hypertension	An enhancement in skin permeation (~2.15 times), compared to control gel; improved reduction in blood pressure
Nano-vesicular lipid carriers	For the delivery of angiotensin II receptor blocker (valsartan)	Improved anti-hypertensive effects; no skin toxicity

Micro-/ Nanosystems	Applications	Advantages/Benefits
Dendrimeric NPs	For selective delivery of liver-x-receptor ligands to atherosclerotic plaque-associated macrophages while limiting hepatic uptake; modulation of atherosclerosis	High reduction in atherosclerotic plaque progression, plaque necrosis, and plaque inflammation; macrophage-specific delivery platforms for targeted transferring anti-atherosclerotic agents to the plaque-associated macrophages to reduce plaque burden

Source: Iravani, S., & Varma, R. S. advanced drug delivery micro- and nanosystems for cardiovascular diseases. Molecules. 2022; 27(18), 5843. https://doi.org/10.3390/molecules27185843.

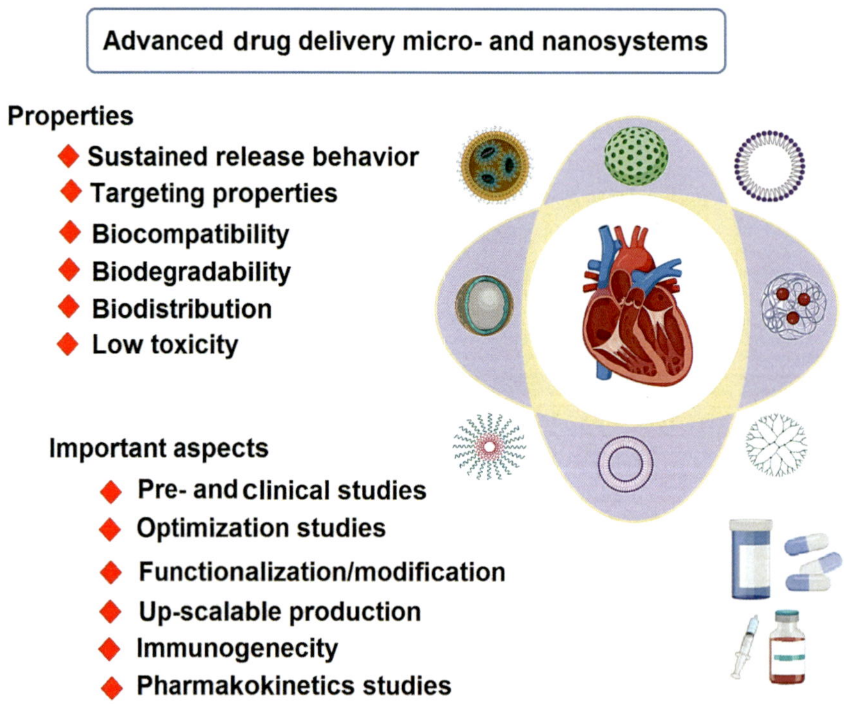

Figure 3.8. *Advanced drug delivery micro- and nanosystems.*

Source: Iravani, S., & Varma, R. S. Advanced drug delivery micro- and nanosystems for cardiovascular diseases. Molecules. 2022; 27(18), 5843. https://doi.org/10.3390/molecules27185843.

3.4. Impact of Current Trends in Healthcare on DDS

The impact of new technologies on medicine is always changing. The practice of medicine has historically been more of an art than a science, but new findings in the life sciences are changing this. There is a lag time before changes in medical practice become apparent, and groundbreaking discoveries in molecular biology did not immediately affect medicine. While some of these improvements are due to advances in the understanding of the disease, others are the result of advancements in the delivery of pharmaceuticals. The idea of personalized medicine is one of the biggest developments in healthcare.

3.4.1. Personalized Medicine

Simply put, personalized medicine refers to the prescription of particular therapies and treatments that are most appropriate for a given individual. Individualized or individual-based therapy is another name for it. The concept of personalized medicine is predicated on the notion of considering a patient's genotype in addition to other factors when determining their course of treatment. The development of personalized medicines has been made easier by genomic and proteomic technologies, but other technologies are also helping in this endeavor. This personalization process, which is founded on pharmacogenomics and pharmacogenetics, begins during the drug's development phase. Choosing the DDS that is best for a patient is one aspect of personalized medicine.

Understanding the genetic foundation of a disease aids in differentiating between clinically similar conditions because all major diseases have a genetic component. It is more effective to diagnose and treat diseases based on genetic differences in affected individuals rather than just clinical symptoms. One day, medical professionals will be able to subclassify diseases and customize treatments for each patient thanks to the identification of human genetic variations.

Nowadays, molecular terms are used to describe many diseases. Certain flaws can result in multiple disorders, and diseases will no longer be categorized based on symptoms and gross pathology, but rather on their molecular basis. This implies that multiple diseases sharing the same molecular basis can be treated with the same medication. The division of patient populations within the same disease group based on genetic markers and medication response represents another method of reclassifying human diseases.

Improvements in medication delivery, along with other technologies, will be crucial to the growth of personalized medicine. A well-known example is how glucose sensors control how much insulin is released into diabetic patients' bodies. As an advanced drug delivery technique, gene therapy can be tailored to meet the specific needs of each patient.

A Closer Look

Buccal Absorption

Medication held or administered in the buccal region (in the cheek) diffuses through the mucosal surface (the tissues lining the mouth) and directly enters the blood circulation in a process known as buccal absorption. Buccal administration results in a higher bioavailability and a faster onset of action than oral administration because the medication does not transit through the digestive tract, avoids pre-systemic metabolism, and has no first-pass effect.

When a medication is inserted between your gums and cheeks, it dissolves and enters your bloodstream through a process known as buccal absorption. Medication for the buccal and sublingual regions can be found as tablets, sprays, or films.

Sore throat is one of the symptoms where Buccal Absorption is important. Any number of factors, such as changes in the weather, allergies, pollution, colds, or the flu, can cause sore throats at any time. Additionally, people with sore throats look for immediate, efficient, long-term relief. Turkey, as an herbal and ayurvedic supplement, relieves irritation, swelling, itching, and sore throats. It has curcumin, a strong active ingredient that was separated from organic turmeric. It makes use of Buccal Absorption Technology (BAT), which facilitates the direct absorption of curcumin into the bloodstream for quick relief.

The inner lining of the cheek and the floor of the mouth are part of the buccal cavity, which has mucous membranes through which drugs are absorbed. This process is known as buccal absorption. This approach is appealing for some medications because it has a number of benefits over conventional methods like injection or oral ingestion.

The avoidance of first-pass metabolism is a major benefit of buccal absorption. When taken orally, medications travel via the liver and digestive system before entering the bloodstream, where they may experience substantial metabolism, which lowers their bioavailability. On the other hand, buccal absorption enables medications to evade the liver and digestive system, resulting in more stable and elevated blood levels of the drug.

The buccal mucosa has an extensive blood vessel network near its surface, indicating its high vascularization. This makes the drug's surface area much larger and makes it easier for it to enter the bloodstream quickly. Furthermore, the buccal mucosa's thin epithelial layer facilitates effective drug diffusion across the membrane, improving absorption even more.

Numerous factors impact the speed and degree of absorption through the buccal mucosa, such as the drug's physical and chemical properties, the type of formulation used, the pH of the oral cavity, and the presence of enzymes or substances that enhance permeation. Lipophilic medications are typically absorbed more easily through the buccal mucosa, while hydrophilic drugs may need permeation enhancers for better absorption. Buccal absorption is particularly beneficial for drugs with low oral bioavailability, drugs that undergo significant first-pass metabolism, or drugs that require fast action. Examples include nitroglycerin for angina, hormone replacement therapy, and specific antiemetic medications. All things considered, buccal absorption presents a practical and efficient substitute drug administration route with a number of benefits, such as quick onset of action, avoiding first-pass metabolism, and enhanced bioavailability. However, to maximize buccal drug delivery and guarantee therapeutic efficacy, careful evaluation of drug properties and formulation factors is necessary.

Summary

- Drugs may be introduced into the human body by various anatomical routes. They may be intended for systemic effects or targeted to various organs and diseases.
- The oral route of drug administration has been the one used most for both conventional and novel drug delivery.
- Parenteral administration of drugs is now an established part of medical practice and is the most commonly used invasive method of drug delivery.
- Transdermal drug delivery is an approach used to deliver drugs through the skin for therapeutic use as an alternative to oral, intravascular, subcutaneous, and transmucosal routes.
- Drugs have been administered nasally for several years for both topical and systemic effects. Topical administration includes agents for the treatment of nasal congestion, rhinitis, sinusitis, and related allergic and other chronic conditions.
- Nasal drug delivery can be enhanced by reducing drug metabolism, by prolonging the drug residence time in the nasal cavity, and by increasing absorption.
- An accurate estimation of the pharmacokinetics of inhaled therapeutics for systemic delivery is a challenging experimental task.
- Drugs may be delivered to the lungs for local treatment of pulmonary conditions, but here the emphasis is on the use of the lungs for systemic drug delivery.
- The pulmonary route for drug administration is now established for systemic delivery of drugs. A wide range of drugs can be administered by this route but the special attraction is for the delivery of peptides and proteins.
- Drug delivery to the cardiovascular system is different from delivery to other systems because of the anatomy and physiology of the vascular system; it supplies blood and nutrients to all organs of the body.
- Controlled release implies regulation of the delivery of a drug usually by a device. The control is aimed at delivering the drug at a specific rate for a definite period of time independent of the local environments.
- A prodrug is a pharmacologically inert form of an active drug that must undergo transformation to the parent compound in vivo by either a chemical or an enzymatic reaction to exert its therapeutic effect.

References

1. Beck-Broichsitter, M., Dalla-Bona, A. C., Kissel, T., Seeger, W., & Schmehl, T. (2014). Polymer nanoparticle-based controlled pulmonary drug delivery. In K. K. Jain (Ed.), *Drug Delivery Systems: Methods in Molecular Biology*, (Vol. 1141). Springer, New York.
2. Boopathy, A. V., & Davis, M. E. (2014). Self-assembling peptide-based delivery of therapeutics for myocardial infarction. In K. K. Jain (Ed.), *Drug Delivery Systems: Methods in Molecular Biology* (Vol. 1141). Springer, New York.
3. Castle, J. (2014). Ultrasound-directed site-specific gene delivery. In K. K. Jain (Ed.), *Drug Delivery Systems: Methods in Molecular Biology* (Vol. 1141). Springer, New York.
4. Cullis, P. R., & Ramsay, E. (2014). Microfluidic-based manufacture of siRNA-lipid nanoparticles for therapeutic applications. In K. K. Jain (Ed.), *Drug Delivery Systems: Methods in Molecular Biology*, (Vol. 1141). Springer, New York.
5. Cummins, J., Cronin, M., van Pijkeren, J. P., Gahan, C., & Tangney, M. (2014). Bacterial systems for gene delivery to systemic tumors. In K. K. Jain (Ed.), *Drug Delivery Systems: Methods in Molecular Biology*, (Vol. 1141). Springer, New York.
6. De Andres, J., et al. (2014). Intrathecal delivery of analgesics. In K. K. Jain (Ed.), *Drug Delivery Systems: Methods in Molecular Biology*, (Vol. 1141). Springer, New York.
7. De, A., Mishra, S., Garg, S., & Mozumdar, S. (2014). Synthesis of a smart nanovehicle for targeting liver. In K. K. Jain (Ed.), *Drug Delivery Systems: Methods in Molecular Biology*, (Vol. 1141). Springer, New York.
8. Donnelly, R. F., Garland, M. J., & Alkilani, A. Z. (2014). Microneedle-iontophoresis combinations for enhanced transdermal drug delivery. In K. K. Jain (Ed.), *Drug Delivery Systems: Methods in Molecular Biology*, (Vol. 1141). Springer, New York.
9. Farra, R., Sheppard Jr, N. F., McCabe, L., et al. (2012). First-in-human testing of a wirelessly controlled drug delivery microchip. *Science Translational Medicine, 4*(122), 122ra21.
10. Gao, J. Q., & Hu, U. L. (2014). Stem cells as carriers for cancer gene therapy. In K. K. Jain (Ed.), *Drug Delivery Systems: Methods in Molecular Biology*, (Vol. 1141). Springer, New York.
11. Gizurarson, S. (2012). Anatomical and histological factors affecting intranasal drug and vaccine delivery. *Current Drug Delivery, 9*, 566–582.
12. Guarnieri, D., Muscetti, O., & Netti, P. A. (2014). A method for evaluating nanoparticle transport through the blood-brain barrier in vitro. In K. K. Jain (Ed.), *Drug Delivery Systems: Methods in Molecular Biology*, (Vol. 1141). Springer, New York.
13. Gupta, S., Batra, S., & Jain, M. (2014). Antibody labeling with radioiodine and radiometals. In K. K. Jain (Ed.), *Drug Delivery Systems: Methods in Molecular Biology*, (Vol. 1141). Springer, New York.
14. Jain, K. K. (2009). *A Textbook of Personalized Medicine*. Springer Science, New York. Edition 1, 430 pages, 1441907688, 9781441907684
15. Jain, K. K. (2011). *Applications of Biotechnology in Cardiovascular therapeutics*. Springer Science, New York. Edition Number 1, Pages- 350, https://doi.org/10.1007/978-1-61779-240-3.
16. Jain, K. K. (2012). Nanobiotechnology-based strategies for crossing the blood-brain barrier. *Nanomedicine, 7*, 1225–1233.

17. Jain, K. K. (2013). *Applications of Biotechnology in Neurology*. Springer, New York. Edition Number 1, Pages- 638, https://doi.org/10.1007/978-1-62703-272-8.

18. Jain, K. K. (2014). *Cardiovascular Drug Delivery: Technologies, Markets, and Companies*. Jain PharmaBiotech Publications, Basel. pp 1–268

19. Jain, K. K. (2014). *Drug Delivery in Cancer: Technologies, Markets, and Companies*. Jain PharmaBiotech Publications, Basel. pp 1–668

20. Jain, K. K. (2014). *Drug Delivery in CNS Disorders: Technologies, Markets, and Companies*. Jain PharmaBiotech Publications, Basel. pp 1–360

21. Jain, K. K. (2014). *Gene Therapy: Technologies, Markets, and Companies*. Jain PharmaBiotech Publications, Basel.

22. Jain, K. K. (2014). *Nanobiotechnology: Applications, Markets, and Companies*. Jain PharmaBiotech Publications, Basel. pp 1–774

23. Jain, K. K. (2014). *Personalized Medicine: Scientific and Commercial Aspects*. Jain PharmaBiotech Publications, Basel. pp 1–860

24. Jain, K. K. (2014). *Transdermal Drug Delivery: Technologies, Markets, and Companies*. Jain PharmaBiotech Publications, Basel. pp 1–280

25. Jain, K. K. (Ed.). (2010). *Drug Delivery to the Central Nervous System*. Humana, New York.

26. Krishnaiah, Y. S., & Khan, M. A. (2012). Strategies of targeting oral drug delivery systems to the colon and their potential use for the treatment of colorectal cancer. *Pharmaceutical Development and Technology, 17*, 521–540.

27. Lesch, H. P., Kaikkonen, M. U., Pikkarainen, J. T., & Ylä-Herttuala, S. (2010). Avidin-biotin technology in targeted therapy. *Expert Opinion on Drug Delivery, 7*, 551–564.

28. Li, H. Y., & Zhang, F. (2012). Preparation of nanoparticles by spray-drying and their use for efficient pulmonary drug delivery. *Methods in Molecular Biology, 906*, 295–301.

29. Malhotra, M., Tomaro-Duchesneau, C., Saha, S., & Prakash, S. (2014). Intranasal delivery of chitosan-siRNA nanoparticle formulation to the brain. In K. K. Jain (Ed.), *Drug Delivery Systems: Methods in Molecular Biology*, (Vol. 1141). Springer, New York.

30. Mishra, S., De, A., & Mozumdar, S. (2014). Synthesis of a thermoresponsive polymer for drug delivery. In K. K. Jain (Ed.), *Drug Delivery Systems: Methods in Molecular Biology*, (Vol. 1141). Springer, New York.

31. Muzykantov, V. R. (2010). Drug delivery by red blood cells: Vascular carriers designed by mother nature. *Expert Opinion on Drug Delivery, 7*, 403–427.

32. Nguyen, N. T., Shaegh, S. A., Kashaninejad, N., & Phan, D. T. (2013). Design, fabrication and characterization of drug delivery systems based on lab-on-a-chip technology. *Advanced Drug Delivery Reviews, 65*(11–12), 1403–1419.

33. Salomon, J. J., & Ehrhardt, C. (2012). Organic cation transporters in the blood-air barrier: Expression and implications for pulmonary drug delivery. *Therapeutic Delivery, 3*(6), 735–747.

34. Singh, R. M., Kumar, A., & Pathak, K. (2013). Mucoadhesive in situ nasal gelling drug delivery systems for modulated drug delivery. *Expert Opinion on Drug Delivery, 10*, 115–130.

35. Tajmir-Riahi, H. A., Nafisi, S., Sanyakamdhorn, S., et al. (2014). Applications of chitosan nanoparticles in drug delivery. In K. K. Jain (Ed.), *Drug Delivery Systems: Methods in Molecular Biology*, (Vol. 1141). Springer, New York.

36. Torne, S., Darandale, S., Vavia, P., et al. (2013). Cyclodextrin-based nanosponges: Effective nanocarrier for Tamoxifen delivery. *Pharmaceutical Development and Technology, 18*, 619–625.

37. Yamada, Y., & Harashima, H. (2014). Methodology for screening mitochondrial fusogenic envelopes for use in mitochondrial drug delivery. In K. K. Jain (Ed.), *Drug Delivery Systems: Methods in Molecular Biology*, (Vol. 1141). Springer, New York.

38. Zhang, H., Wang, G., & Yang, H. (2011). Drug delivery systems for differential release in combination therapy. *Expert Opinion on Drug Delivery, 8*, 171–190.

Chapter

PHARMACOKINETICS AND PHARMACODYNAMICS

4

Contents

Introduction

The study of the time course of drug absorption, distribution, metabolism, and excretion is currently known as pharmacokinetics. Pharmacokinetic principles are applied in clinical pharmacokinetics to ensure safe and efficient drug therapy for each patient.

Improving a patient's medication therapy's efficacy and lowering its toxicity are the main objectives of clinical pharmacokinetics. By establishing robust relationships between drug concentrations and their pharmacologic reactions, pharmacokinetic principles can now be applied by clinicians to real-world patient scenarios.

It would be helpful to keep an eye on this concentration because a drug's effect is frequently correlated with its concentration at the site of action. Drug receptor sites are either widely dispersed throughout the body or are not usually accessible to human observation, making it impractical to measure drug concentrations directly at these locations. Digoxin, for instance, is believed to have receptor sites inside the myocardium. Of course, we are unable to measure the drug concentration in this tissue directly. On the other hand, we can quantify the amount of drug in blood or plasma, urine, saliva, and other readily extracted fluids. The consistent correlation between the concentration of a drug in plasma and its concentration at the receptor site where it acts as a therapeutic agent is known as kinetic homogeneity. Drug concentration variations at the receptor site and in other tissues are reflected in variations in plasma drug concentrations. The concentration of the drug in most tissues will rise in proportion to the increase in plasma drug concentration.

In the same way, a drug's concentration in tissues will drop if its plasma concentration does. This idea is demonstrated as a simplified plot of the drug concentration versus time profile following an intravenous drug dose.

For the presumptions made in clinical pharmacokinetics, the quality of kinetic homogeneity is crucial. It serves as the basis for determining both toxic and therapeutic plasma drug concentrations. That is, we assume that when we study a drug's concentration in plasma, the concentrations in plasma directly correspond to the concentrations in tissues where the drug is intended to modify the disease process (e.g.the brain in cases of Parkinson's disease or the bone in cases of osteomyelitis). However, not all drugs will fit under this assumption.

Orientation and Directional Terms

Term	Definition	Illustration
Absorption	The first stage of pharmacokinetics where medications enter the body and travel from site of administration into the body's circulation.	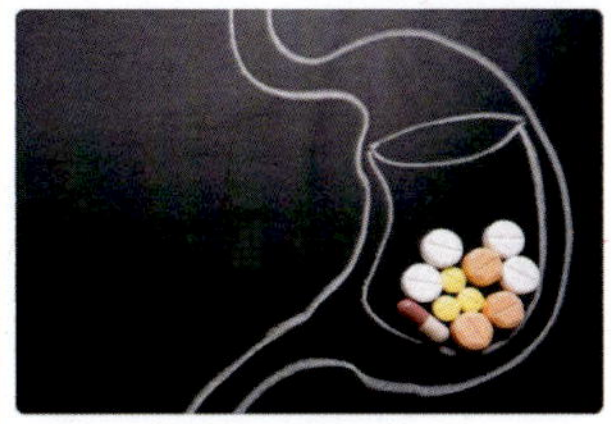
Blood-brain barrier	A barrier preventing the entry of molecules	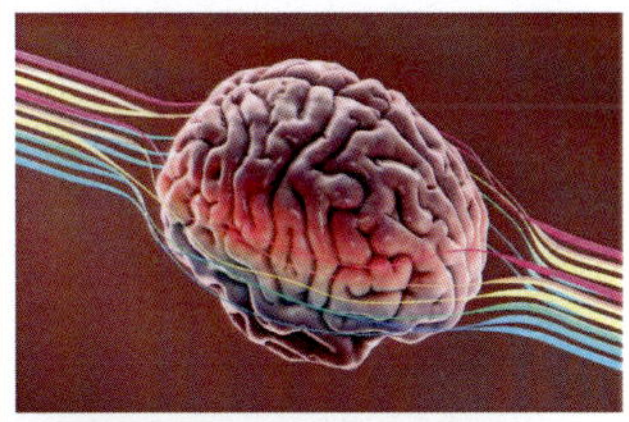
Pharmacodynamics	Drug effects and mechanisms	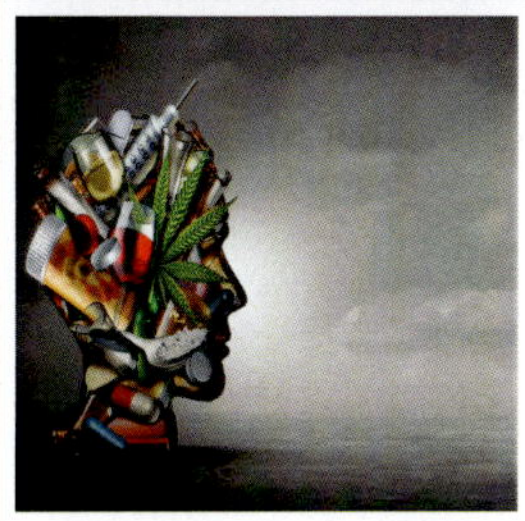
Pharmacokinetics	The study of how the body absorbs, distributes, metabolizes, and eliminates drugs.	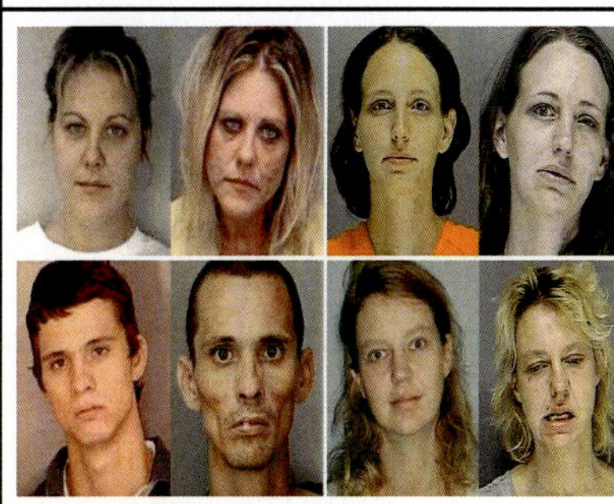
Pharmacogenetics	Genetics in influencing drug responnse	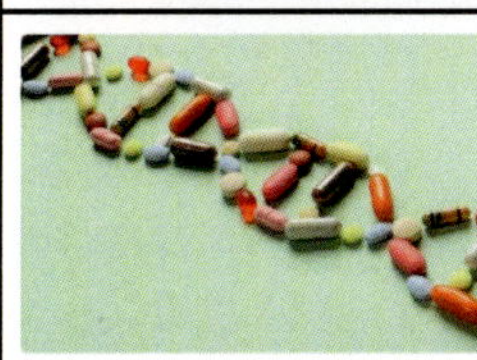
Protein Binding	Binding influences the efficacy of a drug	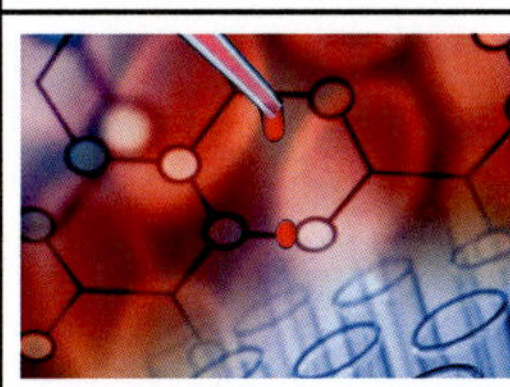

4.1. Pharmacokinetics – Examining the Interaction of Body and Drug

The term pharmacokinetics refers to the four phases of drug metabolism, excretion, distribution, and absorption. Substances that are administered to the body and cause a physiological reaction are referred to as drugs. Within the human body, medications go through four basic stages: absorption, distribution, metabolism, and excretion. ADME is a common acronym for this entire process.

The first phase of pharmacokinetics, known as absorption, happens when drugs enter the body and move from the site of administration into the bloodstream. The second phase of pharmacokinetics is distribution. It is the method by which medicine is absorbed by the body. The breakdown of a drug molecule takes place during metabolism, which is the third stage of pharmacokinetics. The last phase of pharmacokinetics is called excretion, and it describes the body's removal of waste.

Researchers with a focus on pharmacokinetics must also consider time as a factor in how drugs act in the body. It is impossible for scientists to see where a medicine is going or how long it will stay active. To make up for this, they employ mathematical models and exact measurements of blood and urine to ascertain the distribution of drugs and the amount of drug (or breakdown product) that is left over after the body processes them. Additional markers, like hepatic enzyme levels in the blood, can be used to estimate the amount of a drug that will be absorbed.

Because the interactions between drugs and body molecules are a sequence of chemical reactions, chemistry principles are also applied in the study of pharmacokinetics. It is vital to comprehend the chemical interactions that occur between pharmaceuticals and biological settings, like the bloodstream and the greasy cell surfaces, toestimate the amount of a drug that the body will metabolize.

Pharmacodynamics is the study of how drugs work in the body and how they do it. Drugs have distinct affinities, or how strongly they bind to drug-receptor sites, as they pass through the bloodstream. The lock and key system that is created between drugs and receptor sites (refer to Figure 4.4) influences how drugs function and whether they remain in the bloodstream after administration. The general term for this idea is drug bioavailability (Figure 4.1).

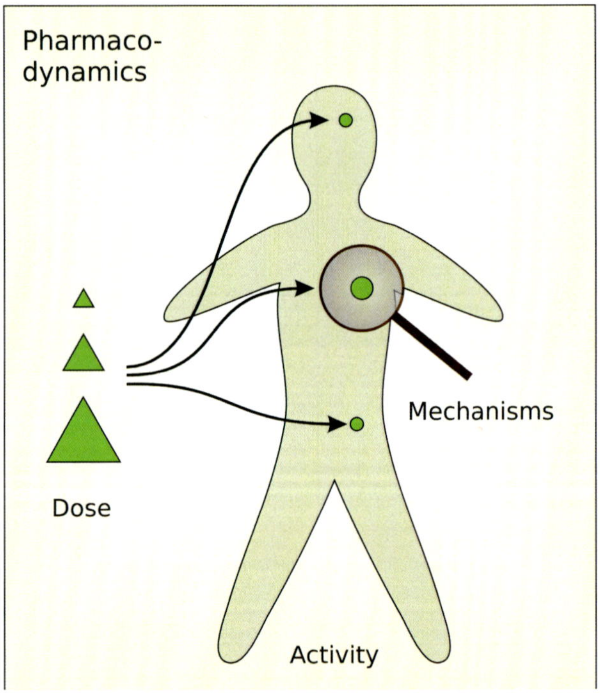

Figure 4.1. *Pharmacodynamics.*

Source: By Scivit – Own work, CC BY 4.0, https://commons.wikimedia.org/w/index.php?curid=89573356.

When creating and packaging medications, chemists and pharmaceutical scientists pay close attention to a drug's bioavailability. No matter how well a medication functions in a lab simulation, the human body will not always respond to it in the same way, so each patient's unique reaction to the medication must be taken into account. A person's specific genetic composition may have a substantial influence on how they react to a drug, even though many drug responses may be predicted. Pharmacogenetics is the study of how a person's genetic makeup influences how they react to medications.

4.2. Absorption, Distribution, Metabolism, and Excretion (Adme) of Drugs

The four processes a drug goes through in the body are absorption, distribution, metabolism, and excretion (ADME).

- **Absorption:** The drug enters the bloodstream
- **Distribution:** The drug moves from one location in the body to another
- **Metabolism:** The drug is broken down
- **Excretion:** The drug is removed from the body

4.2.1. Absorption

Absorption is the term for the initial phase of pharmacokinetics. The biological membrane allows the drug to enter the bloodstream through absorption when it is administered through a site or route.

4.2.1.1. Factors Affecting Drug Absorption

It is the study of variables affecting a drug's rate and degree of absorption and release from its different physicochemical characteristics and dosage forms, as well as the therapeutic effect that results from its administration.

The rate and total amount of drug absorbed is dependent upon many factors, which are:

- **Biological Factors**
  - **Passage of Drug through Body Membranes:** For a medication to have the intended effect, it must travel to the site of action and stay there for a specific amount of time, regardless of the route or form of administration. Drug molecules must pass through one or more lipoidal membranous barriers with varying pore sizes to reach the site of action. Higher water partition coefficient substances are more easily able to pass through natural membranes than lower values. Natural substances such as glucose, bile salts, and amino acids easily cross bodily membranes despite having molecules that are too big.
  - **Site of Absorption:** The stomach, intestines, colon, or mouth (for buccal administration) are the primary locations of absorption. Only the buccal cavity or under the tongue will contain certain vasodilators (such as nitroglycerine) and hormones that can pass through the buccal mucosal wall. It prevents gastrointestinal interactions and has a quick start of action. The stomach's absorption is influenced by pH, gastrointestinal motility, and gastric emptying. For instance, most of the activity

of benzylpenicillin is lost if it is left in the stomach for an extended period of time.

- **Presence of Food and Other Salts:** In general, food slows down the rate at which medications like tetracycline are absorbed in the gastrointestinal tract (GIT); however, when griseofulvin is given with fatty meals, absorption is increased. The primary reason why bile salts have a positive impact on drug absorption is because of their surface activity.
- **Routes of Administration:** The drugs are mostly given by oral route. The other routes of administration of drugs in relation to absorption are being discussed here.
- **Parenteral Administration:** This route is applicable for drugs which are inactivated by gastrointestinal tract or absorption is poor when given orally or there is an urgency for fast response in small dose.
- **Inhalational Administration:** The absorption of drug takes places through lungs and the absorbing membrane is very thin and surface area is quite large. The lipid soluble drugs are readily absorbed from the nasal mucosa, as these drugs diffuse more rapidly.
- **Topical Administration:** It is employed for local action in the form of ointments, creams, jellies etc., for its antiseptic and local anesthetic action. The lipid soluble drugs penetrate the skin easily and rapidly.
- **Rectal Administration:** The drug is also administered rectally in the form of suppositories and enema preparations which are absorbed from the colon.

- **Physico-chemical Factors:** Lipid solubility, dissolution rate, salt from complexation, viscosity, and drug stability in the GIT are the physico-chemical parameters influencing absorption.
  - **Lipid Solubility Dissociation Constant and pH:** The stomach's weak acid (pH = 1.0; acidic) drug solution will take on a more unionized form, making it more lipid soluble and easier for the stomach to absorb. A weak base solution in the stomach is most unabsorbable because it is more ionized. g. Five nine. The intestinal pH is high, which facilitates the absorption of weak bases.
  - **Dissolution Rate:** When given, all medications, whether in suspension or solid dosage form, first transform into drug solutions in bodily fluids. Therefore, a significant factor influencing the rate of absorption is the dissolution rate. It is highly likely that a drug's absorption will be dissolution rate limited if it is absorbed from solution more quickly or completely.
  - **Viscosity:** Viscosity limits the dissolution rate and thereby affect the rapid absorption,

e.g., aqueous solution of sodium salicylate is absorbed faster than its suspension form.

- **Pharmaceutical Factors**
  - These factors primarily relate to the different drug dosage forms. Whether they are in the form of an aqueous solution, suspension, powder, tablet, capsule, or something else determines how well they are absorbed.
  - **Aqueous Solutions:** The aqueous solution absorbs the fastest. However, most drugs are not intended to be used in aqueous solutions unless absolutely necessary in certain preparations due to their poor stability, limited solubility, and packaging issues.
  - **Solid Forms**: Powders, Capsules, Tablets: When drug is given in the form of powder its absorption is largely dependent upon particle size, interaction with other diluents and dissolution rate. The micronized powder gives much higher concentration in blood as compared to ordinary powder and tablets. The absorption of capsule is also dependent on their type, e.g., hard capsule and soft capsule. The hard capsule dissolves much more readily in gastrointestinal tract as compared to soft capsules. After swallowing, the tablet first disintegrates into granules and primary solid particles and then into solution by dissolution for absorption. The absorption of any tablets is dependent on its disintegration and dissolution time, which may be affected by adding certain pharmaceutical additive, e.g., dissolution can be increased by increasing the starch content, binders can retard the dissolution as they delay disintegration.

4.2.1.2. Bioavailability

Any medication's rate and degree of absorption are referred to as its bioavailability. This is primarily used to characterize a drug's biological availability from a preparation and is computed/determined based on the drug's concentration or presence rate in different bodily fluids, such as blood, urine, etc.

It can also be used to denote a measurement of the quantity and rate at which a medicine is administered and circulated broadly.

4.2.1.3. First-Pass Effect

The gastrointestinal (GI) tract may experience markedly reduced absorption of a medication when it is taken orally or enterally. Protein-based drugs, for instance, can be swiftly rendered inactive by enzymes as they travel through the duodenum and stomach when they enter the GI tract. If a portion of the medication enters the bloodstream from the colon and is absorbed, liver enzymes may break down some of it while allowing the remaining portion to enter the general circulation. The fraction of the medication that reaches the bloodstream will either circulate freely or act at a receptor site or it will become protein-bound, rendering it inactive. The first-pass effect is the whole process that lowers the amount of active medication that is in a person's circulation. Prescribers and nurses who administer medications must be aware that multiple doses of an oral medication may be required before sufficient free drug remains active in the circulation to produce the intended effect, due to the first-pass effect.

4.2.1.4. Alternate Routes

By administering medication via different routes to the GI tract, the first-pass effect can be circumvented. One can administer medication by transdermal, nasal, inhalation, injection, or intravenous means, among other methods, which circumvent the first-pass effect. By entering the bloodstream directly or through absorption through the skin or lungs, alternative methods of medication administration avoid the first-pass effect. For instance, intravenous (IV) administration of painkillers allows for the immediate release of the drugs into the bloodstream, where they are then distributed to individual body tissues.

There are additional possible considerations when using alternative medication routes. For instance, injections hurt a lot and split the skin, which is a crucial infection-prevention barrier. Additionally, they may result in localized side effects, be expensive and challenging to administer on a daily basis, or contribute to erratic variations in the blood levels of medications.

The main advantage of using an alternative method—transdermal application of medication—is that it delivers the drug gradually and steadily straight to the bloodstream, bypassing the liver. Figure 4.5 shows a client applying a transdermal patch on their own. Transdermal medications enter the bloodstream through the skin's intricate network of tiny capillaries, veins, and arteries. For this reason, transdermal drug delivery is especially helpful when a medication needs to be applied over an extended period of time to control symptoms. For instance, a scopolamine patch can prevent motion sickness during a cruise vacation, a nitroglycerin patch is used to prevent chronic chest pain, and transdermal application of fentanyl, a pain medication, can effectively manage pain over a few hours. Transdermal patches have a number of benefits, but one major disadvantage is that only very small drug molecules can pass through the skin and into the body. For certain medications, this means of application is not appropriate. (Figure 4.2).

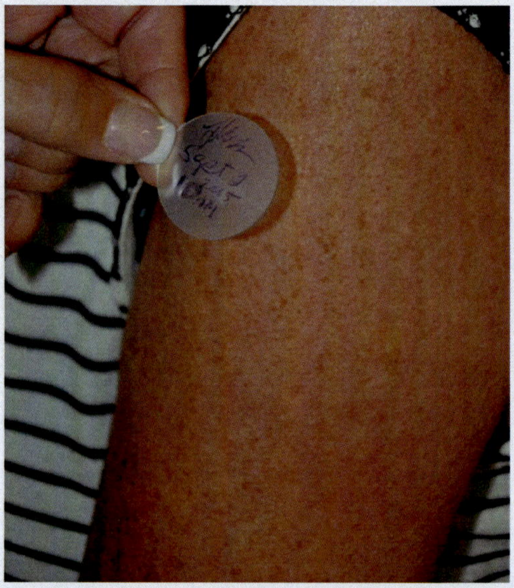

Figure 4.2: *A transdermal patch.*

***Source**: Open Resources for Nursing (Open RN); Ernstmeyer, K., & Christman, E., editors. Nursing Pharmacology [Internet]. 2nd edition. Eau Claire (WI): Chippewa Valley Technical College; 2023. Available from: https://www.ncbi.nlm.nih.gov/books/NBK595000/.*

Another option for quick drug delivery that avoids the liver is to inhale medications through the mouth or nose. Figure 4.6 shows a client using an inhaler on their own. Nasal steroid medications are frequently prescribed for allergy and sinus problems, and metered-dose inhalers have been a mainstay of asthma therapy for many years (Figure 4.3).

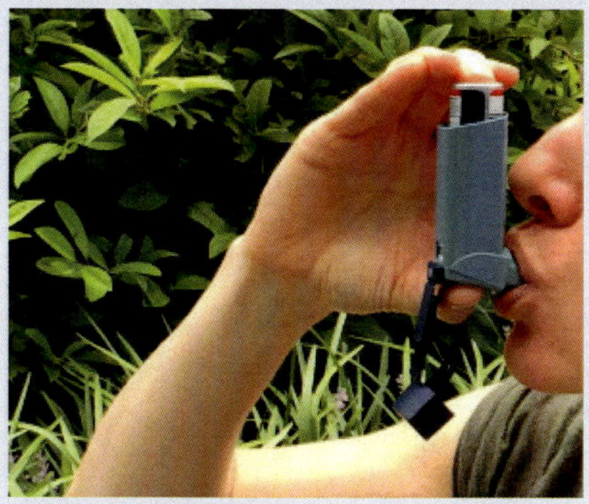

Figure 4.3: *An inhaler.*

Source: Open Resources for Nursing (Open RN); Ernstmeyer, K., & Christman, E., editors. Nursing Pharmacology [Internet]. 2nd edition. Eau Claire (WI): Chippewa Valley Technical College; 2023. Available from: https://www.ncbi.nlm.nih.gov/books/NBK595000/.

4.2.1.5. Emerging Discoveries and Recent Developments

Currently, researchers are looking into different drug delivery strategies, like inhaling powdered insulin. One type of inhaled insulin that the Food and Drug Administration (FDA) has approved to help with blood sugar control is called Afrezza®. This technology is based on cutting-edge applications of engineering and chemistry to produce insulin particles that are precisely the right size for absorption. If the insulin particles are too big, they may become lodged in the lungs; if they are too small, they will be exhaled.

4.2.1.6. Life Span Considerations

- **Neonate & Pediatric:** The way neonates and pediatric clients absorb gastric differs from adults. In babies, the stomach's acid-producing cells are underdeveloped until about one to two years old. Furthermore, their gastric emptying may be slowed due to irregular peristalsis. Children and infants have an immature liver, leading to reduced first-pass elimination and potentially higher levels of drugs in the blood.
- **Older Adult:** Due to the natural aging process, older adults may experience reduced blood flow to tissues in the GI tract. This can lead to changes in stomach pH, affecting the absorption of some medications. Additionally, older clients may have fluctuations in plasma proteins, which could impact the drug levels of medications that bind tightly to proteins.

When peripheral circulation is reduced in older patients with reduced cardiac output, subcutaneous and intramuscular injections should be taken into consideration as well because this can lead to decreased medication absorption. Adults also frequently have reduced subcutaneous fat as they get older, which affects how well transdermal patches absorb medication because proper absorption of the patches depends on sufficient subcutaneous fat stores.

4.2.2. Distribution

Distribution is the process that makes up the second stage of pharmacokinetics. A drug's dispersion throughout the blood and tissues of the body is known as distribution. A medication will move from vascular spaces to tissues once it has been absorbed or administered directly, where it will interact with receptors to produce its desired effect.

Because they bind more firmly to one particular receptor site and consistently cause or block an action, drugs are primarily made to have one effect. On the other hand, if the medication binds to locations other than the target tissue, it may have unintended consequences and side effects. It may be necessary to stop taking the medication as a result of these side effects, which can range from acceptable to intolerable. For instance, if someone takes ibuprofen (Advil) to relieve pain in a sore leg muscle, they may experience a side effect of stomach irritation in addition to the pain being relieved.

Many physiological factors, including blood flow, tissue variations, plasma protein binding, the blood-brain barrier, and the placental barrier, affect how a drug is distributed throughout the body.

4.2.2.1. Blood Flow

Medication is carried by the bloodstream throughout the body by the circulatory system. Numerous factors, including reduced blood flow from dehydration, blocked vessels from atherosclerosis, constricted vessels from uncontrolled hypertension, and weaker heart muscle pumping from heart failure, can impact blood flow and the delivery of medication. For instance, because atherosclerosis has blocked blood vessels in the legs and feet, it may be difficult for an antibiotic to travel through the blood vessels all the way to the infected area of a diabetic client's toe when treating an infection.

4.2.2.2. Tissue Differences

The tissues (such as the lungs, kidneys, liver, and brain) with the highest density of blood vessels and the highest blood flow rates experience the fastest distribution. Low blood flow is the result of distribution occurring least quickly in tissues (like fat) with fewer blood vessels. Still, lipophilic medications (i.e., medications that disintegrate in lipid environments) distribute into adipose tissue in obese individuals at a disproportionate rate.

Capillary permeability varies depending on the tissue. The liver and kidney's capillaries are porous, which increases permeability. Due to the tight junction between capillary endothelial cells and the blood-brain barrier, distribution rates into the central nervous system are either nonexistent or much slower than in other regions.

4.2.2.3. Protein-Binding

A drug dissolves in plasma water and becomes partially free once it enters the bloodstream, but it also binds to proteins in some amounts. This is significant because only drugs that are free and unbound will enter tissues from the bloodstream and interact with receptors to produce the initial effects of a drug. The other part of the medication that attaches itself to proteins is dormant during this time. These bound forms can make up 95–98% of the total for a number of drugs.

As the medication is released gradually and has a prolonged effect, protein binding may also serve as a reservoir. The quantity of free drug that is easily absorbed by tissues as well as the protein binding that releases the drug gradually should both be taken into account when analyzing drug distribution.

One of the most significant proteins in blood is albumin. Liver disease and malnutrition are two conditions that can lower albumin levels. Because of the consequent effect on protein-binding and distribution, patients with low albumin levels may not experience the desired effects of medication as prescribed.

The competition between drugs for plasma binding can also affect the drugs' effects. Aspirin and warfarin, for instance, are anticoagulants that compete with one another for the same site on plasma proteins. When both medications are given at the same time, there will be more unbound medication, which will intensify their effects and raise the patient's risk of bleeding.

Think of travelers at a bus stop heading to their destination as an analogy for how protein binding impacts the dispensing of medications.

For an illustration of a bus connected to this analogy, see Figure 4.7. Numerous travelers (i.e., pharmaceutical molecules) wish to board the bus. Everybody wants to arrive at their destination (i.e., receptor sites) and looks for a place to sit. Stronger passengers (drug molecules with higher protein-binding capacity, for example) take all the seats first. Some passengers are left at the bus stop and are "free" to move about or walk to their destination when there aren't enough seats on the bus. Similarly, non-protein-bound "free" drug molecules flow freely through the bloodstream. In this analogy, the "free" passengers have the option of traveling straight to their destination or making stops along the way. Similar to this, when "free" drug molecules bind to receptors in the body, they cause the first intended or inadvertent effects. Furthermore, the medication molecules attached to proteins are eventually released and attach to the receptor sites, just like the passengers who had seats on the bus and later got off at their destination.

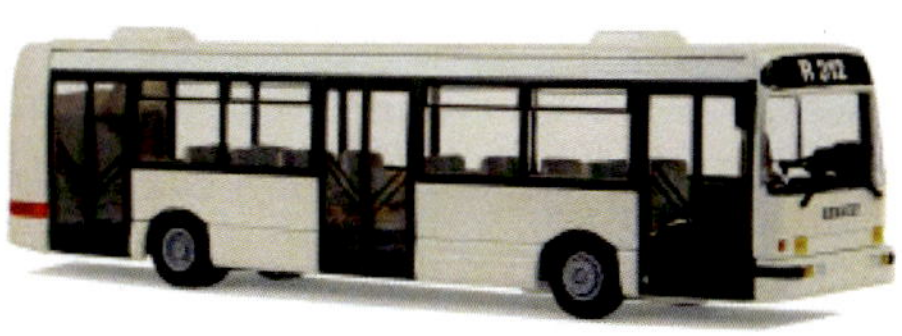

Figure 4.4: *The seats on a bus and protein binding.*

Source: Open Resources for Nursing (Open RN); Ernstmeyer, K., & Christman, E., editors. Nursing Pharmacology [Internet]. 2nd edition. Eau Claire (WI): Chippewa Valley Technical College; 2023. Available from: https://www.ncbi.nlm.nih.gov/books/NBK595000/.

4.2.2.4. Blood-Brain Barrier

Drugs intended for the central nervous system—the brain and spinal cord—face an even more formidable obstacle than protein binding: they need to cross the blood-brain barrier, an almost impenetrable barrier. This barrier is made of a densely packed network of capillaries that shields the brain from potentially harmful agents like viruses and poisons. Only specific drugs with a "carrier" or composed of lipids (fats) can pass through the blood-brain barrier.

Researchers have figured out how to get drugs past the blood-brain barrier. For instance, carbidopa and levadopa are two medications combined to make the brand-name drug Sinemet®. The purpose of carbidopa is to transport the drug levadopa through the blood-brain barrier to the brain, where it transforms into dopamine to alleviate Parkinson's disease symptoms.

As a side effect, some drugs unintentionally cross the blood-brain barrier and affect a person's central nervous system function. Diphenhydramine, for instance, is an antihistamine that is used to lessen allergy symptoms. But it can also depress the central nervous system, pass through the blood-brain barrier, and have the adverse effect of making you drowsy. This drowsy side effect might be helpful for someone who has trouble falling asleep, but it can be troublesome for someone who is trying to go about their daily activities.

4.2.2.5. Placental Barrier

The blood-placental barrier controls the transfer of molecules between the fetal and maternal circulation to safeguard the developing embryo. The placenta connects the mother and fetus. Drug transporters play a role in the passage of drugs through the placenta, potentially influencing the fetus's access to drugs. Certain drugs are known to pass through the placenta, and some medications can seriously harm the developing fetus. Many drugs, however, have not been thoroughly investigated in expectant patients, and it is unknown how they may affect the developing fetus.

Because of this, whenever medication is given to a client who is pregnant or may become pregnant, it is crucial to take into account the possible effects on the fetus. If medication is able to be given to the fetus, nurses are essential in alerting the healthcare provider to any possible safety concerns. Nurses should never give medication to a client who is pregnant or may become pregnant without first consulting a current, evidence-based drug reference.

4.2.2.6. Life Span Considerations

- **Neonate & Pediatric:** Children and infants have lower fat content due to higher total body water content. Furthermore, the ability to bind proteins is reduced, and the blood-brain barrier is growing, which permits more medications to pass through and into the central nervous system.
- **Older Adult:** Generally speaking, older adults have higher body fat percentages than younger adults when they have the same body mass index. Because of this extra body fat, many medications that build up in fatty tissues may take longer to take effect. Additionally, there is a drop in serum albumin, which increases the amount of the active free drug in the blood. For these distribution-related reasons, many older adult clients need smaller medication dosages.

4.2.3. Metabolism

A process called metabolism breaks down a drug once it has been absorbed and distributed throughout the body, allowing the body to excrete it. Various bodily systems chemically change drugs to produce compounds that are easier to excrete.

The intestines and liver neutralize medications that are swallowed or otherwise given to the gastrointestinal system; this process is referred to as the "first-pass effect.". Furthermore, the liver metabolizes anything that enters the bloodstream—be it through the skin, injection, inhalation, swallowing, or production by the body itself. The liver is depicted in Figure 4.8. We refer to these changes in composition as "biotransformations.". The liver's enzymes carry out the biotransformations that occur there.

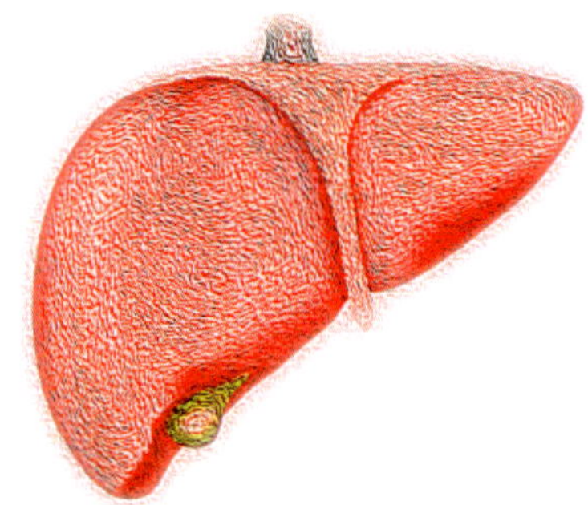

Figure 4.5: *The liver.*

Source: Open Resources for Nursing (Open RN); Ernstmeyer, K., & Christman, E., editors. Nursing Pharmacology [Internet]. 2nd edition. Eau Claire (WI): Chippewa Valley Technical College; 2023. Available from: https://www.ncbi.nlm.nih.gov/books/NBK595000/.

Biotransformations occur by mechanisms categorized as either Phase I (modification), Phase II (conjugation), and in some instances, Phase III (additional modification and excretion.)

Drugs undergo phase I biotransformations, which change their chemical makeup. Numerous metabolites—products of enzymatic breakdown—have lower chemical activity than the parent molecule. The liver is known as a "detoxifying" organ as a result. When the anxiety drug diazepam is converted to desmethyldiazepam and then to oxazepam, it is an example of a Phase I biotransformation.

Similar physiological and psychological effects of diazepam are produced by both of these metabolites.

Phase I biotransformations can occasionally convert an inactive medication into an active form known as a "prodrug." Prodrugs increase the efficacy of a medication. They might also be made to prevent specific harmful effects or side effects. Sulfasalazine, for instance, is a drug prescribed for rheumatoid arthritis. It is a prodrug that undergoes Phase I modification to make it active after ingestion.

Phase II biotransformations entail conjugation reactions, which unite the drug molecule with another molecule. Usually, conjugation makes the compound water soluble and pharmacologically inert, facilitating easy excretion. The kidney, liver, lungs, intestines, and other organ systems may go through these processes. The conjugation of oxazepam, the active metabolite of diazepam, with glucuronide to render it physiologically inactive and enable its excretion without additional chemical modification, is an example of Phase II metabolism.

Following Phase II metabolism, Phase III biotransformations may also occur, where the conjugates and metabolites are excreted from cells.

4.2.3.1. Factors Affecting Metabolism

The nature and level of liver enzymes are important aspects of drug metabolism. The two most significant enzymes for medical use are cytochrome P450 and monoamine oxidase. Numerous substances are metabolized by these two enzymes.

Numerous factors can impact the metabolism of drugs. Depot binding is a significant perturber of drug metabolism. Drug molecules bind to inactive sites in the body, a process known as depot binding, which prevents the drug from being metabolized. The duration of action of other medications that are prone to depot binding may also be impacted by this action. For instance, the primary psychoactive ingredient in marijuana, tetrahydrocannabinol (THC), is highly lipid-soluble and depot binds in users' adipose tissue. Weeks after the last use, THC metabolites can be found in urine due to this interaction, which significantly slows down the drug's metabolism.

Enzyme induction is another factor in drug metabolism. The same drug is used repeatedly to induce enzymes. The body adjusts by producing more of the enzyme required for the drug's metabolism as it grows used to the drug's continuous presence. This leads to a state known as tolerance, where patients need ever-higher dosages of some medications to achieve the same result. For instance, patients taking opioid analgesics for an extended length of time may observe a decrease in the effectiveness of their medication.

On the other hand, certain drugs inhibit certain enzymes, increasing the patient's sensitivity to other drugs that are metabolized by those enzymes. For instance, monoamine oxidase inhibitors (MAOIs) are prescribed as antidepressants because they increase the concentration of serotonin and dopamine in the central nervous system by blocking the enzyme that breaks these chemicals down. But when patients taking MAOIs also take other drugs that raise their levels of these chemicals—like cough syrups dextromethorphan—this can lead to issues.

Drugs with similar metabolic pathways can also "compete" for the same binding sites on enzymes, which reduces the metabolism of both drugs. For instance, the cytochrome P450 enzyme is required for the metabolism of alcohol and some sedatives, and there aren't many of these enzymes in the body. Because alcohol molecules occupy the majority of cytochrome P450 enzymes, if a client takes a sedative after consuming alcohol, the sedative will not be metabolized effectively. As a result, there is less excretion and a higher concentration of both medications in the body, which has better effects. Because of this, it can be fatal to combine alcohol with sedatives.

i. **Age**: In general, infants and older (human or animals) tend to be more sensitive to the action of the drugs. The impairment of drug metabolism in the new born infants usually results from a diminished capacity to deactivate drugs and consequently to more prolonged pharmacological action and to increased toxic reactions.
ii. **Nutrition**: Protein or calcium deficiency impairs drug metabolism in animals, due to decreased activity of the microsomal enzymes of the liver. The sleeping time by hexobarbitone is increased as a result of prolonged protein malnutrition.
iii. **Disease Conditions**: Patients with liver disease may exhibit an increased sensitivity of many drugs. Patients with obstructive jaundice, hepatitis, cirrhosis shows reduce ability to synthesize glucuronide and sulfate conjugates.
iv. **Hormonal Effects**: The hormones of adrenal glands, thyroid and pancreas exert various effects on the metabolism of drugs. Administration of ACTH, adrenaline or thyroxine impairs the hepatic microsomal metabolism of drugs.
v. **Genetic Factor – Species Differences**: Species differences in the metabolism of drug may be due to the difference in the rate of metabolism or in their metabolites difference. Certain drugs have been found safe and non-toxic in animals, but when they were tested in human beings severe toxic effects were observed. For example, when sulfanilamide was tested in dog it was found safe and non-toxic, but when it was administered to human being, certain toxic effects like the hematuria, renal failure were observed.

4.2.3.2. Clinical Significance

Nurses need to be aware of the medication's metabolism and excretion schedule when giving it to patients. The majority of the time, a drug's rate of elimination is influenced by its bloodstream concentration. On the other hand, some medications are eliminated at a steady pace that is unaffected by plasma concentrations. For instance, regardless of the bloodstream concentration, the ethanol found in alcoholic beverages is eliminated at a steady rate of roughly 15 mL/hour.

- **Half Life:** The half-life of a drug is the time it takes for 50% of the drug to be removed from the body. This can vary greatly between different drugs. Some drugs have a short half-life and need to be taken multiple times a day, while others have a longer half-life and can be taken just once a day. Figure 4.9 shows how half-life impacts the concentration of medication in the blood over time.

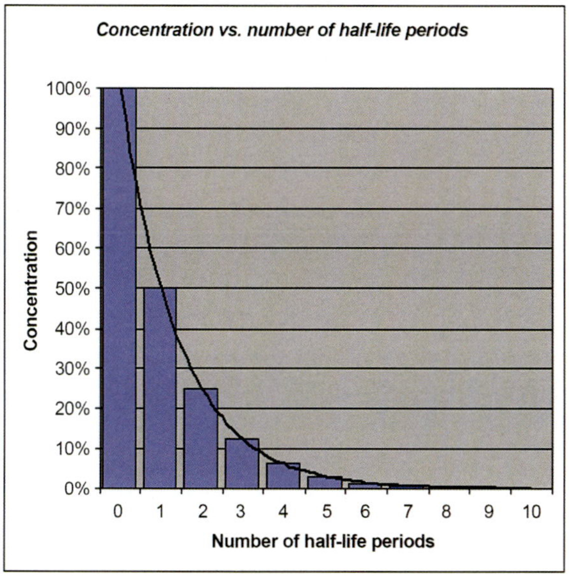

Figure 4.6: *Half-life influences the level of a drug in the blood*

Source: *Open Resources for Nursing (Open RN); Ernstmeyer, K., & Christman, E., editors. Nursing Pharmacology [Internet]. 2nd edition. Eau Claire (WI): Chippewa Valley Technical College; 2023. Available from: https://www.ncbi.nlm.nih.gov/books/NBK595000/.*

The duration of a medication's therapeutic effect is influenced by its half-life. Half-life can be influenced by numerous factors. For instance, if the liver is unable to properly metabolize the medication, it may prolong the half-life. Evidence-based medication references contain information on a given medication's half-life.

Impairment in either system can drastically change medication dosing, dose frequency, expected therapeutic effect, and even whether a specific medication can be used at all, depending on whether the drug is metabolized and eliminated by the liver or kidneys. To avoid medication interactions that could have a serious negative impact on a patient's health and wellbeing, nurses must collaborate with other members of the healthcare team. In particular, if the patient has liver or kidney disease, nurses need to be on the lookout for any indications of a toxic accumulation of metabolites or active medications so they can notify the healthcare provider. In other situations, pharmacists dose and oversee the administration of medications like warfarin and specific antibiotics, keeping an eye on renal function and the drugs' serum levels.

4.2.3.3. Life Span Considerations

- **Neonate & Pediatric: In** newborns and early children, the developing liver produces fewer enzymes. This could lead to the infant or young child's diminished capacity to metabolize drugs. Conversely, once the hepatic enzymes are fully produced, older children may have an increased metabolism and need higher dosages of medication.
- **Older Adult:** In older adults, there may be a marked decrease in liver metabolism. Because of this, dosages ought to be modified following the client's expected metabolic rate and liver function. Older adults may have higher "free" circulating drug concentrations and, consequently, be more susceptible to side effects and toxicities because first-pass metabolism also declines with age.

4.2.4. Excretion

The last phase of a drug's interaction with the body is excretion. The remaining parent drugs and metabolites in the bloodstream are often filtered by the kidney, where a portion undergoes reabsorption back into the bloodstream and the remainder is excreted in the urine. The body has now absorbed, distributed, and metabolized the medication molecules. Waste and byproducts are also expeled by the liver into the bile. The lungs are an additional excretory pathway. For instance, the lungs frequently get rid of substances like alcohol and anesthetic gases. Drugs that don't get absorbed well are eliminated in the stools.

- **Renal Excretion**: The kidneys serve as the primary and major organ for removal of most drugs, which is constituted by the microunits called 'nephron'. Three major processes that are involved in the excretion of drugs through kidneys are: glomerular filtration, tubular secretion and passive diffusion.
- **Pulmonary Excretion**: Volatile lipophilic substances like volatile general anesthetics, ethyl alcohol, paraldehyde are excreted by the lungs. These volatile substances and certain gases that enter the body through the respiratory tract in the form of aerosol are excreted by this route.
- **Biliary Excretion**: Certain drugs are excreted in urine only in small amounts but appear in high concentrations in the bile for example, erythromycin, novobiocin, tetracycline, phenolphthalein etc. The abnormality or any disease related to liver may impair bile secretion which can lead to the accumulation of these drugs

Certain drugs that are secreted by the liver into the bile and then to small intestine are not eliminated out through the feces, so that the drugs will reenter the blood that perfuses the intestine and again carried to the liver (repeatedly reabsorbed from the intestine and re-excreted in the bile) and thereby prolongs the action by the so called 'enterohepatic circulation'.

- **Excretion in Other Body Fluids**:
  - **Sweat and Saliva:** The excretion of drugs through sweat and saliva is primarily dependent upon the diffusion of the non-ionized, lipophilic form of the drug across the epithelial cells of the glands. The compounds like lithium, potassium iodide and heavy metals are present in these secretions.
  - **Milk:** The excretion of drugs into the mother's milk will depend upon the amount of drug in blood, its lipid solubility and the extent of its active excretion. A highly lipid soluble drug should tend to accumulate in milk fat. As milk has a lower pH (6.5), the basic drugs are more concentrated in it. The drugs which are excreted in milk include sulfonamides, penicillin, tetracycline and other antibiotics, morphine, lithium, antithyroid drugs, antineoplastic agents, radioactive iodine etc. So, these drugs should be avoided or breast feeding should be suspended in lactating mothers as these drugs have effect on the infants.

4.2.4.1. Routes of Excretion

Drug excretion has been documented to occur via a variety of pathways, primarily the skin, lungs, alimentary tract, and kidneys. Only a small number of drugs can be expeled through the skin and lungs (mainly volatile substances like ether, chloroform, and ethyl alcohol).

- **Kidney:** The kidneys are the most frequent site of excretion. The majority of waste and drug byproducts are eliminated in the urine as the kidneys filter blood. Some client characteristics, such as age, weight, biological sex, and kidney function, can be taken into account when estimating the rate of excretion. The three primary renal functions—tubular secretion, tubular reabsorption, and glomerular filtration—have well-documented gender differences. Men typically have higher renal clearance than women.

Test results for kidney function include serum creatinine, creatinine clearance, and glomerular filtration rate (GFR). A client's capacity to excrete medication is impacted if their kidney function is compromised, necessitating alterations to drug dosages for safe administration.

Chronic kidney disease is one type of renal disease that can impair drug excretion and lower kidney function. Age-related declines in kidney function make drug excretion less effective, necessitating possible dosage modifications. Drug elimination may also be impacted by other medical disorders that affect kidney blood flow. Heart failure, for instance, can impact the kidney's systemic blood flow, which can lead to a reduction in the filtration and excretion of medications.

- **Liver:** Hepatocytes, or liver cells, actively transport certain medications and their metabolites to bile as the liver filters blood. The gallbladder receives bile before it is transferred via the bile ducts to the small intestine. Certain medications may be partially reabsorbed into the bloodstream by the intestine during this process. Other medications are reabsorbed after being biotransformed, or metabolized, by intestinal bacteria. Feces contain excreted drugs and byproducts/metabolites that have not been absorbed.

The ability of a client to excrete medication is impacted by reduced liver function, necessitating adjustments to drug dosages. The enzymes alanine transaminase (ALT) and aspartate aminotransferase (AST), which the body releases in reaction to liver disease or injury, are measured as part of laboratory tests known as liver function tests.

Diseases that reduce the liver's blood supply can also have an impact on how drugs are metabolized and eliminated. For instance, reduced liver perfusion is caused by shock, hypovolemia, or hypotension, which may necessitate adjusting medication dosages.

- **Other Routes to Consider:** Substances such as drugs and their byproducts/metabolites can also be found in tears, sweat, breast milk, and reproductive fluids like seminal fluid. This may present a toxic risk, such as when a baby is exposed to drugs in breast milk or the residue of the mother's drug consumption. Therefore, before giving medication to a breastfeeding mother, nurses must consult a drug reference and get in touch with a healthcare provider if they have any concerns.

4.2.4.2. Life Span Considerations

- **Neonate & Pediatrics:** The kidneys of infants and young children are immature, having reduced tubular secretion, glomerular filtration, and resorption. They consequently do not eliminate drugs from the body as quickly. The majority of drugs used to treat young patients are dosed according to kilogram weight; a lower dose is typically recommended for these patients. Furthermore, pediatric patients may become toxic more quickly than expected and may have higher levels of free circulating medication. To detect side effects and drug toxicity early on, nurses must carefully monitor infants and children and double-check dosages before giving medications.
- **Older Adults:** As people age, their kidney and liver function frequently decline, which can affect how well they metabolize and excrete drugs. Because of the higher levels of circulating drugs, medication may have a longer half-life and a higher potential for toxicity. Due to these factors, some medications may be avoided or smaller doses may be advised for older clients; this approach is commonly known as "Start low and go slow."
- **Putting It All Together:** Safe medication administration to patients is a serious concern that calls for collaboration between nurses, prescribing physicians, and pharmacists.

4.3. Basic Pharmacodynamic Concepts

The study of drug effects, both physiological and biochemical, and their mode of action is known as pharmacodynamics. Once the medication reaches its site of action, it begins to have pharmacological effects that may eventually have a therapeutic effect, as well as some unfavorable side effects and other effects that might not be clinically significant.

Pharmacodynamics is the study of the relationship between the concentration of a drug at the site of action and the effect that results, encompassing the duration and severity of both beneficial and negative effects. A drug's ability to bind to a receptor determines its effect when it is present at the site of action. Neurons in the central nervous system (i.e., opiate receptors) can reduce pain perception, on the heart muscle to modify the force of contraction, or even inside bacteria to interfere with the upkeep of the bacterial cell wall.

The majority of drugs have an intensity of action that is determined by the concentration at the receptor site (Figure 4.7). However, drug response is also influenced by other factors. Drug effect may be influenced by the density of receptors on the cell surface, the process by which substances known as second messengers (substances inside the cell) carry a signal into the cell, or regulatory factors that manage protein synthesis and gene translation. This multilevel regulation determines whether a person is more sensitive to a drug's effects than another and whether they develop a tolerance to those effects.

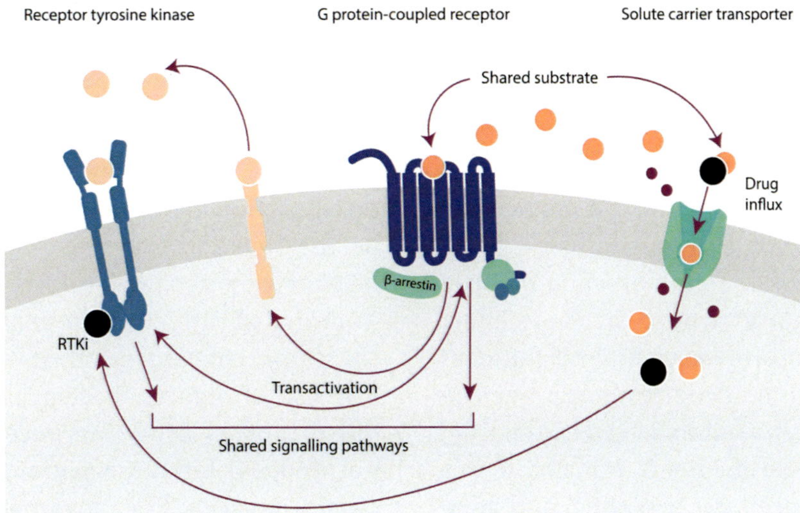

Figure 4.7: *Drug-receptor associations*

Source: Gorostiola González, M., Rakers, P. R. J., Jespers, W., IJzerman, A. P., Heitman, L. H., van Westen, G. J. P. Computational Characterization of Membrane Proteins as Anticancer Targets: Current Challenges and Opportunities. International Journal of Molecular Sciences. 2024; 25(7), 3698. https://doi.org/10.3390/ijms25073698.

Drug concentration at the receptor site and pharmacologic effect are correlated in the most basic examples of drug effect. A maximum effect (E_{max}), if sufficient concentrations are tested, can be found (Figure 4.8). The plotting of the logarithm of concentration against effect reveals that an effect is observed only at a certain concentration, while no greater effect can be achieved above that concentration.

Piclidenoson **Namodenoson**

(A)

Piclidenoson

Receptor	IC_{50} (nM)	K_i (nM)
A_1	>1000	-
A_{2A}	685	560
A_{2B}	47,600	42,300
A_3	0.68	0.47

Namodenoson

Receptor	IC_{50} (nM)	K_i (nM)
A_1	5390	3140
A_{2A}	2090	1170
A_{2B}	No activity	No activity
A_3	0.717	0.661

(B)

Figure 4.8: *Drug effects.*

Source: Fishman, P. Drugs Targeting the A3 Adenosine receptor: Human clinical study data. Molecules. 2022; 27(12), 3680. https://doi.org/10.3390/molecules27123680.

Finding the concentration at which 50% of the maximum effect is attained is one method of comparing the potency of different drugs. The 50 % effective concentration, or EC_{50}, is what is meant by this. When two medications are tested on the same person, the medication that has a lower EC_{50} is thought to be more potent. This implies that a more potent drug requires less of a dose to have the same effect as a less potent drug. However, other significant factors that determine drug response, like the length of the effect, are not indicated by the EC_{50}. The length of time a medicine remains active on a receptor, intracellular signaling, and gene regulation are just a few of the many variables that affect how long an effect lasts. With continued use, some medications may lose some of their effectiveness. It is known as tolerance in this context. Pharmacokinetic factors that lower the concentrations attained with a given dose, such as increased drug metabolism, may be the cause of tolerance. Another possibility is pharmacodynamic tolerance, which is the diminished effect of repeated exposure to the same concentration at the receptor site. The use of opiates to treat chronic pain is an illustration of drug tolerance. With time, it is not unusual for these patients to need higher opiate dosages. The dose-response curve can be used to characterize tolerance.

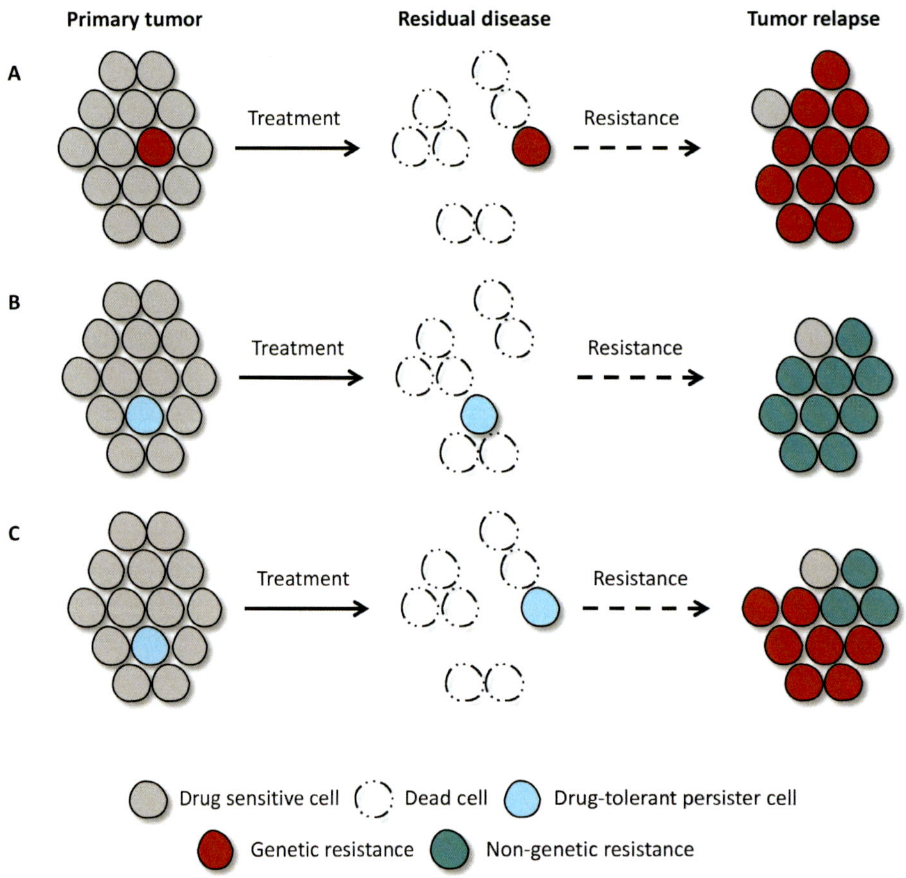

Figure 4.9: *Drug tolerance.*

Source: De Conti, G., Dias, M. H., & Bernards, R. Fighting drug resistance through the targeting of drug-tolerant persister cells. Cancers. 2021; 13(5), 1118. https://doi.org/10.3390/cancers13051118.

Pharmacokinetic and pharmacodynamic factors should be taken into account by the clinician to estimate the likely impact of a given drug regimen. Both are crucial in figuring out the effects of a medication.

4.3.1. Sites and Mechanism of Drug Action

The site of drug action means where a drug acts and mechanism means how the drug acts. Drug which act only at the site of application (i.e., localized region) are termed as local or topically acting drugs for example, ointments, paste, creams and certain other local preparations used externally produce only local effect. The local anesthetics like lignocaine, procaine produce anesthesia (local) in a localized region only.

The second kind of action is systemic, or general, action that occurs after absorption. General anesthetics, for instance, act centrally after absorption, and many medications, including antacids and antibiotics, act systemically.

4.3.2. Effects of Drug Action

The drug may produce their effects by:

i. **Stimulation**: Stimulation is an increase in the selective activity of specialized cells, which increases the secretion from a gland.

ii. **Depression**: It is a reduction/decrease in the activity of specialized cells. For example barbiturates depress central nervous system.

iii. **Irritation**: It is the effect of drugs on the growth, nutrition and morphology of living tissues which induce a gross change in cellular function.

iv. **Replacement**: It includes certain drugs, which are used to replace some missing endogenous component of the body or when the production of endogenous components is reduced.

v. **Bactericidal and Cytotoxic Action**: The bacteriostatic activity which is inhibition of growth and multiplication of bacteria and bactericidal activity, which is bacterial death, is induced by certain types of antibiotics. Cytotoxic action is selective for invading cancer cells and altering them without affecting the host cells.

4.3.3. Factors Modifying Drug Action

It is possible to modify the drug's action quantitatively (by increasing or decreasing it) or qualitatively (by changing the type of response). The factors are:

i. **Age**: In newborn infants, the renal filtration rate is immature, which takes 5 to 7 months to mature. Also, the hepatic drug metabolism capacity is also inadequate (that is why chloramphenicol can produce 'gray baby syndrome'), and due to the higher permeability of blood brain barrier, certain drugs attain high concentration in the Central Nervous System.

The dose of a drug for children is often calculated from adult dose.

$$\text{Child dose} = \frac{\text{Age}}{\text{Age} + 12} \times \text{Adult dose}$$

Children are more susceptible to special adverse effects of drugs and in the elderly, the renal function is on decline and doses of drugs have to be reduced.

ii. **Body Size/Weight**: The average adult dose refers to individuals of medium body build. For obese or lean individuals, doses of drug may be calculated by the formula:

$$\text{Adult dose} \times \frac{\text{Weight (kg)}}{70}$$

Dose can be calculated more accurately by body surface area (BSA).

$$\text{Individual dose} = \frac{\text{BSA(m)}^2}{1.7} \times \text{Average adult dose}$$

iii. **Sex**: Females require lower dose than males. Drugs given during pregnancy can affect the fetus. There are certain physiological changes that take place during pregnancy, which can alter the drug disposal.

iv. **Species and Racial Difference**: In animal species, rabbits are resistant to atropine and rat and mice are resistant to digitalis.

v. Among human beings, blacks require higher and Mongols require lower concentration of atropine and ephedrine to dilate their pupils.

vi. **Genetics**: In certain individuals, the same dose may produce their effect 5–6 times more among others, which is due to their differing rate of drug metabolism.

vii. **Routes and Time of Administration**: The different routes of administration may affect the intensity of drug effect, e.g., magnesium sulfate, when used orally acts as a purgative, in local application it relieves inflammation of wound or boil and when it is used intravenously it causes depression of central nervous system (CNS) and reduce seizures.

The time of administration can also affect drug response, e.g., corticosteroids when taken in morning as single dose cause less adrenal pituitary suppression.

i. **Pathological Conditions**: Several disease conditions also influence the drug disposal and action of drug. For example: bioavailability of drug (having first pass metabolism) is increased due to diminished liver function.

ii. **Tolerance**: Tolerance is a condition when there is a requirement of higher dose of a drug to produce a given response. Tachyphylaxis is the rapid development of tolerance in which there is a marked reduction in response even after repeated doses of a drug.

iii. **Drug Resistance**: It is tolerance of microorganisms to inhibitory action of antimicrobials, e.g., staphylococci to penicillin.

iv. **Other Drugs**: Drugs may modify the response to each other by pharmacokinetic or pharmacodynamic interaction between them.

4.3.4. Drug Receptors

The macromolecular sites known as drug receptors are found inside or on the surface of effector cells, where a particular agonist (ligand/drug) combines to trigger a response. An antagonist has no independent effect; instead, it blocks an agonist's action on a receptor (Figure 4.10).

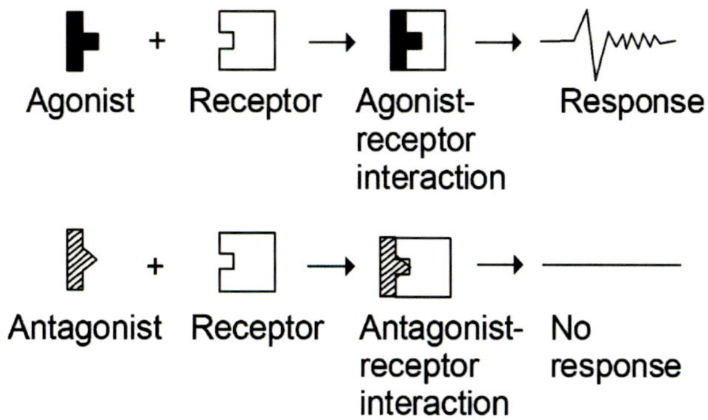

Figure 4.10. *Drug-receptor interactions.*

Source: https://egyankosh.ac.in/bitstream/123456789/38323/1/Unit%202.pdf.

An antagonist only partially fits the receptor site, is unable to produce any pharmacological response, and inhibits the agonist from combining with the receptors, whereas the agonist fully fits (interacts) with the receptor site to produce a pharmacological response.

The term "affinity of the drug" refers to a substance's capacity to bind to a receptor. "Intrinsic activity of the drug" refers to the drug's capacity to elicit a pharmacological response subsequent to its interaction with the receptor; this capacity also establishes the extent of the receptor response. A maximal receptor response is produced by agonists, an intermediate response is produced by partial agonists, and little to no response is produced by antagonists.

4.3.5. Combined Effect of Drugs

4.3.5.1. Synergism

Synergistic drugs are those that act in concert to increase the effects of one given at the same time. When taken together, the medications may act in tandem, or they may each be inert when taken separately. Additive or supradditive synergisms are possible.

- **Additive:** When the effect of two drugs are in the same direction. For example, when aspirin is combined with paracetamol the combined effect is analgesic/antipyretic.

- **Supradditive:** In this the effect of combined therapy is greater than the individual effect of the one drug. For examples when sulfonamide and trimethoprim are combined for antibacterial action.

4.3.5.2. Drug Antagonism

Antagonism is the result of one drug inhibiting or reducing the effects of another. There are three types of antagonism: chemical, where two drugs react chemically to form a biologically inactive compound, physical, where one drug's physical properties can affect another drug's absorption, and receptor, where one drug prevents another drug from binding to the receptor. Drug antagonism can be classified as either noncompetitive or competitive based on the receptor.

4.4. Therapeutic Drug Monitoring

Therapeutic drug monitoring is the process of measuring drug concentrations in plasma using assay techniques, and then interpreting and using the concentration data to create safe and efficient treatment plans. When carried out correctly, this procedure makes it possible to obtain therapeutic concentrations of a drug more quickly and safely than when using empirical dose adjustments. In conjunction with clinical effect observations, it ought to offer the safest method for achieving the best possible drug therapy.

The idea that pharmacologic response and drug concentration at the site of action are closely related underlies the utility of plasma drug concentration data. Studies conducted on patients with particular drugs have yielded information about the therapeutic range, or range of plasma concentrations that is safe and useful in treating particular diseases (Figure 4.11). The medication has the desired effects within this therapeutic range. It is below which there is a higher chance that the therapeutic benefits will not materialize, and above it there may be toxic effects.

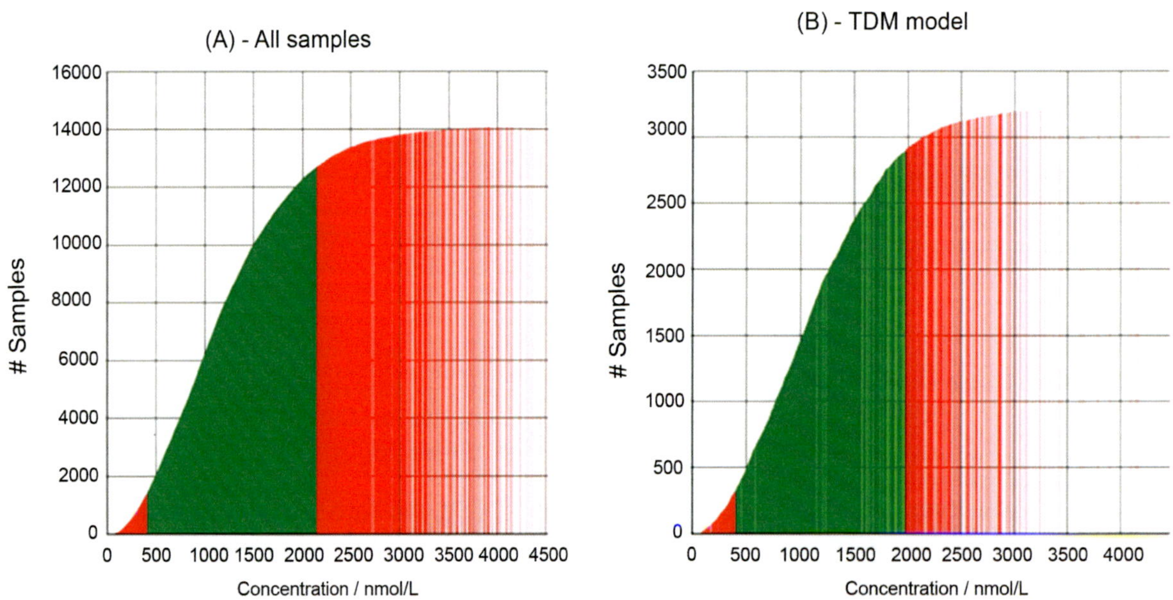

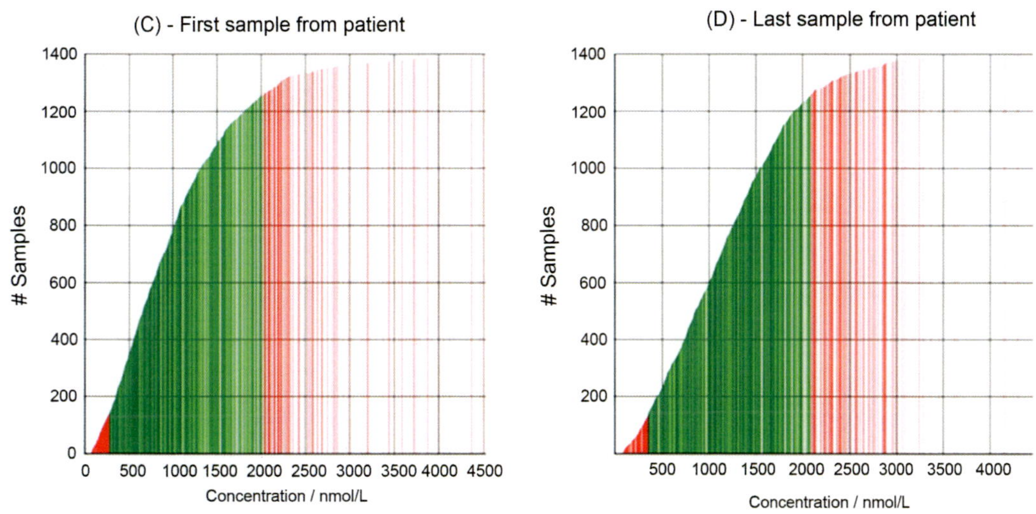

Figure 4.11: *The therapeutic dose.*

Source: Larsen, J. B., Hoffmann-Lücke E, Aaslo, P. H., Jørgensen, N. R., & Greibe, E. Automated Interlaboratory Comparison of Therapeutic Drug Monitoring Data and Its Use for Evaluation of Published Therapeutic Reference Ranges. Pharmaceutics. 2023; 15(2), 673. https://doi.org/10.3390/pharmaceutics15020673.

Subtherapeutic, therapeutic, and toxic drug concentrations are not separated by absolute limits. Because each patient's response to a drug varies, most drugs have a gray area where these concentrations overlap.

When a medication is given to different patients, its pharmacokinetic properties can cause variations in the plasma concentration attained with a given dose. The main causes of this interpatient variability are one or more of the following:

- Variations in drug absorption
- Variations in drug distribution
- Genetic impact
- Disease states impact drug kinetics
- Drug interactions

Therapeutic monitoring using drug concentration data is valuable when:

1. A good correlation exists between the pharmacologic response and plasma concentration. Over at least a limited concentration range, the intensity of pharmacologic effects should increase with plasma concentration. This relationship allows us to predict pharmacologic effects with changing plasma drug concentrations.
2. Wide intersubject variation in plasma drug concentrations results from a given dose.

3. The drug has a narrow therapeutic index (i.e., the therapeutic concentration is close to the toxic concentration).
4. The drug's desired pharmacologic effects cannot be assessed readily by other simple means (e.g., blood pressure measurement for antihypertensives).

The value of therapeutic drug monitoring is limited in situations in which:

1. There is no well-defined therapeutic plasma concentration range.
2. The formation of pharmacologically active metabolites of a drug complicates the application of plasma drug concentration data to clinical effect unless metabolite concentrations are also considered.
3. Toxic effects may occur at unexpectedly low drug concentrations as well as at high concentrations.
4. There are no significant consequences associated with too high or too low levels.

Table 4.1 provides the importance of therapeutic ranges for commonly used medications.

Table 4.1. Therapeutic Ranges and Their Importance: Clinical Implications of Systematic Reviews of Therapeutic Ranges

Clinical Improvement (Lower Limit)	Suspected Adverse Effects (Upper Limit)	Clinical Implication
Better in 'therapeutic' participants compared to subtherapeutic	Higher frequency or severity in supratherapeutic participants compared with therapeutic	No change to clinical practice, therapeutic range is correct
Better in 'therapeutic' participants compared to subtherapeutic	No difference between therapeutic and supratherapeutic participants	Clinicians should aim serum levels above the lower limit. Additional studies to determine accurate upper range may be required
No difference between therapeutic and subtherapeutic participants	Higher in supratherapeutic participants compared with therapeutic	Clinicians should aim for serum levels below the upper limit. Additional studies to determine the lower range may be required

No difference between therapeutic and subtherapeutic participants	No difference between therapeutic and supratherapeutic participants	Existing therapeutic range not related to outcomes of interest. Additional studies to determine optimal therapeutic range and/or if TDM beneficial for this drug/indication/population

Source: Cooney, L., Loke, Y. K., & Golder, S., et al. Overview of systematic reviews of therapeutic ranges: methodologies and recommendations for practice. BMC Med Res Methodol. 2017; 17(1), 84. Published 2017 Jun 2. doi:10.1186/s12874-017-0363-z

4.5. Pharmacokinetic Models

The body's response to a drug can be highly intricate because it affects drug concentrations in tissues and fluids through a variety of processes, including absorption, distribution, metabolism, and elimination. The behavior of a drug in the body must be predicted by simplifying bodily functions. Using mathematical concepts to the various processes is one way to simplify these procedures.

A body model needs to be chosen toapply mathematical concepts. The compartmental model is a fundamental kind of model used in pharmacokinetics. The number of compartments required to characterize the behavior of the drug in the body is the criterion used to classify compartmental models. Models with one, two, and multiple compartments are available. The compartments could represent a collection of related tissues or fluids rather than a single tissue or fluid. The time course of drug concentrations in the body can be predicted using these models.

The reason compartmental models are called deterministic is that the kind of compartmental model needed to explain the pharmacokinetics of the drug is determined by the observed drug concentrations. We will see this idea clearly when we look at one- and two-compartment models.

Simplified body structures are used to build a compartmental model as a representation of the body. Tissues and organs with comparable drug distribution patterns are combined into a single section. For most drugs, distribution into renal tissue is different from distribution into adipose tissue. These tissues might therefore be located in various compartments. The heavily perfused body parts (e.g., liver, kidneys, and heart) frequently exhibit comparable drug distribution patterns, making these regions potentially regarded as a single compartment. The heart, lungs, liver, kidneys, and blood (plasma) are all included in what is commonly referred to as the central compartment, or the highly blood-perfused compartment. There is also the peripheral compartment, which is less well perfused than the central compartment and contains muscle, fat, and cerebrospinal fluid.

The expression of variations in the amount of drug in the body over time is another way that physiological processes are simplified. We refer to these variations over time as rates. The change in the amount of drug in the body as a result of drug elimination over time is described by the elimination rate. The premise of most pharmacokinetic models is that elimination remains constant over time.

Any model's predictive power for drug concentrations in tissues and fluids determines its value. The simplest model that can predict changes in drug concentrations over time with the greatest accuracy is usually the one to use. A more complex model (two or more compartments) is not required if a one-compartment model is adequate to predict plasma drug concentrations (and those concentrations are of most interest to us). However, to forecast tissue drug concentrations, more sophisticated models are frequently needed.

4.5.1. Compartmental Models

In clinical practice, the most commonly utilized model is the one-compartment model. Using a visual representation helps with model structuring. Straight arrows are used to represent drug transfer rates, and an enclosed square or rectangle is used to represent the compartment. All that indicates that a drug has been placed in that compartment is the arrow pointing into the box. Additionally, the drug is exiting the compartment as indicated by the arrow coming out of the box.

With just one compartment, this model is the most basic. Every bodily fluid and tissue is regarded as belonging to this compartment. Moreover, it is presumed that a drug dose distributes instantly throughout the entire body after being given.

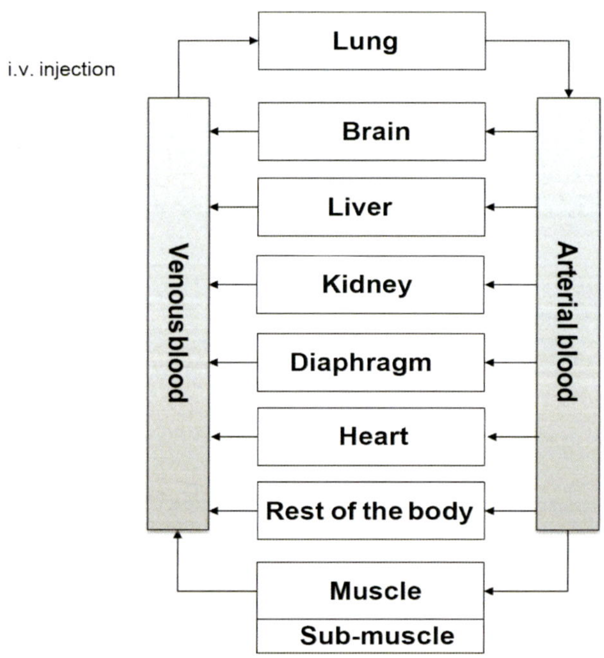

Figure 4.12: *A physiologically based pharmacokinetic (PBPK) model for the description of drug pharmacokinetics in anatomically relevant tissues and organs. Here, the drug is administered as a bolus dose into the venous blood compartment.*

Source: Kok-Yong, S., & Lawrence, L. (2015). Drug Distribution and Drug Elimination. InTech. doi: 10.5772/59929.

Even after an intravenous bolus is administered, some medications do not instantly spread to every part of the body. An intravenous bolus dose is given over a very brief period of time. Rapid drug distribution through the bloodstream and to highly perfused organs like the kidneys and liver is a common distribution pattern. The medication then spreads to other bodily tissues, albeit more slowly. Two compartments in the model could represent this drug distribution pattern. To keep things in balance, the drug alternates between these compartments.

4.5.2. Volume of Distribution

Until now, we have spoken of the amount of drug (X) in a compartment. If we also consider the volume of the compartment, we can describe the concept of drug concentration. Drug concentration in the compartment is defined as the amount of drug in a given volume, such as mg/L:

$$\text{concentration} = \frac{\text{amount of drug in body}}{\begin{array}{c}\text{volume in which}\\ \text{drug is distributed}\end{array}} = \frac{X}{V} \tag{4.1}$$

Volume of distribution (V) is an important indicator of the extent of drug distribution into body fluids and tissues. V relates the amount of drug in the body (X) to the measured concentration in the plasma (C). Thus, V is the volume required to account for all of the drug in the body if the concentrations in all tissues are the same as the plasma concentration:

$$\text{volume of distribution} = \frac{\text{amount of drug}}{\text{concentration}}$$

A large volume of distribution usually indicates that the drug distributes extensively into body tissues and fluids. Conversely, a small volume of distribution often indicates limited drug distribution.

The volume of distribution does not reflect the tissues or fluids that the drug distributes into; rather, it indicates the extent of distribution. Even though the volume of distribution of two drugs is equal, one drug may concentrate in adipose tissues while the other may distribute mainly into muscle tissues. Table 4.2 displays the approximate volumes of distribution for a few commonly used medications.

Table 4.2. The Volumes of Distribution of a Few Examples

Drug	V_d (L)
Warfarin	8
Gentamicin	18
Digoxin	440
Diazepam	80
Nortriptyline	1700
Chloroquine	> 15000

Source: Kok-Yong, S., & Lawrence, L. (2015). Drug distribution and drug elimination. InTech. doi: 10.5772/59929.

Certain tissues should have substantially higher drug concentrations than plasma when V is many times the body's volume. The plasma volume is the smallest possible volume in which a drug can distribute.

Since the body is mostly made of water, let's first visualize the body as a fluid-filled tank to demonstrate the idea of volume of distribution. We can add a known amount of material to the tank and measure the substance's concentration in the fluid to determine the tank's volume. If the amount of substance (X) and the resulting concentration (C) is known, then the volume of distribution (V) can be calculated using the simplified equations:

$$X = VC \quad \text{or} \quad C = \frac{X}{V} \quad \text{or} \quad V = \frac{X}{C}$$

where, X = amount of drug in body; V = volume of distribution; and C = concentration in the plasma.

As with other pharmacokinetic parameters, volume of distribution can vary considerably from one person to another because of differences in physiology or disease states. Something to note: The dose of a drug (X_0) and the amount of drug in the body (X) are essentially the same thing because all of the dose goes into the body.

Important presumptions have been made in this example, including the occurrence of instantaneous distribution and its equal distribution throughout the tank. Elimination does not occur in the closed tank. This illustration is comparable to a one-compartment model of the body following an intravenous bolus. One complicating factor, though, is that the drug is being eliminated from the body the entire time it is there. Therefore, the concentration used to determine the tank's volume would be continuously changing if we were to think of the body as a tank with an open outlet valve (Figure 4.13).

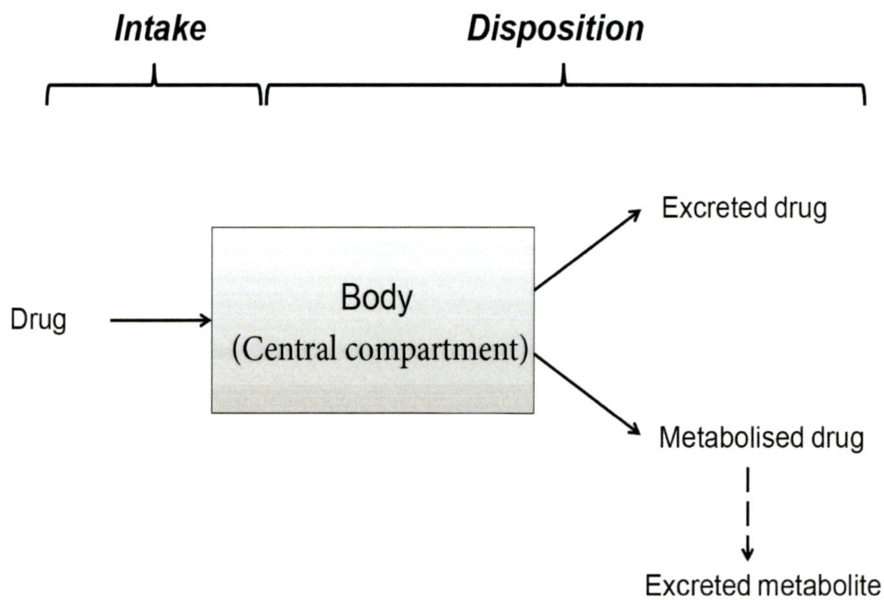

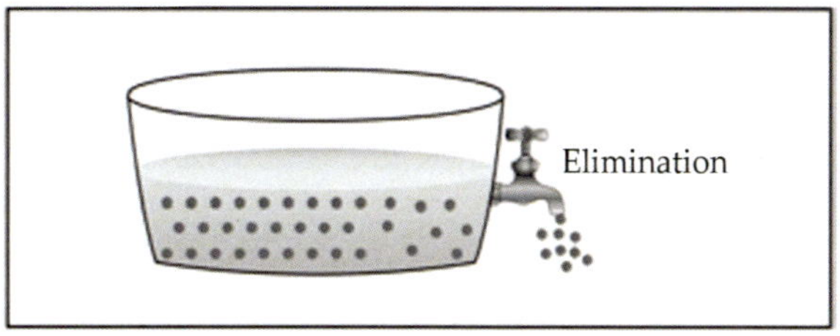

Figure 4.13. *Drug elimination model.*

Source: Kok-Yong, S., & Lawrence, L. (2015). Drug distribution and drug elimination. InTech. doi: 10.5772/59929.

To estimate a drug's volume of distribution in a patient, we can utilize the relationship between volume, amount of drug administered, and resulting concentration found in Equation 4.1. A volume of distribution can be computed by administering a medication at a known dose and measuring the amount of the drug that is achieved in the plasma. However, changes brought about by drug elimination must be considered in the concentration used for this estimation.

For example: If 100 mg of drug X is administered intravenously and the plasma concentration is determined to be 5 mg/L just after the dose is given, then:

$$\text{volume of distribution } (V) = \frac{\text{dose}}{\text{resulting concentration}} = \frac{X_0}{C} = \frac{100\text{ mg}}{5\text{ mg/L}} = 20\text{ L}$$

4.5.3. Plasma Drug Concentration versus Time Curves

When a drug is continuously measured in the plasma following an intravenous bolus dose using the one-compartment model, and the drug concentrations are plotted against the time of acquisition, a curve is the outcome. Take note that this plot is a curve, and that at time zero (t_0), immediately following the dose, the plasma concentration is at its highest.

Measuring drug concentrations typically requires obtaining a limited number of plasma samples due to cost constraints and patient convenience in clinical settings. We can forecast the plasma drug concentrations for the times when we don't have samples using these known values. It is uncommon to take more than two samples in clinical settings following a dose.

Many sources of error can arise when predicting drug concentrations from known concentrations. However, some errors can be avoided if we are aware of the assumptions that went into the predictions. When we examine the one-compartment system, these presumptions are brought to light.

The knowledge that the concentrations are all on a straight line rather than a curve makes it simpler to predict the plasma concentrations mathematically. Plotting the plasma drug concentration's natural logarithm (ln) against time allows for this conversion to be achieved for the majority of drugs. Essentially, the curve plot is transformed into a straight line by utilizing the natural log of the plasma drug concentration.

The natural log of plasma drug concentration versus time plot yields a straight line only for drugs with a one-compartment distribution and first-order elimination processes. First-order elimination happens when the quantity of a drug in the body at a given time determines how much of it is eliminated from the body in that same time frame.

Plotting the actual concentration and time values on semilogarithmic (or semilog) paper, a unique graph paper that automatically adjusts for the logarithmic relationship by changing the distance between lines on the y-axis, is an alternative to calculating the natural log values. Instead of being evenly spaced, the y-axis lines are related logarithmically within each log cycle (or multiple of 10). Thus, a straight line is produced when the actual plasma drug concentration values are plotted against the time values. The values on the x-axis are not logarithmically converted; instead, they are spaced evenly. (The word semilogarithmic denotes the conversion of only one axis). 0.1 through 1, 1 through 10, 10 through 100, or any series with a 10-fold difference in the range of values can all be represented by the numbers on the y-axis.

Visual inspection or, more precisely, linear regression techniques can be used to draw a straight line through a set of known plasma concentration versus time points plotted on semilog paper. A mathematical technique called linear regression is used to identify which line best represents a group of plotted points.

This line allows us to forecast drug concentrations in plasma at times when measurements are not available (Figure 4.14).

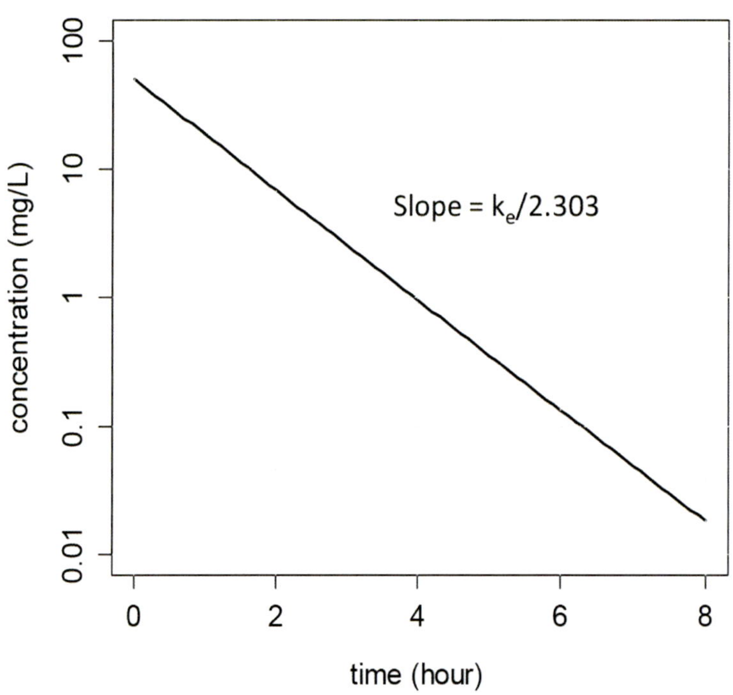

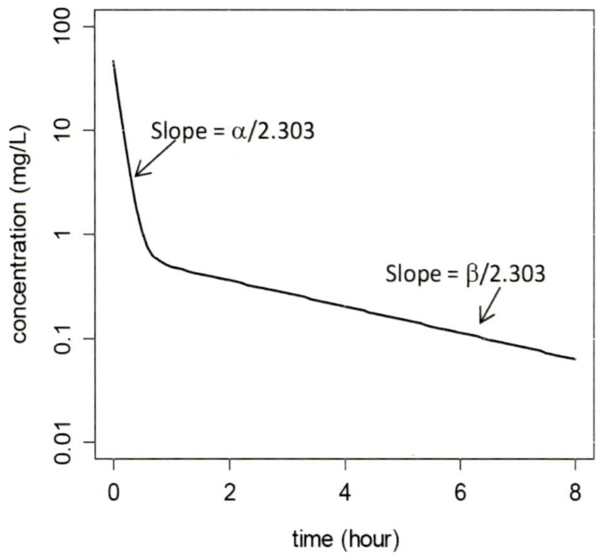

Figure 4.14: *Plasma concentration versus time profiles following i.v. bolus administration on a semi-logarithmic graph for a drug exhibiting a one-compartment model (upper panel) and a two-compartment model (lower panel). For the two-compartment model, the slopes α and β denote the rates of combined distribution plus elimination, and elimination, respectively, of the drug from the central compartment.*

Source: Kok-Yong, S., & Lawrence, L. (2015). Drug distribution and drug elimination. InTech. doi: 10.5772/59929.

A Closer Look

Adverse Drug Reactions / Drug Toxicities

Adverse drug reaction may be defined as 'any response to a drug which is noxious (injurious) and unintended, and which occurs at doses of an appropriately given drug used in man for prophylaxis, diagnosis or therapy excluding therapeutic failures.'

Adverse drugs reactions are not rare and have increased in number, which may be due to irrational use of multiple drug therapy, availability of most of the drugs as OTC (over the counter) i.e., without prescription and self-medication by the patients.

Adverse effects can be based on the pharmacodynamics of the drug, i.e., side effects (occur at therapeutic dose of the drug), toxic effects (occurs at overdose or poisoning) and drug withdrawal symptoms (i.e., withdrawal of narcotic drugs) and secondly, the effects which are individual to individual like drug allergy (hypersensitivity to drugs), idiosyncracy. Other types are teratogenicity (drug causing fetal abnormalities), carcinogenicity (drug causing cancer), iatrogenicity (drug induced diseases).

- **Side Effects:** These are undesirable and unavoidable pharmacological effect of the drug, which occur at therapeutic dose. These unwanted effects of many drugs are based on their pharmacological actions.
- **Toxic Effects:** Toxic effects develop due to excessive pharmacological action of drug, which may be due to overdose or continuous use of drug for prolonged period. The overdose toxicity occurs when the high dose of drug is required for the specific treatment or the drug is taken accidentally or with the intention of suicide. The effects are predictable and dose related.
- **Hypersensitivity (Drug Allergy):** Drug allergy is a cell-mediated immune reaction producing symptoms, which are unrelated to the pharmacological effects of the drug. It results from previous sensitization to the drug itself or a particular chemical with similar structure.
- **Teratogenicity:** Teratogenicity is derived from the word 'teratos' mean 'monster.' teratogens may act directly on the fetus, e.g., thalidomide and anticancer drugs act directly on the fetus, or act indirectly on placenta, e.g., vitamin a, 5-ht.

It is clear that the major fetal damage occur by drug when it is taken in early pregnancy (i.e., first 2–9 weeks when organogenesis takes place.)

The teratogenic drugs can affect different stages of pregnancy i.e.

- At fertilization and implantation stage (i.e., conception to 3 weeks).
- Organogenesis period (3 to 9 weeks), and
- In growth and development period (i.e., after 9 weeks).

- **Carcinogenicity:** Certain drugs affect the genes and structural changes in the chromosomes. The drugs that cause cancer are called as carcinogenic drugs, for example, oral contraceptives increase the incidence of benign liver tumors, vaginal adenocarcinomas in the female offsprings of women who have taken stilboesterol during her pregnancy for abortion purpose.

- **Idiosyncrasy:** It is genetically determined abnormal reactivity to a drug. The abnormal reactions to the drug are precipitated sometime because of genetically determined total absence or reduced activity of some enzyme in the body of the recipient.
- **Poisoning:** Poison is a substance which endangers life due to its toxic reaction/ poisoning on certain vital functions in the body. The poisonous substances may be the toxins, very high doses of drug, industrial chemicals/gases, household chemical like insecticides-DDT, BHC, etc. For the treatment of poisoning, a selective antidote (which antagonizes the action) may be given.

- **Management of Poisoning**: Some general guidelines have been given for the management of poisoning. These guidelines are aimed at prevention of further exposure to the poisonous substance, alleviation of the symptoms of poisoning and maintenance of the vital body functions. The guidelines can be summarized as follows:
- Maintain a clear airway/adequate ventilation (for inhaled poisons).
- Washing the eyes and other surface of the body (for local poison entering from the surface).
- Gastric lavage (with hypertonic saline solution, apomorphine injection for ingested poison).
- Activated charcoal (to bind the unabsorbed drug) 10–30 g in suspension in 200 ml water.
- Identify the poison and specific antidotes should be given.
- Maintenance of blood pressure and other related body function by fluid infusion, pressor agents, depending upon the condition of the patient.
- The nonspecific antidotes are also given, for example anticonvulsants in convulsions.
- Forced diuresis by furosemide, mannitol etc., and altering the urinary pH–increasing the pH of urine favors ionization of acidic drugs like salicylates, phenobarbital etc., whereas reducing the pH favors ionization of basic drugs like pethidine, amphetamine etc.
- Haemodialysis and hemoperfusion which is a passage of blood through a charcoal or adsorbent resin column may be instituted, depending upon the patient's condition.

Summary

- Pharmacokinetics is the term that describes the four stages of absorption, distribution, metabolism, and excretion of drugs. Drugs are medications or other substances that have a physiological effect when introduced to the body. There are four basic stages a medication goes through within the human body: absorption, distribution, metabolism, and excretion. This entire process is sometimes abbreviated as ADME.
- The first stage of pharmacokinetics is known as absorption. Absorption is the entry of the drug into the blood via the biological membrane from the site/route of administration.
- The second stage of pharmacokinetics is the process known as distribution. Distribution is the process by which a drug is dispersed throughout the body's blood and tissues. After a drug enters systemic circulation by absorption or direct administration, it will pass from vascular spaces to tissues where a drug-receptor interaction will occur, creating the effect of the drug.
- After a drug has been absorbed and distributed throughout the body, it is broken down by a process known as metabolism so that it can be excreted from the body. Drugs undergo chemical alteration by various body systems to create compounds that are more easily excreted.
- The excretion of drugs has been known to take place through different routes mainly kidneys, skin, lungs and alimentary tract. Only a few drugs are eliminated through the skin and via the lungs (only for volatile drugs like chloroform, ethyl alcohol, ether etc.).
- Pharmacodynamics refers to the relationship between drug concentration at the site of action and the resulting effect, including the time course and intensity of therapeutic and adverse effects. The effect of a drug present at the site of action is determined by that drug's binding with a receptor. Receptors may be present on neurons in the central nervous system (i.e., opiate receptors) to depress pain sensation, on cardiac muscle to affect the intensity of contraction, or even within bacteria to disrupt maintenance of the bacterial cell wall.
- The drug receptors are macromolecular sites that are situated on the surface or inside the effector cells with which specific agonist (ligand/drug) combines to produce its response. Antagonist prevents the action of an agonist on a receptor, but does not have any effect of its own.
- Therapeutic drug monitoring is defined as the use of assay procedures for the determination of drug concentrations in plasma, and the interpretation and application of the resulting concentration data to develop safe and effective drug regimens. If performed properly, this process allows for the achievement of therapeutic concentrations of a drug more rapidly and safely than can be attained with empiric dose changes. Together with observations of the drug's clinical effects, it should provide the safest approach to optimal drug therapy.

References

1. Fernandez, E., Perez, R., Hernandez, A., Tejada, P., Arteta, M., & Ramos, J. T. (2011). Factors and mechanisms for pharmacokinetic differences between pediatric population and adults. *Pharmaceutics, 3*(1), 53–72. https://doi.org/10.3390/pharmaceutics3010053.
2. Lambert, D. G. (2004). Drugs and receptors. *Continuing Education in Anaesthesia Critical Care & Pain, 4*(6), 181–184. https://doi.org/10.1093/bjaceaccp/mkh050. Retrieved 2023-01-15.
3. Lees, P., Cunningham, F. M., & Elliott, J. (2004). Principles of pharmacodynamics and their applications in veterinary pharmacology. *Journal of Veterinary Pharmacology and Therapeutics, 27*(6), 397–414. https://doi.org/10.1111/j.1365-2885.2004.00620.x. PMID: 15601436.
4. Li, X., Martinez-Lozano Sinues, P., Dallmann, R., Bregy, L., Hollmén, M., Proulx, S., Brown, S. A., Detmar, M., Kohler, M., & Zenobi, R. (2015). Drug pharmacokinetics determined by real-time analysis of mouse breath. *Angewandte Chemie International Edition, 54*(27), 7815–7818. https://doi.org/10.1002/anie.201503312. hdl:20.500.11850/102558. PMID: 26015026.
5. Liu, L., & Liu, X. (2019). Contributions of drug transporters to blood-placental barrier. *Advances in Experimental Medicine and Biology, 1141*, 505–548. https://doi.org/10.1007/978-981-13-7647-4_11.
6. Ruiz-Garcia, A., Bermejo, M., Moss, A., & Casabo, V. G. (2008). Pharmacokinetics in drug discovery. *Journal of Pharmaceutical Sciences, 97*(2), 654–690. https://doi.org/10.1002/jps.21009. PMID: 17630642.
7. Vauquelin, G., & Charlton, S. J. (2010). Long-lasting target binding and rebinding as mechanisms to prolong in vivo drug action. *British Journal of Pharmacology, 161*(3), 488–508. https://doi.org/10.1111/j.1476-5381.2010.00936.x. PMC: 2990149. PMID: 20880390.
8. Vijay. (2003). Predictive software for drug design and development. *Pharmaceutical Development and Regulation, 1*(3), 159–168.

Chapter

CHEMOTHERAPY AND DRUG ACTION

5

Contents

Introduction

Chemotherapy is a cancer treatment method that differs significantly from radiation therapy and surgery. Chemotherapy has four uses: palliative, adjuvant, neoadjuvant, and primary treatment. Chemotherapy employs chemical agents (anti-cancer or cytotoxic drugs) to interact with cancer cells toeradicate or control the growth of cancer, as opposed to physically removing a tumor or a portion of it. Chemotherapy is used as an adjuvant treatment following surgery to either eliminate microscopic cancer cells or reduce the risk of cancer recurrence.

Chemotherapy is frequently applied as a post-adjuvant therapy. Chemotherapy, when used as a neoadjuvant treatment, is intended to decrease the tumor's size and/or bulk to facilitate surgical resection.

Chemotherapy affects both types of cells because it is unable to differentiate between cancerous and normal cells. Unpleasant side effects are caused by chemotherapeutic agents' toxicity to normal cells. Chemotherapy is valuable, though, because cancer cells are specifically selected for death by chemotherapeutic agents as opposed to healthy host cells. Chemotherapy rarely causes permanent damage to normal tissues because they can regenerate and heal themselves.

Inhibiting DNA repair can enhance chemotherapy because the term "chemotherapy" has come to refer to the broad use of intracellular poisons to prevent mitosis (cell division) or cause DNA damage. The term "chemotherapy" implies a broad category of drugs that are more focused on blocking extracellular signals (signal transduction). Hormonal therapies are the development of treatments with particular molecular or genetic targets that block signals from classic endocrine hormones (mainly estrogens for breast cancer and androgens for prostate cancer) that promote growth. Targeted therapy, on the other hand, refers to different inhibitions of growth signals, such as those connected to receptor tyrosine kinases.

Importantly, because medications are injected into the bloodstream, they can theoretically treat cancer at any anatomic site in the body. This makes drug use—whether it be for hormonal therapy, targeted therapy, or chemotherapy—a form of systemic therapy for cancer. Systemic therapy is frequently used in conjunction with other cancer treatment modalities such as radiation therapy, surgery, or hyperthermia therapy that are considered local therapy (i.e., treatments whose efficacy is limited to the anatomic area where they are applied).

Orientation and Directional Terms

Term	Definition	Illustration
Good Clinical Practice (GCP)	Good clinical practice (GCP) is an international quality standard, which governments can then transpose into regulations for clinical trials involving human subjects.	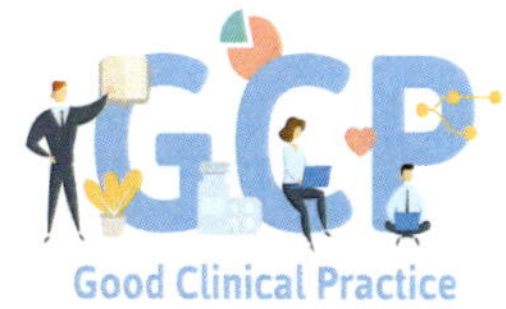
Hormone therapy	Hormone therapy is used to treat cancers that use hormones to grow, such as some prostate and breast cancers. Hormone therapy is a cancer treatment that slows or stops the growth of cancer that uses hormones to grow. Hormone therapy is also called hormonal therapy, hormone treatment, or endocrine therapy.	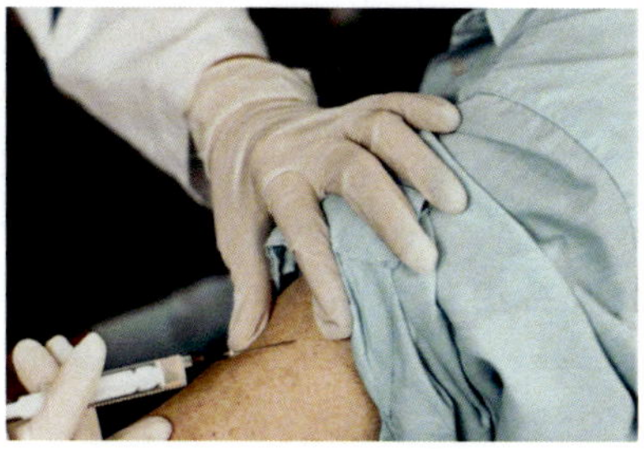
Antimicrobial agent	Infections and diseases may be caused by different types of organisms like bacteria, fungi, and viruses, etc., in humans and animals. The drug used to prevent the pathogenicity of microorganisms is called an antimicrobial agent.	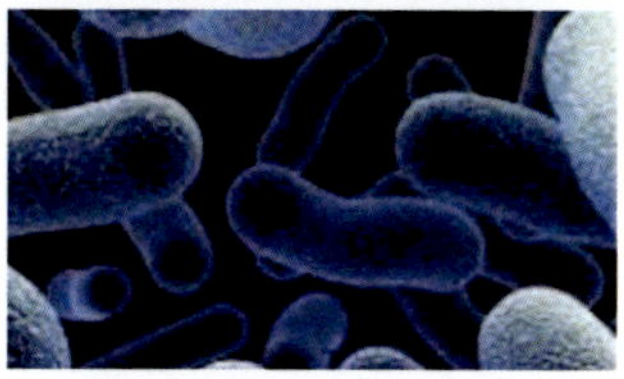
Lipopolysaccharides (LPS)	Lipopolysaccharides (LPS) are important outer membrane components of gram-negative bacteria. They are large amphipathic glycoconjugates that typically consist of a lipid domain (hydrophobic) attached to a core oligosaccharide and a distal polysaccharide.	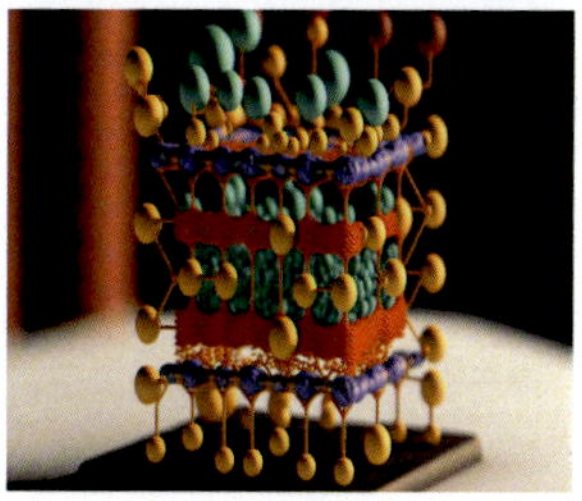
Antimicrobial Peptides	Antimicrobial peptides (AMPs), also called host defense peptides (HDPs) are part of the innate immune response found among all classes of life. Fundamental differences exist between prokaryotic and eukaryotic cells that may represent targets for antimicrobial peptides.	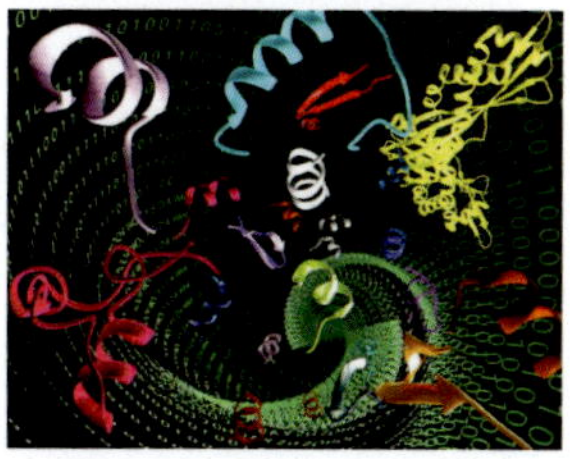

5.1. Principles of Chemotherapy

One type of treatment called chemotherapy uses medications to kill cancer cells. Unlike surgery or radiation therapy, which focuses on particular areas of the body, this treatment is systemic, meaning it affects the entire body. Chemotherapy medications function by obstructing the growth and division of cancerous cells. Chemotherapy has the potential to kill cancer cells, but it can also damage healthy cells that divide quickly, including those in the bone marrow, digestive system, and hair follicles. As a result, side effects like nausea, hair loss, and weakened immune system may result. There are several ways to administer chemotherapy, including intravenously, orally, or through injections. Depending on the kind and stage of the disease, it's frequently used in conjunction with other cancer treatments.

5.1.1. The History of the Development of Chemotherapy

Any drug or chemical treatment used to treat any disease is referred to as chemotherapy. Malignancy is treated with cytotoxic, or anti-neoplastic, chemotherapeutic agents.

The discovery of cytotoxic chemotherapy at the start of the 20th century completely changed the way that cancer was treated, particularly when it came to spreading illnesses like leukemia. The discovery that certain chemicals acted primarily on rapidly dividing cells, including cancer cells, was crucial to the development of cytotoxic chemotherapy. It was observed that soldiers exposed to nitrogen gas during World War I experienced abnormally low white cell counts. In the 1940s, nitrogen mustard—a byproduct of nitrogen gas—was first applied as an anti-cancer remedy. Many of the cytotoxic medications used today were unintentionally found while creating medications for different uses, while some were created expressly to disrupt metabolic processes.

5.1.2. Cell Cycle

A basic understanding of the normal cell cycle is essential to comprehending the principles and mechanisms of chemotherapy. The cell cycle consists of multiple successive phases and is an ordered sequence of events. The cell cycle allows for self-reproduction, the replacement of damaged or dead cells, and the addition of new cells during tissue growth.

Somatic and reproductive cell division are the two types, and they serve different purposes. All cells, with the exception of germ cells used in reproduction, divide during somatic cell division. In somatic cell division, a nuclear division process known as mitosis causes each cell to duplicate its contents and split into two identical cells. The two primary phases of the cell cycle are the mitotic (M) phase, which occurs when the cell is dividing, and the interphase, when the cell is not dividing.

5.1.2.1. Interphase

During this fast-growing phase, the cell duplicates its DNA. G1, S, and G2 are the three phases of interphase. DNA synthesis is the focus of the S phase, and breaks or disruptions in DNA replication occur during the G phase.

1. **G1 Phase:** The G^1 phase is the time interval or space that exists between the S phase and the mitotic stage. The synthesis of RNA and protein makes the cell metabolically active and ready for the synthesis of DNA. This phase can extend up to 10 hours, although some cells stay in it longer and are referred to as being in the G^0, or resting, phase.
2. **S Phase:** A cell is committed to dividing once it reaches this stage.

The S phase lasts for about eight hours and occurs between G^1 and G^2. DNA replicates during this stage of DNA synthesis, guaranteeing that the genetic material forming the two newly formed cells is the same.

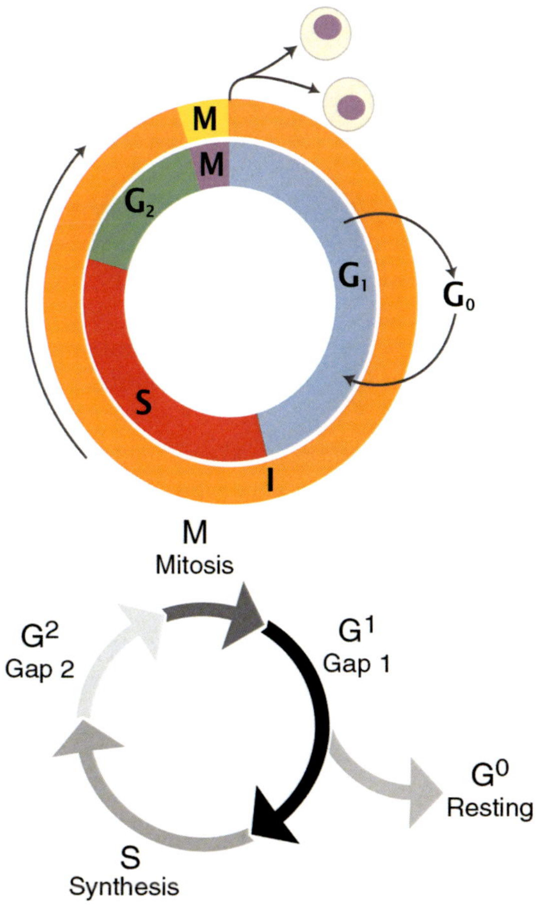

Figure 5.1. *The cell cycle.*

Source: By Cell_Cycle_2.svg: *Cell_Cycle_2.png: Original uploader was Zephyris at en.wikipediaderivative work: Beaoderivative work: Histidine (talk) - Cell_Cycle_2.svg, CC BY-SA 3.0, https://commons.wikimedia.org/w/index.php?curid=12800954.

3. **G2 stage:** This is the interval that separates the S phase from mitosis, the process that produces two daughter cells. This stage could go on for four or six hours. Enzymes and other proteins are synthesized as cells continue to grow and get ready to divide.

5.1.2.2. M phase (Mitosis)

The nucleic and cytoplasmic division that occurs during this phase yields two daughter cells that are identical to one another. Prophase, metaphase, anaphase, and telophase are the four distinct phases that make up this process, which ends in cytokinesis, or the division of cytoplasm into two new cells.

The sequence of events in the cell cycle is shown in Figure 5.1:

$$G^1 \text{ Phase} \rightarrow \text{S phase} \rightarrow G^2 \text{ phase} \rightarrow \text{M phase}$$
$$\text{(Mitosis)} \rightarrow \text{Cytokinesis} \rightarrow \text{two new cells}$$

The ability of cancer cells to proliferate uncontrollably is a defining feature. Cytotoxic chemotherapy affects both cancer cells and other quickly proliferating cells by interfering with cell division at different stages of the cell cycle. Thanks to this understanding, medications that either act only at a particular point in the cell cycle (cell cycle phase-specific) or that have an effect at every stage of the cell cycle (cell cycle non-phase-specific) can now be developed. Chemotherapeutic agents that do not target specific cell cycles, such as platinum compounds and alkylating agents, can also be successful in treating quiescent G_0 cells. This class of medications has proven especially successful in treating slow-growing tumors.

5.1.2.3. Cell Cycle Time

Any cancer treatment plan's main goals are to keep the patient alive and eradicate the tumor while causing the least amount of disturbance to regular cell activity. Tumors are known to grow steadily and progressively; this pattern is influenced by factors such as cell cycle time, growth fraction, and cell loss. Chemotherapy is more effective against cells that divide quickly. It appears that cancer cells go through a fast-paced, proliferative phase in which they cycle from mitosis to mitosis very quickly. Depending on the type of cell, a cycle can take anywhere from 24 to 120 hours to complete.

Cellular proliferation is known to be influenced by age and developmental stage. Children and young adults have more body tissues with dividing cell populations due to their growth, which helps to explain why pediatric cancers seem to respond better to chemotherapy and are more vulnerable to its potentially harmful side effects.

5.1.3. Growth Fraction

The percentage of cells undergoing division at any given time is represented by the growth fraction. A high percentage of cells divide during the early stages of tumor development, when the bulk of the tumor is small, and tumors can grow twice as large very quickly. As tumors get larger, there is less room for growth and a compromised supply of blood, oxygen, and nutrients. The doubling time is shortened during this period due to the low cell growth fraction and slowed cycle time. When tumors reach this stage, chemotherapy may be less effective because it is more effective against rapidly dividing cells. It is believed, however, that by achieving an initial tumor reduction—either by chemotherapy, radiotherapy, or surgery—it might be possible to increase both the cell growth fraction and the cell cycle time. To replenish the lost bulk, this would activate trigger mechanisms on the cell surfaces to attract new cells into the cycle. Chemotherapy can then again be effective against smaller tumors after this is accomplished. Therefore, it can be inferred that doubling times can differ significantly amongst tumor types and that tumors that are sensitive to chemotherapy tend to grow more quickly than slower-growing tumors that are less sensitive to the drug.

5.1.4. Pharmacokinetics and Pharmacodynamics

Pharmacokinetics is the study of how drugs enter, travel through, and are metabolized and excreted from the body. Therefore, pharmacokinetics is crucial to the effective use of chemotherapy for cancer. Even when a particular cytotoxic agent is known to be effective against certain tumors, the agent may still not elicit a response. Choosing the right dosage, timing, and delivery method for a patient requires knowledge of how their body responds to a given medication. A patient's response to therapy may vary depending on a number of factors, including changed organ function. Cytotoxic drug pharmacokinetic behavior has not been thoroughly studied for children, but new methods have made it more important to measure different drug concentrations through pharmacokinetic studies.

The study of the connection between drug concentration and drug effect is known as pharmacodynamics. As a result, administering a specific medication as an infusion or bolus may be able to produce entirely different toxic or therapeutic effects.

The toxic and anti-tumor effects of chemotherapy are closely related, so there may not be much of a difference between an effective and toxic dose. Therefore, the goal of any chemotherapeutic regimen is to achieve the strongest anti-tumor effect at a tolerable level of toxicity.

Comprehending these two tenets underscores the significance of meticulous and consistent patient monitoring before every therapeutic phase, enabling dosage adjustments as needed.

5.1.5. Protocol Development and Clinical Trials

Since childhood cancer is extremely uncommon, multi-institutional trials conducted within a cooperative group—which could be national or international—are the best way to look for better treatments. Within the United Kingdom, the Children's Cancer and Leukemia Group (CCLG) oversees the coordination of trials. A 70% cure rate for all childhood cancers is the product of this research efforts. The benefit of multi-institutional collaboration is faster patient accrual, which enables the drawing of trustworthy conclusions more quickly. Trial coordination minimizes redundancy and enables quick assessment of novel medications and delivery methods.

5.1.5.1. Clinical trials

There are only a few conditions where treatment is believed to be completely effective, providing an opportunity for significant advancements. Enhancements to recommended treatments can be identified through participation in a clinical trial, which is a carefully planned study aimed at determining the best treatment for individuals with a specific condition.

A protocol document contains a description of every clinical trial. This protocol will include details about the goal, plan, and execution of the study, such as which patients qualify, what treatments will be assessed, and how each patient's reaction will be assessed. To assess how well a patient responds to a particular treatment plan, trial data will be examined. The amount of time until death or relapse can be used to gauge the patient's outcome. Many childhood cancer trials seek to lower treatment morbidity while preserving efficacy as outcomes improve.

All research involving human participants must adhere to strict regulations. The European Union Directive on Good Clinical Practice (GCP) was enforced in May 2004 as a global standard for ethical and scientific quality in trials with human subjects. GCP applies to all individuals involved in clinical trials, regardless of whether they work in the pharmaceutical field or academia. Noncompliance with GCP regulations is considered a criminal offense. These rules have specifically impacted personnel conducting clinical trials for childhood cancer treatment, necessitating additional training and adherence to standardized operating procedures.

Clinical trials fall into three phases:

1. Phase I to determine an acceptable drug dosage
2. Phase II to provide evidence of efficacy of treatment
3. Phase III to compare efficacy/side effects with those of other drugs/ treatments

1. **Phase I Studies:** The initial human trials are known as phase I studies. These could be thought of as toxicity screening studies, in which a novel medication is tested in labs and then given to humans to find the highest dose that can be tolerated and any toxicities that are dose-limiting. The first human trials are conducted on adults; however, since children's tolerance patterns for chemotherapy drugs differ from adults', it is not possible to accurately extrapolate the pediatric dose from the adult trials' outcomes. Pediatric patients are eligible to enroll in phase I trials only if they have not responded to traditional treatments. Pharmacokinetic information is routinely gathered through repeated blood and urine sampling to ascertain the new drug's patterns

of absorption, bioavailability, and excretion.

2. **Phase II Studies:** These seek to ascertain the new drug's possible effectiveness in treating various cancer types. A statistically defined number of children with various relapsed or refractory cancers are administered the maximum tolerated dose, and their response is tracked. A phase II study's objective is to determine which medications, for a particular tumor type, need more research.
3. **Phase III Studies:** Phase III studies refer to the extensive multicenter or international randomized trials in childhood cancer that most children in the UK will be enrolled in at the time of diagnosis. A lot of kids will either receive brand-new medications or previously used medications in a different combination or dosage. These novel components are typically used in conjunction with standard therapy to assess whether the new treatment is superior to the standard one or whether a significant survival benefit is obtained by adding them to the prior "best known" treatment.

5.1.6. Considerations when Planning Chemotherapy Treatments

5.1.6.1. Drug Resistance

Patients undergoing chemotherapy exhibit a wide range of therapeutic responses and unacceptable toxicities. Certain cancer cells exhibit an innate or acquired resistance to antimicrobial agents.

Several mechanisms of drug resistance in cancer cells have been identified:

- decreased drug uptake by the cell;
- increased efflux (flow outwards) of drug out of the cell;
- detoxification of drugs in the cell secondary to metabolic changes;
- increased DNA repair;
- alterations in the structure of drug receptor sites or targets;
- decreased sensitivity to apoptosis (programmed cell death);
- multidrug resistance gene from genetic mutation following exposure to particular chemotherapeutic agents.

The multidrug resistance (MDR) gene is present in resistant malignant cells. The MDR gene is present from the beginning in cases of intrinsic resistance, but in acquired resistance, the gene results from a genetic mutation that occurs after chemotherapy exposure. The cell surface of these resistant cells contains a protein known as P-glycoprotein. As an efflux pump, this protein quickly pushes through and removes the chemotherapeutic agents from the cell, halting the therapeutic effect of the drugs.

5.1.6.2. Toxicities

The cytotoxic effect of chemotherapy drugs is the same for both malignant and healthy cells. Cell toxicity frequently has dose limitations and restrictions. To prevent toxicities that could endanger life or patients' quality of life, normal cells must have time to heal in between treatments. This will ensure that patients are satisfied with their care both now and down the road. The harmful effects of chemotherapy on normal cells can lead to unacceptable toxicities even in the presence of drug resistance.

Most cytotoxic medications share many toxicities, including alopecia, nausea and vomiting, and myelosuppression. Most of the time, these acute toxicities are curable. Certain medications also have distinct toxicities that target particular tissues or organs, such as anthracycline-associated cardiotoxicity. Numerous of these distinct toxicities build up over time and can even be irreversible.

When a disease is in its palliative stages and the goal of treatment is no longer to cure it, great care must be taken to ensure that the toxic side effects of any prescribed treatments are carefully weighed against an achievable quality of life. Toxicology that was considered appropriate during active therapy might not be acceptable to the child who is dying.

5.1.7. Treatment Approaches

For every patient, a cure and a higher quality of life are the ultimate goals of treatment. To accomplish this, a variety of treatment modalities will be employed.

- **Single Agent Versus Combination:** Combination medication regimens have long been known to dramatically raise the likelihood of total remission. This is so that drug resistance to individual agents can be overcome through combination regimens. To minimize treatment-related morbidity, it is customary to choose medications with distinct toxic effects when treating a given tumor.
- **Adjuvant Chemotherapy:** Adjuvant chemotherapy is a term that is occasionally used to refer to treatment that is administered in addition to other forms of treatment, like radiotherapy or surgery. This works especially well for patients with solid tumors, for example, who have a high chance of relapsing at metastatic sites.
- **Neo-adjuvant Chemotherapy:** This phrase refers to chemotherapy administered to decrease the bulk of the tumor and allow for less invasive surgical or radiotherapeutic procedures, before final localized therapy, such as radiotherapy or surgery. When chemotherapy is applied in this manner, micrometastases can also be treated earlier. Additionally, it is feasible to determine which chemotherapy drugs work best for a given patient and their specific tumor.
- **Dose-intensive Regimes:** Making sure that medications are given at the highest possible drug intensity is one strategy to combat drug resistance. There are two methods for achieving dose intensification. It is feasible to maintain the cytotoxic assault on malignant cells while allowing bone marrow recuperation by switching between myelotoxic and non-myelotoxic medications, administered at the neutropenic nadir. Another strategy is to give colony-stimulating factors along with intense chemotherapy to shorten the course of marrow aplasia.
- **Combination chemotherapy:** Combining drugs may increase their effectiveness against cancerous cells, though the exact reason for this effect is still unknown. Because tumor cells do not go through the cell cycle simultaneously, it is crucial to choose antitumor agents that act at distinct phases

of the cell cycle. Any regime's goal is to kill as many tumor cells as possible while avoiding undue toxicity. When possible, drugs with distinct toxicities will be selected; however, in cases where overlapping toxicities—such as bone marrow depression—cannot be avoided, dosage reductions or longer intervals between cycles may be required.

- **Reducing Doses:** Many of the advancements in the treatment of childhood cancers can be attributed to high-dose therapies. Randomized trials are currently being carried out to determine whether certain children can receive treatment at lower dosages without compromising effectiveness. For instance, the ongoing trial aims to identify low-risk children for acute lymphoblastic leukemia by examining minimal residual disease at different stages of the induction phase of treatment. The primary goal is to lessen the risk of infertility and secondary cancers linked to alkylating agents, as well as the cumulative, dose-related cardiotoxic effects of the anthracyclines. It is hoped that by lowering the overall dosages administered, switching to less toxic equivalents of effective medications, and, when feasible, staying away from anthracyclines and alkylating agents entirely, the ideal balance between effective treatment and low toxicity can be reached. Children taking part in these studies will need to have their responses closely monitored so that, if needed, their treatment can be adjusted back to standard therapy.
- **Chemoprotective agents:** Cytotoxic chemotherapy has a lot of undesirable side effects and is very toxic. Alopecia and other unpleasant side effects, like nausea and vomiting, can be treated and do not pose a serious threat to health. Although bone marrow depression can be fatal, it is typically curable, particularly with dose modifications. Certain toxicities, such as the cardiotoxic effects of anthracyclines, have the potential to be fatal and can permanently harm healthy cells. Thus, there has been a lot of interest in creating medications that could prevent the harmful effects of chemotherapy while still having antitumor effects. These developments include methotrexate (folinic acid), ifosfamide (mesna), and doxorubicin (liposomal preparations and cardio-protective agents) as well as rescue and chemoprotective drugs.
- **Administration Schedules:** The potential benefits of extended drug administration to reduce toxicity are being investigated. Slow administration over several days is believed to decrease the toxicity associated with peak serum levels of certain drugs like anthracyclines. However, the advantages of these longer regimens over shorter infusions have not been proven, as prolonged infusion time may amplify other side effects like mucositis.

5.2. Antimicrobial Agents

Chemotherapy, the medical treatment for infectious diseases brought on by bacteria, viruses, fungi, and parasites, depends heavily on antimicrobial agents. These substances either kill or stop the growth of microorganisms by focusing on particular parts or functions that are necessary for their survival.

5.2.1. Mechanisms of Action of Antimicrobial Agents

There are six basic mechanisms of antimicrobial agents presented below:

1. Inhibition of microbial cell wall synthesis.
2. Inhibition of microbial cell membrane function.
3. Inhibition of microbial protein synthesis.
4. Inhibition of microbial DNA synthesis.
5. Inhibition of microbial RNA synthesis.
6. Inhibition of microbial metabolic pathways.

5.2.1.1. Inhibition of Microbial Cell Wall Synthesis

The cell wall is a crucial component of microorganisms that determines the shape of the cell. Moreover, the cell wall inhibits cell lysis and makes it easier for extracellular proteins like adhesins to be anchored due to the high cytoplasmic osmotic pressure. With so many antimicrobial drugs in clinical use, bacterial cell wall synthesis may now be the target field most frequently exploited for antimicrobial production. The components of the machinery involved in cell wall synthesis are attractive targets for antimicrobials because they have no counterparts in human biology. This provides intrinsic objective selectivity. The successive late steps in cell wall synthesis consist of the cytoplasmic synthesis of building blocks known as MGP subunits, which are N-acetyl muramic acid (M) linked to N-acetyl glucosamine (G) with an attached pentapeptide (P) side chain. Following translocation through the cytoplasmic membrane to the exterior, or periplasmic space, of the cell is made possible by the attachment of the MGP subunit to the lipid II molecule. The MGP subunits are then put together into a linear backbone by transglycozylase enzymes, which catalyze glycosidic bonds between the M and G components of the subunits. An immature peptidoglycan structure is made up of MGP subunits that are linearly connected. After that, transpeptidase enzymes function to cross-link pentaglycine bridges to the peptide side chains. During this process, the peptide side chain's terminal two D-alanines are cleaved to produce the mature, lattice-like peptidoglycan that gives the bacterium its shape and osmotic stability. The most commonly used antibiotics that stop cell wall biosynthesis are β-lactams, like cephalosporins and penicillins. These β-lactam antibiotics efficiently inhibit bacterial transpeptidases through direct interaction. Because β-lactams are transpeptidase inhibitors and prevent the maturation of peptidoglycan, these enzymes are also known as penicillin-binding proteins (PBPs). They can do this because of the β-lactam moiety's stereochemical similarity with the D-alanine-D-alanine substrate. In the presence of the medication, transpeptidases form a deadly covalent penicilloyl enzyme complex that aids in inhibiting the typical transpeptidation reaction. This leads to the formation of weakly cross-linked peptidoglycan, which renders the developing bacteria highly vulnerable to cell lysis and eventual death.

5.2.1.2. Inhibition of Microbial Cell Membrane Function

In essence, biological membranes are the building blocks of lipids, proteins, and lipoproteins. Diffusion barriers for water, ions, nutrients, and transport systems are provided by the cytoplasmic membrane. Nowadays, the majority of healthcare professionals believe that membranes are made of a lipid matrix through which uniformly distributed globular proteins can pass through the lipid bilayer. Several antimicrobial agents have the potential to cause membrane disarray. These substances fall into three groups: neutral, cationic, and anionic. The two most well-known substances are colistemethate (polymyxin E) and polymyxin B. Many antimicrobial agents rely on the cytoplasmic membrane as a crucial barrier.

Certain antimicrobial agents may work by increasing membrane permeability, which facilitates the passage of other compounds as well as the antimicrobial agents. Antibacterial cationic agents, hydrophobic compounds, like polymyxin B, and enhanced permeability of the outer membrane to lysozyme have been identified. These antimicrobial agents first work by rupturing the outer membrane's structure, which permits the cell to bind to other substances and impedes specific metabolic processes.

There are several cell-damaging properties of Polymixin B:

i. The surface charge, lipid composition and membrane structure are disturbed;

ii. The K^+ gradient on the cytoplasmic membrane is dissipated; and

iii. The cytoplasmic membrane is depolarized. One of the key factors regulating bacterial exposure to polymixin B is the permeability of the external membrane to lipophilic compounds.

The packing order of lipopolysaccharides (LPS) is altered in the presence of polymixin B because it is bulkier than the inorganic divalent cations it replaces. Many molecules become more permeable to the outer membrane as a result, and polymixin B uptake—also known as "self-promoted" uptake—is also encouraged.

5.2.1.3. Inhibition of Microbial Protein Synthesis

Inhibiting the synthesis of bacterial proteins (ribosome function) is how many different classes of antimicrobial agents function. This group of drugs includes oxazolidinones, aminoglycosides, macrolides, tetracyclines, ketolides, lincosamides, streptogramins, and chloramphenicol. Together with cytoplasmic factors, ribosomes drive the synthesis of microbial proteins. These factors bind temporarily to particles during the initiation, elongation, and termination phases of the process. The 70S particles found in microbial ribosomes are made up of two 50S and 30S subunits that combine during the beginning of protein synthesis and split during the end. Antimicrobial agents interfere with the function of either ribosomes or cytoplasmic factors in bacterial protein synthesis, blocking different steps in the process. The majority of inhibitors that attach to the 30S ribosomal subunit disrupt initiation, but some also disrupt the pairing of the AA-tRNA anticodon with the mRNA codon, impairing elongation. The steps in the elongation process interact with elongation factors that are momentarily attached to ribosomes at specific stages of the cycle or with inhibitors that bind to the 50S ribosomal subunit.

Aminoglycosides work by binding to specific ribosomal subunits. Aminoglycoside-type medications have the ability to misread and induce the formation of aberrant, non-functional complexes, which can then combine with other binding sites on 30S ribosomes to kill bacteria. The aminoglycosides of aminocylitol are closely associated with the antimicrobial agent streptomycin. It attaches itself to a specific ribosome protein and exhibits bacteriostatic, but not bactericidal, properties. Other substances that bind to 30S ribosomes are tetracyclines. These substances usually prevent aminoacyl tRNA from attaching to the bacterial ribosome's A site. Tetracycline is bacteriostatic for these agents because of its transient binding. However, a variety of bacteria, including mycoplasmas and chlamydias, are highly beneficial agents that are inhibited. The ribosomal subunit of 50S is inhibited by three main classes of medications. Chloramphenicol is a bacteriostatic agent that inhibits both gram-positive and gram-negative bacteria. It inhibits the formation of peptide bonds by attaching itself to a peptidyltransferase enzyme on the 50S ribosome. Large lactone ring compounds known as macrolides attach to 50S ribosomes and tend to hinder peptidyltransferase translocation, reaction, or both. The most important macrolide is erythromycin, which inhibits gram-posi Mycoplasma. Newer drugs like azithromycin and clarithromycin are more effective than erythromycin against many of these pathogens. Clindamycin is the most significant liginoid that has a comparable site of activity. Typically, lincinoids and macrolides are bacteriostatic; they only prevent the synthesis of new peptide chains.

5.2.1.4. Inhibition of Microbial DNA Synthesis

DNA synthesis, mRNA transcription, and cell division all require reactions. DNA topoisomerase enzymes are divided into two groups, I and II, based on whether they catalyze reactions involving the transient breakage of either (type I) or both (type II) strands of DNA. Protein translation and cell replication depend on the topological state of DNA, which is controlled by topoisomerases inside cells. DNA gyrase is a type II DNA topoisomerase that negatively supercoils DNA when ATP is present. Additionally, this enzyme untangles DNA knots, relaxes negatively supercoiled DNA, and contributes to the decatenation and catenation reaction of a double-stranded DNA circle in the absence of ATP. Because of this, the enzyme is essential for practically all cellular processes involving duplex DNA, such as transcription, recombination, and replication. It is specific to the prokaryotic kingdom and vital to the survival of the organism. Thus, DNA gyrase continues to be a desirable and ideal target for antibacterial medications. Quinolones are the most potent antimicrobial agents that target DNA gyrase. The compounds came from nalidixic acid, a naphthyridone that was unintentionally found as a by-product during the synthesis of chloroquine.

Quinolones are distinct inhibitors of DNA gyrase. Quinolones inhibit DNA gyrase reactions, specifically the breakage-reunion reaction by interacting with subunit A (GyrA). This includes supercoiling and relaxation, which involve DNA breakage and reunion. Nalidixic acid and oxolinic acid, the first-generation quinolones, have comparatively weak antimicrobial activity. However, a number of powerful antimicrobial agents have been produced as a result of the synthesis and development of fluoroquinolones over many generations, including norfloxacin and ciprofloxacin (second generation), levofloxacin (third generation), and moxifloxacin and gemifloxacin (fourth generation). In addition to type II topoisomerases, the majority of bacterial pathogens also contain topoisomerase I (Topo I), an additional essential topoisomerase. Since Topo I differs from Gyrase and Topoisomerase IV in both architecture and mechanism, it is a promising candidate for the discovery of novel antibacterial chemotypes.

5.2.1.5. Inhibition of Microbial RNA Synthesis

By binding the DNA-bound and highly-effective transcription RNA polymerase to the β-subunit, rifamycins inhibit DNA-dependent transcription. The β-subunit is found in the channel created by the RNA polymerase-DNA complex, which is where the freshly synthesized RNA strand emerges. Because rifamycins can sterically inhibit the initialization of nascent RNA strands, it is evident that RNA synthesis must not have advanced past the addition of two ribonucleotides. Note that rifamycins are not thought to function by preventing the elongation stage of RNA synthesis; however, a new class of RNA polymerase inhibitors based on the CBR703 compound may prevent elongation by altering the enzyme allosterically.

5.2.1.6. Inhibition of Microbial Metabolic Pathways

Trimethoprim and sulfonamides disrupt folic acid metabolism in the microbial cell by competitively inhibiting the biosynthesis of tetrahydrofolate, which functions as a carrier of one-carbon fragments and is necessary for the final synthesis of DNA, RNA, and bacterial cell wall proteins. Unlike mammals, bacteria and protozoan parasites usually do not have a transport mechanism that allows them to remove preformed folic acid from their host. While some of these species can use exogenous thymidine, most of them must synthesize folic acid to avoid requiring folic acid metabolism. Sulfonamides competitively inhibit pteridine synthetase's ability to convert pteridine and p-aminobenzoic acid (PABA) to dihydrofolic acid. Pteridine synthetase is more receptive to sulfonamides than is PABA. When trimethoprim is bound to bacterial dihydrofolate reductase, it inhibits tetrahydrofolate synthesis. This affinity is 10,000–100,000 times greater than that of the mammalian enzyme.

5.2.2. Mechanisms of Resistance to Antimicrobial Agents

Antimicrobial resistance is, in general, the ability of an organism to withstand the effects of an antimicrobial agent to which it was previously susceptible. Antibiotic-resistant *P. aeruginosa* bacteria-related nosocomial infections have become a significant concern in clinical care settings due to the increasing production of MDR strains, which are resistant to at least three antibiotics. Since its outer membrane has a low permeability (1/100 of that of the outer membrane of *E. coli*), *P. aeruginosa* demonstrates inherent resistance to a range of antimicrobial substances (including the β-lactam and penem classes of antibiotics). Their intrinsic resistance is also caused by many other mechanisms, such as the efflux system, which drives antibiotics out of the bacteria in the cell, and the synthesis of inactivating enzyme antibiotics. On the other hand, this bacterium is an extremely versatile pathogen that can adjust to its surroundings. The mediated response strengthens bacterial resistance to antibiotics and promotes bacterial survival when exposed to selective pressure from antibiotics.

P. aeruginosa strains have been shown to develop and become resistant to antibiotics during antimicrobial therapy, confirming the development of antibiotic resistance during host colonization in CF patients. Research has demonstrated a direct correlation between an increase in ciprofloxacin applications and the emergence of ciprofloxacin-resistant strains. Thus, another factor linked to the rise in MDR-*Psedomonas aeruginosa* is the overuse of antimicrobial agents. This acquired resistance can result from the over-expression of endogenous β-lactamases or efflux pump, or it can be caused by the acquisition of the resistance gene through horizontal gene transfer. It can also occur during the mutational event of antibiotic therapy.

5.2.2.1. Resistance to β-lactam

β-lactam antibiotics are necessary to inhibit the synthesis of the bacterial peptidoglycan cell wall. This class includes monobactam, carbapenem, cephalosporin, and penicillin. These classes include imipenem, meropenem, doripenem (carbapenems), aztreonam (monobactam), ceftazidime (third-generation cephalosporin), cefepime (fourth-generation cephalosporin), and piperacillin and ticarcillin (penicillin). The most potent β-lactam that is frequently used to treat *P. aeruginosa* is β-lactam. Due to resistance to β-lactam mediated by β-lactamases, these enzymes break the amide bond of the β-lactam ring, making the antimicrobial ineffective. This drug inactivation may be the cause of either the expression of acquired or endogenous β-lactamases. The substrate specificity of the hundreds of β-lactamases that have been identified to date sets them apart. Amber's molecular classification system divides beta-lactamases into four main groups that are known to exist in *P. aeruginosa*: A-D. Classes A, C, and D inactivate β-lactams through their serine-residue catalytic activity, whereas class B, also known as metallo-β-lactamases (MBLs), need zinc to function.

5.2.2.2. AmpC β-lactamase (Cephelosporinase)

Specifically, the emergence of endogenous β-lactamases, like chromosomal cephalosporinase (AmpC β-lactamase). Numerous β-lactam antibiotics, including imipenem, benzyl penicillin, and narrow-spectrum cephalosporin, can be induced in *P. aeruginosa*. Of course, *P. aeruginosa*is susceptible to ceftazidime, aztreonam, and carboxypenicillins; however, it can acquire resistance due to a mutation in the gene that causes an excess of AmpC β-lactamase. The enzyme is typically expressed at a "low-level," where resistance to aminopenicillins and the majority of early cephalosporins is established. According to Bush et al., *P. aeruginosa* produces an inducible chromosome-coded AmpC β-lactamase (cephalosporinase), which is the first functional group and a member of the Ambler-based molecular class C.

Nonetheless, when β-lactams (particularly imipenem) are present, the chromosomal cephalosporin production can multiply 100–1000 times. AmpC cephalosporinase function is not inhibited by β-lactamase inhibitors used in clinical practice, such as clavulanic acid, sulbactam, and tazobactam. The gene ampC encodes the β-lactamase of ampC. AmpC gene induction involves many genes, including ampR, ampG, and ampD. A positive transcriptional regulator that is required for the induction of β-lactamase is encoded by AmpR. The second gene involved is AmpG, a transmembrane protein that serves as a permease for 1,6-anhydromurapeptides, which are known to be the signal molecules responsible for ampC's induction. The cytosolic amidase of N-acetyl-anhydromuramyl-L-alanine, which is encoded by the third gene, ampD, hydrolyzes 1,6-anhydromurapeptides and suppresses the expression of ampC. The cytoplasmic membrane protein that functions as the sensory transducer molecule required for induction is encoded by the ampE gene, which is located on the fourth chromosome. Commercially available β-lactam does not inhibit the activity of this AmpC β-lactamase, except avibactam.

5.2.2.3. Class A Carbenicillin Hydrolyzing β-Lactamases

In P, four β-lactamases (PSE- of Pseudomonas-specific enzyme) that hydrolyze carbenicillin were found. aeruginosa: CARB-3, CARB-4, PSE-1 (CARB-2), and PSE-4 (CARB-1). These enzymes have a substrate profile that includes cefsulodine, carboxypenicillins, and ureidopenicillins. They are classified as β-lactamases in molecular class A. These enzymes are members of molecular class A and functional group 2c. This β-lactamase can be inhibited by commercially available β-lactam inhibitors, such as clavulanic acid, tazobactam, and sulbactam.

5.2.2.4. Resistance to Aminoglycoside

Aminoglycosides are a class of microbial inhibitors of protein synthesis that work by attaching to the bacterial 30S ribosomal subunit and preventing the start of protein synthesis. Transferable aminoglycoside modifying enzymes (AMEs), low outer membrane permeability, active efflux, and, in rare instances, target modification are the mechanisms by which Pseudomonas develops resistance to aminoglycosides.

5.2.2.5. Aminoglycoside-Modifying Enzymes

By combining the antibiotic molecule with a phosphate, adenyl, or acetyl radical, AMEs render the aminoglycoside inactive. As a result, modified antibiotics reduce the bacterial cell's (30S ribosomal subunit) affinity for binding to its target. Three types of aminoglycoside altering enzymes (AMEs) are involved in aminoglycoside alteration: aminoglycoside phosphoryl transferases (APHs), aminoglycoside adenylyl transferases (also called nucleotidyltransferases) (AADs or ANTs), and aminoglycoside acetyltransferases (AACs). The AMEs that *P. aeruginosa* most frequently expresses are listed below. The *P. aeruginosa* strain is resistant to gentamicin, tobramycin, and netilmicin. It is also known by the resistance codes AAC(69)-II, AAC(3)-I, and AAC(3)-II. Additionally, strains (69)-I, (69)-II, (69)-I, (69)-I, and ANT(29)-I are resistant to tobramycin and gentamicin.

The following AMEs are most commonly expressed by *P. aeruginosa*: AAC(69)-II (resistant to gentamicin, tobramycin and netilmicin), AAC(3)-I (resistant to gentamicin), AAC(3)-II (resistant to gentamicin, tobramycin and netilmicin), (69)-I (resistant to tobramycin, netilmicin and amicacin) and ANT(29)-I (resistant to tobramicin and gentamicin).

5.2.2.6. Low Outer Membrane Permeability

A mechanism known to confer resistance to various antibiotic forms, such as aminoglycosides, β-lactams, and quinolones, is membrane impermeability or reduced permeability. For example, isolates with cystic fibrosis that are continuously exposed to antibiotics frequently exhibit this resistance mechanism. Membrane impermeability can result from many processes, including modifications to lipopolysaccharide (LPS), changes to membranous proteins involved in substratum absorption, and inactivation of enzymatic complexes involved in the energetic membrane required for transport system activity.

5.2.2.7. Active Efflux Pumps

Low membrane permeability and active efflux pumps are partly caused by P. aeruginosa's innate resistance to several antibiotic classes. The antibiotic resistance-related efflux systems of *P. aeruginosa* are members of the resistance-nodulation-division (RND) family. There are four main efflux systems that have been described that confer resistance to multiple antibiotics: MexAB-OprM, MexCDOprJ, MexEF-OprN, and MexXY-OprM.

These systems consist of three proteins:

i. the efflux pump protein found in the cytoplasmic membrane (MexB, MexD, MexF and MexY),
ii. the pore-acting outer membrane protein (OprM, OprJ and OprN) and
iii. A protein in the periplasmic space that bridges the cytoplasmic and outer membrane proteins (MexA, MexC, MexE and MexX).

MexAB-OprM and MexXY-OprM are active in both natural and acquired resistance, while only the other two mechanisms are seen in cumulative resistance.

When these efflux systems are overexpressed, acquired resistance is seen as a result of mutations in the regulatory systems, which can be brought on by antibiotic pressure and confer resistance to all antibiotic classes. Exposure to a single antibiotic can result in resistance to several antibiotic classes that are substrates of these efflux systems.

Quinolones are an essential trigger factor that can produce cross-resistance to the efflux systems of several major antibiotic classes, such as aminoglycosides and β-lactams, for pseudomonal therapy. They are substrates of all efflux systems. It is known that efflux systems provide a moderate level of resistance, but they usually work in tandem with other resistance mechanisms to contribute to the high-level resistance seen in *P. aeruginosa*.

5.2.2.8. Target modification

Bacteria can develop resistance to aminoglycosides because of the drug's low affinity for the bacterial ribosome. 16S rRNA methylation through target modification can accomplish this. In the case of *P. aeruginosa*, several 16S rRNA methylases have been identified: RmtA, which was initially observed in clinical isolates of the bacteria resistant to aminoglycosides and which gave resistance to all aminoglycosides administered parenterally, such as amicacin, tobramycin, isepamicin, kanamycin, arbecacin, and gentamicin; secondary 16S rRNA methylases include RmtB, ArmA, and RmtD.

5.2.2.9. Resistance to fluoroquinolones

The bacterial chromosome gene that codes for topoisomerase 1 V or DNA gyrase can be mutated to cause resistance to fluoroquinolones, or the drug can be successfully transported outside of the cell. Within the motif of the quinolone-resistant determinative region (QRDR), which is thought to be the enzyme's active site, gyrA and gyrB genes are susceptible to Topoisomerase 1 V mutations. This results in modified topoisomerase II with a low affinity for quinolone molecules due to changes in the amino acid sequences of subunits A and B. Point mutations in the parC and parE genes, which encode the ParC and ParE enzyme subunits, modify topoisomerase IV, a secondary target.

The over-expression of efflux includes other types of fluoroquinolone tolerance in Pseudomonas. Mutations in the nalB, nfxB and nfxC genes, resulting in overexpression of MexA-MexB-OprM, MexC-MexD- OprJ and MexE- MexF-OprN fallowing efflux.

5.2.2.10. Biofilm-mediated resistance

A biofilm is a collection of microorganisms that attach themselves to one another on a surface, either living or dead, and are embedded in an extracellular polymeric matrix (EPS) made up of the substances the microorganisms produce on their own, such as proteins, metabolites, eDNA, and exopolysaccharides. When it comes to antimicrobial agents and the host immune response, microbial cells cultivated in biofilms are less sensitive than cells grown in free aqueous suspension.

When bacteria form a biofilm, they can become less susceptible to antibiotics, even if they lack protective mutations in their intrinsic resistance.

The general mechanisms of biofilm-mediated resistance that shield bacteria against antibiotic attack include the induction of an adaptive stress response, the differentiation of persistent cells, and the prevention of antibiotic penetration by an altered microenvironment that promotes slow biofilm cell growth.

P. aeruginosa causes long-term lung infections in patients with cystic fibrosis by forming biofilms on lung epithelial cells with the help of DNA, proteins, and exopolysaccharides. The regulation of biofilm formation by *P. aeruginosa* is complex and relies on quorum sensing systems such as GacS/GacA and RetS/LadS, as well as exopolysaccharides and cdi-GMP. Quorum sensing is a communication method between bacterial cells that controls gene expression in response to changes in cell population. *P. aeruginosa*has three quorum sensing systems that contribute to mature biofilm formation. During biofilm formation, *P. aeruginosa* undergoes various physiological and phenotypic changes, such as transitioning to a mucoid phenotype with increased alginate production, enabling biofilm colony formation. The flagellum of *P. aeruginosa* plays a key role in initiating biofilm formation through swarming and twitching motility. However, *P. aeruginosa* decreases flagellum expression after attaching to a surface and may lose it permanently due to genetic mutations, evading immune detection and phagocytosis.

5.3. Novel Alternative Antimicrobial Therapy for P. aeruginosa Treatment

Antibiotic abuse and overuse, which can result in unfavorable side effects and the emergence of bacterial strains resistant to drugs, is a developing public health concern. Furthermore, the synthesis of novel antibiotics is timely and extremely constrained. Therefore, it is very desirable to develop novel therapeutic approaches to treat *P. aeruginosa* infections, and over the past ten years, there has been increased interest in this area. These novel therapeutic approaches include the use of iron chelation, nanoparticles, probiotics, phage therapy, antimicrobial peptides, and vaccine strategies. They also involve the inhibition of quorum sensing.

5.3.1. Antimicrobial Peptides

Antimicrobial peptides (AMPs), also known as host defense peptides, are produced by a variety of species, including animals and bacteria, and they have broad antimicrobial activity. The mode(s) of operation of AMPs are not fully understood. Most people agree that AMPs attack the cytoplasmic membrane, which results in cell death. Along with their antimicrobial activity, AMPs have also been demonstrated to have anti-biofilm and immunomodulatory qualities. Because of their broad-spectrum activity, AMPs have been suggested as a potential substitute for conventional antibiotics in the treatment of bacterial infections. They also have low levels of host toxicity, quick killing kinetics, and low levels of mediated resistance. Numerous peptides with antimicrobial properties, such as GL13 K, LL-37, T9W, NLF20, cecropin P1, indolicidin, magainin II, nisin, ranalexin, melittin, and defensin, have shown potent antimicrobial activity against *P. aeruginosa* through direct bactericidal effects or disruption of biofilms. Furthermore, certain AMPs have shown to work in concert with conventional antibiotics to combat a variety of bacteria, including *P. aeruginosa*, by promoting antibiotic absorption, interfering with the formation of biofilms, or suppressing bacterial quorum. For example, it has been demonstrated that GL13 K plus tobramycin increased the clearance of *P. aeruginosa* biofilm. Zheng and colleagues found that the minimum inhibitory concentration of cecropin A2 against clinical isolates of *P. aeruginosa* was lowered eight times when combined with tetracycline in vitro.

5.3.2. Phage Therapy

Bacteriophages are viruses that infect and kill bacteria by causing lysis. Phages were first identified in 1915 by the British bacteriologist Frederick Twort. A similar discovery was made independently in Paris two years later by Félix D'Herelle, who also introduced the idea of phage therapy. Phage therapy was abandoned in several countries with the introduction of antibiotic therapy, but it has continued to be developed in Eastern European countries, including Warsaw, Poland, and Tbilisi, Georgia. The phage cocktails available in Georgian and Russian pharmacies contained antipseudomonal phages, as demonstrated by shotgun metagenome sequencing. Few case reports from Belgium and the US have documented the successful treatment of MDR *P. aeruginosa* infections, but this approach is not widely recognized in the West. Replication at the infection site, high precision in targeting bacteria without harming commensal flora, fewer side effects compared to other therapies, bactericidal activity against antibiotic-resistant bacteria, and ease of administration are just a few advantages of phage therapy. Phages have been studied extensively as a potential antibiotic substitute for treating *P. aeruginosa* infections. As many as 137 distinct phages that target the Pseudomonas genus have been described. The effectiveness of phages against persistent P. *aeruginosa* infections has been investigated in numerous in vitro and in vivo investigations. For example, it has been demonstrated that co-cultivating phage PA709 with the clinical strain *P. aeruginosa* 709 dramatically lowers its viability. According to another study, administering P3-CHA bacteriophage intranasally to mice given a deadly dose of Paeruginosa strain CHA significantly increased the mice's survival rate and decreased the amount of bacteria in their lungs.

Phage therapy also has the advantage of allowing for the genetic modification of phages to act as carriers of antimicrobial agents, which increases the effectiveness of treatment. Although phages have demonstrated efficacy against bacterial infection in vitro and in animal models, there have been relatively few phage therapy clinical trials conducted thus far. This is due to a number of factors, such as inadequate stability of phage preparations, safety concerns regarding post-treatment phage clearance and impurity, ignorance of the complete phage mechanism of action, and bacterial resistance to phage growth. Phages have been used in clinical trials to treat *P. aeruginosa* infections in patients with burn wounds, venous leg ulcers, and otitis; during these trials, no unfavorable reactions were noted.

5.3.3. Quorum Sensing Inhibition

Bacteria can control gene expression according to cell density through a process called quorum sensing. Quorum sensing is a mechanism used by *P. aeruginosa* to regulate virulence and biofilm formation. The production of the signal molecules for N-acyl homoserine lactone (AHL), N-(3-oxododecanoyl)-L-homoserine lactone (3O-C12-HSL), and N-butanoyl-L-homoserine lactone (C4-HSL) is carried out by the two main *P. aeruginosa* quorum-sensing systems, Las and Rhl. The virulence factors, namely elastase, proteases, pyocyanin, lectins, rhamnolipids, and toxins, are expressed and biofilms are formed when 3O-C12-HSL and C4-HSL bind to and activate their respective RhlR and LasR cognate transcription factors. Together with the LasI-LasR and RhlI-RhlR systems, it has also been reported that the third *P. aeruginosa* quorum-sensing system, PQSMvfR, promotes the formation of biofilms. This mechanism controls the pqsABCDE operon, which in turn controls the transcriptional regulator MvfR, also known as PqsR, and the development of the 2-heptyl-3-hydroxy-4-quinolone, or *P. seudomonas* quinolone signal (PQS). Furthermore, the formation of biofilms has been linked to the PqsA and PqsD proteins.

One method that shows promise for treating *P. aeruginosa* infections is quorum sensing inhibition. This strategy has a low chance of bacterial resistance developing and can stop or lessen the formation of biofilms, which lowers bacterial virulence. Furthermore, the scope of this strategy is limited, making it impossible for it to have any unintentional inhibitory effects on beneficial bacteria. Quorum sensing inhibitors for the Las and Rhl systems can be natural or synthetic, and they can degrade AHLs, reduce AHL synthase activity, prevent AHL from developing, or compete with AHL receptor binding. The use of quorum sensing inhibitors to treat *P. aeruginosa* infections has been the subject of extensive research in recent years. Typically present in plants, algae, and lichens, the carotenoid zeaxanthin, for instance, inhibited the formation of biofilms in *P. aeruginosa* by binding to the quorum sensing signal receptors, lasR and RhlR, and preventing the expression of virulence genes, lasB and rhlA. A class of naturally occurring plant metabolites known as flavonoids has demonstrated the ability to function as LasR and RhlR antagonists, thereby significantly reducing their capacity to bind to the *P. aeruginosa* promoters of genes regulated by quorum sensing.

5.3.4. Iron Chelation

In addition to being necessary for bacterial growth, iron is also involved in many other cellular functions like electron transport, DNA replication, and electricity production. Human sputum from CF patients was found to have a significantly higher iron content than that of healthy individuals, suggesting that a higher iron intake may contribute to long-term CF lung infections. Pyoverdine and pyochelin siderophores are used by *P. aeruginosa* to extract iron from the extracellular milieu. Therefore, reducing the amount of extracellular iron or interfering with the ability of *P. aeruginosa* to absorb iron is one way to combat infections caused by this bacteria. Numerous researches have connected iron metabolism to the etiology of persistent infections, suggesting that iron chelators and analogs could be useful therapeutic agents against *P. aeruginosa*. For instance, it has been reported that iron chelators such as 2,2′-dipyridyl (2DP), diethylenetriamine pentacetic acid (DTPA), and EDTA inhibit *P. aeruginosa* growth and biofilm formation; these chelators are more effective in anaerobic environments.

The US FDA has approved gallium as a medication for the treatment of cancer-associated hypercalcemia because it is a nonredox iron III analog that acts as an iron replacement in several biological processes, disrupting the metabolism of bacterial iron. Kaneko and associates. found that by lowering the uptake of bacterial iron and suppressing the synthesis of pyoverdine mediated by the transcriptional regulator PvdS, gallium was able to inhibit the growth of *P. aeruginosa*, prevent the formation of biofilms, and exhibit excellent bactericidal activity in vitro. Furthermore, it has been discovered that gallium efficiently eradicates *P. aeruginosa* in mouse infection models.

5.3.5. Nanoparticles

Nanoparticles are currently being used extensively to treat a wide range of diseases, including cancer and bacterial infectious diseases. Nanoparticles are tiny materials with a large surface area to mass ratio and a size of less than 100 nm that have been used in numerous chemical, biological, and biomedical applications. The antimicrobial activity of the nanoparticles is attributed to their high membrane penetration, potential to disrupt biofilm formation, multiple antimicrobial mechanisms, and potent antibiotic carrier capabilities. Metallic and antimicrobial agent-loaded nanoparticles have been studied extensively for the prevention of *P. aeruginosa* infections. For instance, silver nanoparticles are potent antimicrobial agents that produce silver ions that inhibit bacterial enzymatic systems, including DNA synthesis. When applied to clinical strains of *P. aeruginosa*, silver nanoparticles have demonstrated significant antimicrobial effects, effectively eliminating the bacteria and preventing its growth in vitro. Furthermore, silver nanoparticles have shown minimal cytotoxicity to mammalian cells, though further in vivo studies are needed to confirm this.

As previously mentioned, antimicrobial agents like antibiotics can be delivered to bacteria via nanoparticles. Kwon and associates created porous silicon nanoparticles that included membrane-interacting peptides and a unique antimicrobial peptide fused with a synthetic bacterial toxin. To improve the survival rate and bacterial clearance, this engineered nanoparticle was found to be effective in a mouse model of lung infection caused by *P. aeruginosa*. Furthermore, it has been discovered that the efficiency of both antibiotics and nanoparticles is significantly increased when they bind to the surfaces of the latter. When it comes to killing ampicillin-resistant *P. aeruginosa* isolates in vitro, silver ampicillin-attached nanoparticles outperform silver ampicillin-attached nanoparticles in this regard.

5.3.6. Probiotic as an Alternative Antimicrobial Therapy

Living microorganisms known as probiotics have health benefits when consumed in the right amounts. Most probiotic bacteria (e.g., Lactobacillus and Bifidobacterium) are gram-positive, and their main roles involve the regulation and maintenance of intestinal tract health. The greatest number of probiotics are found in the intestines of human hosts. Improved nutrient synthesis, host immune system differentiation, and infection tolerance are all attributed to the commensal intestinal microbiome. *P. aeruginosa* was tested against the probiotic *Pediococcus acidilactici* HW01 that decreased the production of protease and rhamnolipids, decreased pyocyanin development, and decreased formation of biofilms on the surface of stainless steel. Another study carried out by Moraes and colleagues demonstrated the efficacy of *Bifidobacterium bifidum* and *Lactobacillus brevis* against *S. aureus* biofilms grown on titanium discs. The findings showed a decrease in *S. aureus* growth on titanium discs when both probiotics were used, but *L. brevis* was shown to have the greatest inhibitory effect on biofilm formation.

5.3.7. Vaccine Strategy

A vaccine strategy's basic idea is to prevent infection until a vaccine can be made. The goal of vaccine development is to stop and lessen *P. aeruginosa* infections. There isn't currently an approved vaccination against this infection, though. Pathogenesis-causing bacterium *P. aeruginosa* antigens elicit strong immune responses. LPS O-antigen, polysaccharide protein conjugates, outer membrane proteins OprF and OprI, type III secretion system portion PcrV, flagella, pili, DNA, live-attenuated *P. aeruginosa* vaccine candidates could include both *P. aeruginosa* and entire killed cells. Out of all the possible *P. aeruginosa* vaccines, only the flagella vaccine and the recombinant vaccine IC43, which contains OprF and OprI, were tested in phase III clinical trials on patients with cystic fibrosis. Potential candidates for *P. aeruginosa* vaccines include LPS O-antigen, polysaccharide protein conjugates, outer membrane proteins OprF and OprI, type III secretion system portion PcrV, flagella, pili, DNA, live-attenuated *P. aeruginosa*, and entire killed cells. Out of all the possible Paeruginosa vaccines, only the flagella vaccine and the recombinant vaccine IC43, which contains OprF and OprI, were tested in phase III clinical trials on patients with cystic fibrosis.

Due in part to the pathogen's capacity to change its phenotype under a variety of environmental circumstances, clinical trials have shown that the current *P. aeruginosa* vaccines are not very effective. In the lungs of CF patients, for instance, *P. aeruginosa* strains suppress the expression of highly immunogenic virulence factors like LPS O-antigen, type III secretion systems, flagella, and pili. Furthermore, compromised host defense mechanisms frequently lessen the effectiveness of vaccinations. The lung microenvironment in CF patients has become a significant obstacle to effective vaccination because of the altered mucus layer, impaired phagocytosis, dysregulated inflammatory responses, including aberrant cytokine and chemokine production, and reduced phagocyte recruitment.

5.4. Combining Immunotherapy and Targeted Therapies in Cancer Treatment

Targeted therapies function by obstructing vital biochemical pathways or mutant proteins that are necessary for the proliferation and survival of tumor cells1. In molecularly defined patient subsets, these medications can halt the progression of tumors and cause remarkable regressions. In fact, 76% of patients with chronic myelogenous leukemia experienced rapid induction of full cytogenetic responses upon treatment with imatinib, the first small molecule targeted agent. Additional oncoproteins, such as the epidermal growth factor receptor (EGFR), BRAF, KIT, HER2, and anaplastic lymphoma kinase (ALK), that are essential for tumor maintenance were discovered through further investigations into the underlying genetic pathways driving tumor proliferation. Like imatinib, small molecule inhibitors of these kinases have produced remarkable tumor responses in a subset of patients; however, because drug-resistant variants have emerged, regressions are frequently followed by the onset of progressive disease. Secondary mutations in the targeted protein or compensatory modifications in the targeted pathway that get around the drug-mediated inhibition are typically involved in resistance. As a result, although targeted therapies can cause significant tumor regressions, their overall clinical benefit is often limited by their short half-lives.

Simultaneously with these developments in identifying carcinogenic pathways, the recent victories of sipuleucel-T in Phase III clinical trials confirmed that immunotherapy can also increase the longevity of cancer patients4. Sipuleucel-T is an autologous dendritic cell (DC) vaccine that aims to stimulate T cells specific for prostatic acid phosphatase (PAP), a protein that is overexpressed in prostate carcinoma cells. It was recently approved by the US Food and Drug Administration (FDA) for use in metastatic, castration-resistant prostate cancer. While the exact mechanism of action of sipuleucel-T is still being investigated, treatment with this medication extends median survival by four months while posing little toxicity. An essential inhibitory signal for activated T cells is blocked by the antibody ipilimumab, which is directed against cytotoxic T lymphocyte antigen 4 (CTLA4). This enhances T cell responses and accelerates the destruction of tumors. Recently approved by the FDA, ipilimumab improves overall survival compared to standard care and, most notably, results in durable benefits (more than 2.5 years) for 15–20 % of treated subjects. It can be used as first-line or second-line therapy for patients with advanced melanoma. Although the majority of inflammatory toxicities are easily treated with medical intervention, blocking CTLA4 with antibody drugs is linked to a notable incidence of these side effects.

The clinical outcomes pertaining to ipilimumab demonstrate how immunotherapy can elicit enduring responses through the development of anti-tumor memory. Long-term disease control may be achieved by the heightened immune response, even though antibody treatment usually ends in a few months. The unusual pattern of clinical response with ipilimumab, which occasionally shows extended periods of stable disease or even an initial period of tumor growth before stabilization, may also be explained by a dynamic host reaction. Furthermore, ipilimumab-induced immune responses may broaden over time and diversify reactivity to several tumor-associated antigens. Despite these benefits, a significant drawback of ipilimumab is the comparatively small percentage of patients who experience clinical responses. The strong immunosuppressive effects of well-established tumors may be partially to blame for this deficiency, especially since many cancers are discovered late in life when large lesions have already developed.

The strengths and weaknesses of immunotherapy and targeted agents have been analyzed, and the results point to potential complementary roles for both treatments in the management of cancer, as well as potential synergistic effects from combinatorial therapy. Targeted therapies may provide a favorable window for immunotherapy to achieve more potent cytotoxicity because they can cause rapid tumor regressions, which in turn reduce tumor-associated immunosuppression. Furthermore, by ending oncogene "addiction," targeted therapies may enhance anti-tumor immune responses by inducing tumor senescence and promoting T cell-mediated immune clearance. Furthermore, if simultaneous DC activation can be elicited, the massive discharge of antigenic debris following tumor cell death could aid in vaccination in situ. Hence, immunotherapy may combine the potent tumor responses from targeted therapy into long-lasting, robust remissions. In these cases, sustained host responses that target several antigens may lower the likelihood of potentially fatal drug-resistant clones.

Targeted therapies have the potential to directly alter immune responses in addition to killing tumor cells. Certain immune cell populations, such as forkhead box P3 (FOXP3)$^+$ regulatory T cells (Tregs) and myeloid derived suppressor cells (MDSCs), that inhibit cytotoxic T lymphocytes (CTLs), for instance, may become less active as a result of certain targeted therapies. Other specific drugs could improve the presentation of DC tumor antigen and boost the priming of CTLs that are specific to tumors. Additionally, certain targeted treatments may make tumor cells more vulnerable to immune-mediated destruction. The complex interaction between immunotherapy and targeted agents can affect the overall anti-tumor effects and toxicity profiles of the combined treatments. Some of the parameters that may affect this interaction include timing, dosage, and sequence. Advances in the integration of targeted therapies with immunotherapy should come from a deeper comprehension of the effects these medicines have on particular molecular pathways in immune cells.

5.4.1. Activating a Multi-Faceted Immune Response against Tumor Cells

To date, the majority of single agents that target specific stages in the host anti-tumor response have been used in the clinical evaluation of immunotherapy. Since the induction, potency, and persistence of host responses are reflective of the intricate interactions between various immune cells and advancing tumors, it is unlikely that monotherapies will effectively target the primary mechanisms obstructing anti-tumor immune responses in all patients. Indeed, the successful completion of multiple immune processes is probably necessary for the generation of clinically effective anti-tumor reactions. Preclinical research suggests that combinations of treatments that focus on different stages of tumor immunity may work in concert to produce stronger and longer-lasting responses that lead to long-lasting tumor destruction (Figure 5.2).

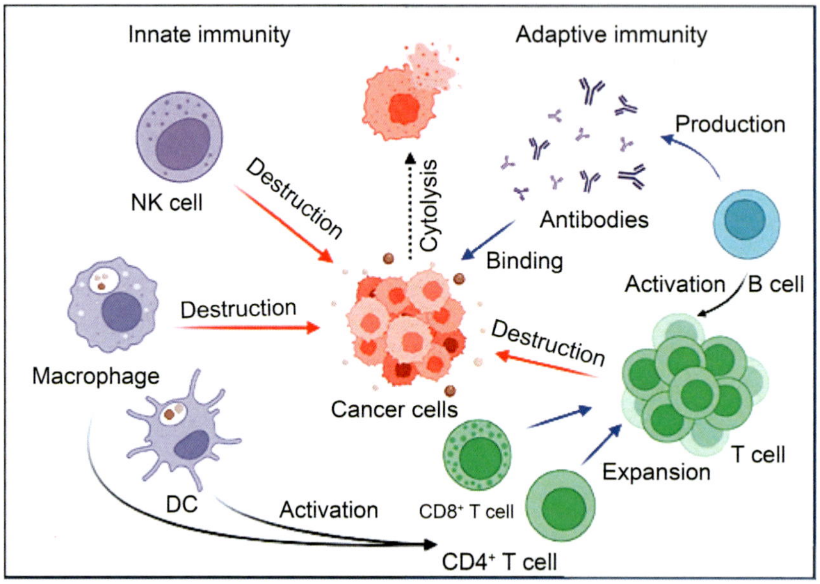

Figure 5.2. *The generation of potent anti-tumor immune responses requires multiple steps.*

Source: Prokopeva AE, Emene CC, Gomzikova MO. Antitumor Immunity: Role of NK Cells and Extracellular Vesicles in Cancer Immunotherapy. Current Issues in Molecular Biology. 2024; 46(1):140–152. https://doi.org/10.3390/cimb46010011.

Antigen-presenting cells, particularly DCs, are required to first enumerate tumor antigens, process them into major histocompatibility complex (MHC) class I and II pathways, and then display the resulting peptide epitopes in an immunogenic context to stimulate $CD4^+$ T cells and $CD8^+$ T cells, typically in a regional lymph node, to generate potent anti-tumor immunity. Although during tumor formation this process seems relatively inefficient, it can be effectively stimulated with a range of cancer vaccination strategies. Second, the T cell receptor (TCR; which determines specificity) and various costimulatory molecules must work together to promote the differentiation of tumor-specific T cells into effector cells. While costimulatory signals are delivered through multiple transmembrane proteins of the B7 and tumor necrosis factor receptor (TNFR) families, as well as receptors for some cytokines, such as interleukin-12 (IL-12), the TCR (and associated CD4 or CD8) engages MHC-peptide complexes presented on DCs. Other activating receptors under active research include 4–1BB (also known as CD137 and TNFRSF9), OX40 (also known as TNFRSF4), and glucocorticoid induced TNFR related protein (GITR; also known as TNFRSF18). In addition to the costimulatory molecule CD28, which binds B7–1 (also known as CD80) and B7–2 (also known as CD86) on DCs. Costimulation can be improved by antagonistic antibodies to these molecules, boosting anti-tumor immunity.

Third, negative regulatory signals that cause tolerance programs like fatigue or anorexia or stifle T cell activation must be avoided. Two important negative costimulatory molecules that are expressed on activated T cells are CTLA4 and programmed death 1 (PD1). Antibody blockade of PD1, like ipilimumab, has been shown to have encouraging anti-tumor effects in early clinical testing and to increase T cell function. Finally, the induced anti-tumor response needs to be able to defeat various immunosuppressive networks that may be fueled by regulatory cell populations and soluble factors in the tumor microenvironment.

5.4.2. Targeted Therapies Display Immunomodulatory Effects

Over the past 20 years, significant progress has been made in our understanding of the molecular biology of cancer. Numerous studies have revealed important pathways underlying the development and upkeep of tumors, leading to the development of well-thought-out medications that may inhibit these circuits. It's interesting to note that several of the targeted pathways are also important for immune cell development, activation, differentiation, and function. As a result, a few of the targeted substances exhibit significant immunomodulatory qualities. Targeted agents can, like more conventional immunotherapies, affect many different aspects of the immune response: they can strengthen tumor antigen presentation and T cell priming; they can improve T cell activation, effector function, and differentiation; they can sensitize tumor cells to immune effector cell killing; and they can counteract tumor-mediated immune suppression. These actions give rise to the intriguing possibility that the host may play a role in some way in the anti-tumor efficacy of targeted therapies.

5.4.3. Targeted Therapies may Augment Tumor Antigen Presentation and T Cell Priming

DCs play a crucial role in activating anti-tumor T cells by internalizing antibody-antigen immune complexes through their Fc receptors. Monoclonal antibodies, such as trastuzumab and cetuximab targeting HER2 and EGFR, respectively, aid in DC[2] uptake of tumor antigens, leading to the stimulation of tumor-specific $CD4^+$ and $CD8^+$ T cells. These antibodies not only inhibit oncogenic signaling but also enhance tumor antigen presentation by forming immune complexes, ultimately boosting the generation of tumor-specific T cells. Studies have shown that patients treated with trastuzumab exhibit a strong T-cell response and improved clinical outcomes. Animal experiments have further demonstrated that the effectiveness of HER2 antibodies depends on Fc receptors and $CD8^+$ T cells, resulting in the production of more tumor-specific T cells compared to control groups (Figure 5.3).

These changes in antigen presentation caused by monoclonal antibodies point to a possible cooperative relationship with cancer vaccines. Mice that received both a cancer cell vaccine and HER2 antibodies in a transgenic mouse model of breast cancer showed noticeably longer survival than either treatment alone. When compared to either agent alone, the combination therapy boosted DC expression of costimulatory molecules like CD40, CD80, and CD86, increased DC uptake of the cancer vaccine cells, and increased tumor-specific T cell responses. In line with these results, a recent Phase I/II clinical trial using a HER2 peptide vaccine in combination with trastuzumab revealed that 70% of patients showed signs of "epitope spreading," which is the targeting of HER2 peptides not included in the vaccine along with other tumor-associated antigens. These results imply that cytokines released by vaccine-activated T-cells may aid in DC trafficking, phagocytosis, activation, and priming of additional tumor-specific T-cells. Increased survival was also correlated with enhanced T cell reactivity as determined by the enzyme-linked immunosorbent spot (ELISPOT) assay.

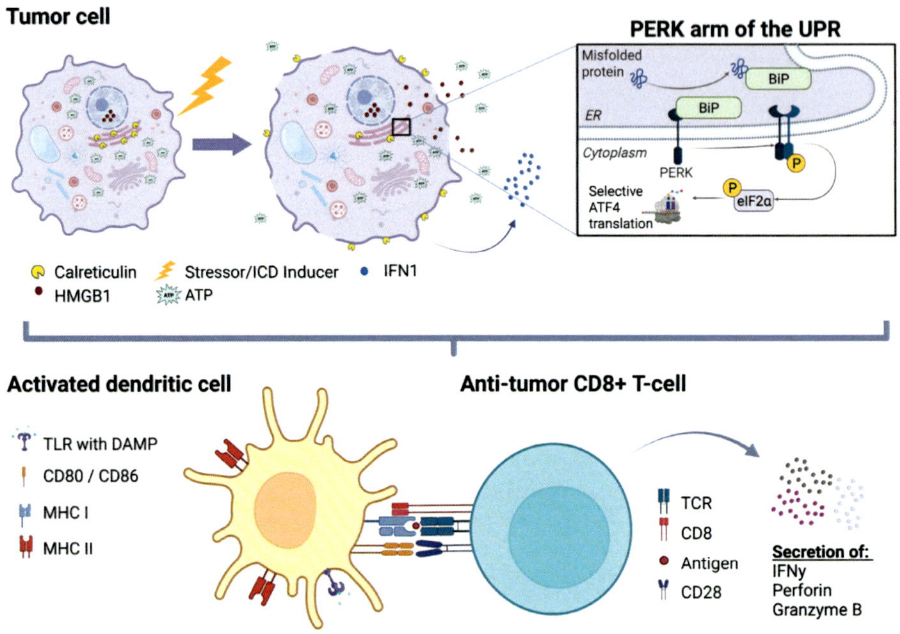

Figure 5.3. *Targeted agents may boost DC priming and the activities of tumor-specific T cells.*

Source: Pelka S, Guha C. Enhancing immunogenicity in metastatic melanoma: Adjuvant therapies to promote the anti-tumor immune response. Biomedicines. 2023; 11(8):2245. https://doi.org/10.3390/biomedicines11082245.

Combinatorial strategies with other approaches to enhance T cell activation seem promising, as HER2 antibody therapy increases T cell priming. In vitro models, agonistic 4–1BB antibodies or PD1 blocker antibodies combined with HER2 antibodies produced better tumor growth control than either treatment alone. Comparing the combination of HER2 antibodies and systemic IL-12, a Th1 polarizing cytokine that stimulates natural killer (NK) and cytotoxic T cells, with either treatment alone, the combination also increased tumor necrosis and decreased tumor progression. These findings are supported by a Phase I clinical trial that combined systemic IL-12 with trastuzumab and paclitaxel and demonstrated increased NK cell activation and pro-inflammatory cytokine production, interferon-γ (IFNγ), which stimulates multiple immune cell types and is correlated with clinical responses.

Additionally, DC priming is facilitated by the EGFR antibody cetuximab to enhance tumor immunity. Cetuximab stimulated DC opsonization of tumor cells and associated maturation, with increased expression of MHC class II, CD40, CD80, and CD86 in an in vitro study using colon cancer cell lines. Compared to DCs incubated with tumor cells only, those incubated with cetuximab and tumor cells more successfully primed tumor-specific T cells. Cetuximab also promotes complement-dependent cytotoxicity (CDC) and NK cell antibody-dependent cellular cytotoxicity (ADCC), which may improve tumor cell death even more. These findings have led to the current Phase II clinical trial's evaluation of cetuximab in conjunction with an allogeneic pancreatic cancer cell vaccine that secretes the immune-stimulating cytokine granulocyte-macrophage colony stimulating factor (GM-CSF).

5.4.4. Enhancing T-Cell Responses and Differentiation with Targeted Therapies

Although DCs play a critical role in initiating the initial anti-tumor T cell response, it is imperative to sustain T cell activation and facilitate their differentiation into memory T cells to attain a durable anti-tumor effect. This is also associated with a longer duration of overall patient survival. Numerous targeted treatments alter T cell growth and reactivity to tumor antigens, which makes them appealing options for possible immunotherapy synergy.

For more than ten years, rapamycin, an mTOR inhibitor, has been used in clinical settings as an immunosuppressant. The role of the mTOR pathway in the regulation of various immune cells has been thoroughly studied. Recent data, however, points to the possibility that mTOR inhibitors may occasionally stimulate T cells. Animals treated with rapamycin demonstrated increased early expansion of $CD8^+$viral specific T cells, increased effector-to-memory T cell differentiation, and improved re-activation, function, and survival of memory T cells in a lymphocytic choriomeningitis virus (LCMV) mouse model of acute viral infection. Similar results were seen in non-human primates administered a live-attenuated viral vaccine and mice given a non-replicating virus vaccine, indicating a new therapeutic use for mTOR inhibitors.

Recent studies have assessed the application of mTOR inhibitors in the context of cancer immunotherapy based on these findings. In the B16 melanoma and RENCA renal cell carcinoma mouse models, respectively, the combination of temsirolimus (a derivative of rapamycin) and cancer vaccination with an HSP90 adjuvant and tumor-specific proteins gp100 and CA9 strongly inhibited tumor growth. Notably, compared to animals receiving either treatment alone, animals receiving temsirolimus and the vaccines developed notably more tumor-specific T cells. In a different mouse model of metastatic renal cancer, the agonistic CD40 antibody plus the mTOR inhibitor AZD8055 led to increased intra-tumoral infiltration of $CD8^+$ T cells, DC, and macrophages as well as better disease control than either treatment alone. However, it should be noted that when agonistic CD40 antibody was combined with another mTOR inhibitor (rapamycin), there was no synergy observed. This suggests that changes in drug design or possibly dosage may result in different immune properties.

mTOR inhibitors affect $FOXP3^+$ Tregs in addition to their stimulatory effects on effector and memory T cells. When administered before an immune stimulus, such as a vaccine, mTOR inhibitors may increase the number of Tregs; however, when administered continuously after immune stimulation, mTOR inhibition may impede both Tregs and T cell effectors equally. Moreover, a quick recovery in the Treg population following tonic blockade may result in the release of mTOR inhibition, which would tilt the ratio of T effectors to Tregs in favor of immunosuppression. These findings suggest that to optimize anti-tumor effects, careful consideration should be given to the timing, dose, sequence, and cycling of mTOR inhibitors in conjunction with immunotherapy.

Another significant oncogenic pathway that could affect T cell differentiation is wnt signaling. GSK3β, or glycogen synthase kinase, is a key player in the Wnt signaling pathway. Inhibitors of GSK3β have the potential to reduce tumor cell viability both in vitro and in vivo, as this protein has been linked to the promotion of tumor growth in numerous gastrointestinal malignancies. Remarkably, a recent study connected memory T-cell differentiation to this pathway. After being exposed to the GSK3β inhibitor TWS119 and stimulated with peptide-loaded DCs, transgenic T cells underwent differentiation into "Tscm" cells, which exhibit characteristics similar to those of stem cells. Unlike classical central memory (Tcm) and effector memory T-cells (Tem), these "Tscm" are different. Tscm cells had low basal rates of division, but they were self-renewing and quickly gave rise to effector and central memory T cells in response to stimulation. Tscm cells exhibited strong tumor regression following adoptive transfer into tumor-bearing mice, while transferred effector or central memory T cells displayed reduced anti-tumor activity, most likely as a result of their lower survival rate. Further research on GSK3β inhibitors in conjunction with immunotherapies is warranted, considering the critical role that long-lasting T cell generation plays in attaining sustainable tumor control.

Similar to agonistic antibodies directed against members of the TNFR superfamily expressed on T cells, such as OX40, GITR, 4–1BB, and others, targeted therapies may also act as costimulatory agents. In this context, antagonists of the inhibitor of apoptosis proteins (IAPs) are particularly interesting. IAP inhibitors were first created to offset IAPs' function of preventing caspase activation and making cancer cells more susceptible to death stimuli. It was discovered that IAP inhibitors unintentionally imitated T-cell costimulatory signaling. These substances had little effect on resting T cells, but when TCRs were engaged, they significantly raised T cell activation, which led to an increase in cytokine production and proliferation. Due to the fact that cIAP1 (also known as BIRC2) and cIAP2 (also known as BIRC3) are important negative regulators of NF-κB inducing kinase (NIK; also known asMAP3K14), these stimulatory effects involved triggering non-canonical nuclear factor-κB (NF-κB) signaling. Tumor cell vaccines and IAP antagonists together produced a larger reduction in tumor growth and more potent anti-tumor T cell responses in a pre-clinical mouse model of melanoma than either treatment alone. These results imply that the effects of vaccination and possibly other T cell immunotherapies may be enhanced by IAP inhibitors.

5.4.5. Targeted Therapies may Sensitize Tumor Cells to Immune-Mediated Destruction

Even though T cells are capable of killing tumor cells effectively, cytotoxic T cells must interact with their specific tumor targets in order for the lytic pathway to be carried out. Tumor cells may therefore evolve escape strategies to elude T cell lysis, such as decreasing MHC class I expression to evade identification or upregulating anti-apoptotic proteins to fend off cytotoxic regimens. To enhance immune-mediated tumor destruction, targeted agents may mitigate these tactics.

Appropriate for the treatment of multiple myeloma, boratezomib is a strong proteasome inhibitor that, at least partially, impairs the viability of tumor cells by causing misfolded proteins to accumulate, which triggers the unfolded protein response. Apart from these effects on cell autonomy, bortezomib also modifies tumor cells' susceptibility to immune attack. Bortezomib may reduce peptide loading and MHC class I expression because the proteasome produces peptide epitopes for MHC class I molecules. This makes tumor cells more vulnerable to NK cells, whose activation is typically inhibited by MHC class I molecules. Additionally, FAS (also known as TNFRSF6) and the TNF-related apoptosis-inducing ligand (TRAIL) receptor DR5 (also known as TNFRSF10B) may be expressed more prominently on the surface of tumor cells by boretisomib, which would enhance the cytotoxicity of natural killer cells. Furthermore, by upregulating the expression of NOXA, a BH3 protein that sequesters strong anti-apoptotic proteins like myeloid cell leukemia sequence 1 (MCL1), bortezomib may make tumor cells more susceptible to lysis. Finally, bortezomib may increase the basal activity of caspase 8 and granzyme B in tumor cells, thereby increasing susceptibility to apoptosis.

In a study using a pre-clinical model of HPV-induced disease, combining bortezomib with an HPV E7-based vaccine resulted in extended stable disease, in contrast to using either treatment alone which had minimal effects. The improved survival was linked to bortezomib-treated tumor cells becoming more susceptible to killing by E7-specific CTLs. Additionally, mice that received the combination therapy had higher E7-specific CTL responses in their splenocytes compared to those who received only one treatment, indicating that bortezomib may enhance T cell priming and activation.

A second class of targeted agents that increase tumor cells' susceptibility to immune-mediated destruction is known as PI3K-AKT pathway inhibitors. These agents work by partially disrupting anti-apoptotic signaling. When AKT was activated, tumor cells with an inducible expression cassette of AKT showed increased resistance to T cell death in comparison to non-induced cells; this involved an upregulation of MCL1 expression. In related research, AKT upregulation was seen in a tumor cell line selected for immunotherapy resistance as opposed to wild-type sensitive cells, and this was linked to increased levels of cIAP1 and 2, BCL-2, and BCL-XL. By reducing the expression of these anti-apoptotic proteins, AKT inhibitors made the tumor cells more vulnerable to in vivo T cell death. These results collectively imply that PI3K-AKT inhibitors may work in concert with certain immunotherapies, though further research is necessary to determine how these medications affect T and NK cell function.

Increasing the concentration of tumor antigens is an additional strategy to improve T cell tumor killing. In this regard, a surprising connection was recently found between the expression of T cell antigens in melanoma and BRAF inhibitors. The BRAF-V600E mutation, which is found in about half of patients with metastatic disease, encourages constitutive activation of the MAPK pathway in malignant melanoma, which fuels tumor growth. Recently approved for the treatment of BRAF mutant melanomas, vemurafenib is a specific BRAF inhibitor that increases the expression of well-defined T cell targets such as gp100 (also known as PMEL), tyrosinase-related protein 1 (TYRP1), TYRP2, and MART1. These findings were supported by the fact that, in comparison to controls, MART1 and gp100 specific T cells produced more IFNγ and were more responsive against melanoma cells treated with BRAF inhibitors. The BRAF inhibitors did not seem to affect T cell activation and differentiation, at least not in vitro. More research is needed to determine the effects of MEK inhibitors on T cell function and melanoma antigen expression. These inhibitors may be used in conjunction with vemurafenib to lessen drug resistance caused by MEK activation.

Inhibitors of heat shock protein 90 (HSP90) offer an extra tactic to boost the expression of tumor cell antigens. A significant chaperone, HSP90 aids in the proper folding of numerous client proteins, including several oncoproteins. Misfolded proteins can accumulate and be broken down into short peptides, which can then be attached to MHC class I molecules. This process is facilitated by HSP90 inhibitors. The sensitivity of tumor cells to adoptive T cell transfer in vivo and CTL-mediated lysis in vitro is enhanced by the antigen presentation effects of HSP90 inhibitors.

HSP90 inhibitors and DNA vaccines were also successfully used in experimental models to slow the growth of tumors and increase patient survival; however, these benefits were reversed when an antibody that depletes $CD8^+$ T cells was administered, indicating that $CD8^+$ T cells play a crucial role in the destruction of tumors.

HSP90 inhibitors increase the production of stress molecules like NKG2D ligands in Hodgkin's lymphoma and multiple myeloma. These proteins on the cell surface can activate NK cells and support CD8+ T cells, which helps to enhance tumor immunity. Similarly, HDAC inhibitors also boost NKG2D ligand expression, indicating that these medications may enhance immune cell killing of tumor cells through a common mechanism.

5.4.6. Targeted Therapies May Dampen Tumor-Induced Immunosuppression

The tumor immunosuppressive microenvironment is a major barrier to anti-tumor T cell therapeutic efficaciousness. Numerous mechanisms could be at play, such as the generation of inhibitory cytokines like transforming growth factor-β (TGFβ) and IL-10, the expression of negative costimulatory ligands like PDL1, and the existence of populations of regulatory lymphocytes and myeloid cells. Finding substances that weaken these suppressive networks could significantly improve the effectiveness of immunotherapies.

Although its effects on angiogenesis are the most well-known, vascular endothelial growth factor A (VEGF-A) also exhibits strong immunoregulatory properties. Among these effects are those that prevent DCs from maturing and encourage MDSC growth. During DC differentiation, the addition of bevacizumab—a monoclonal antibody that neutralizes VEGF—increased the induction of T-cell responses. On the other hand, when bevacizumab was added to mature DCs, its effects were minimal, indicating that VEGF might have a specific window of function during DC development. These findings show that, in comparison to unloaded DCs, DCs loaded with multiple myeloma cell lysates (which contain VEGF-A) had lower levels of costimulatory molecules and a decreased capacity to stimulate T cells. However, these suppressive effects were lessened by bevacizumab. VEGF-A blockade increased NF-κB activation but inhibited STAT3 signaling, leading to a decrease in IL-10 levels but an increase in IL-12. Compared to either monotherapy, VEGF-A antibody plus adoptive T cell transfer increased tumor infiltration, slowed tumor growth, and extended survival in the B16 melanoma model. Pre-treatment of the animals before cell transfer increased the effects of VEGF-A blockade, which may indicate that the transferred T cells were more successfully localized to the tumor microenvironment.

The immunostimulatory effects of small molecule inhibitors that target VEGF receptor (VEGFR) signaling are similar. Sunitinib, a multi-tyrosine kinase inhibitor that inhibits VEGFR function, was given to mice model colon cancer; the mice showed a decrease in the number and function of MDSC and Treg in the tumor microenvironment as well as systemically. As a result, sunitinib increased the cytotoxicity and IFN-γ production of tumor-infiltrating T cells, but it also decreased the expression of PDL-1, PD1, and CTLA4. In addition, regimens combining sunitinib, IL-12, and an agonistic 4–1BB antibody produced better overall survival than those containing just one or two of these drugs. When compared to either drug alone, the combination of sunitinib and a DC vaccine improved survival in a B16 melanoma model. Given that sunitinib was most effective when given in conjunction with vaccination, it is possible that small molecules that block VEGF, similar to antibodies, are most crucial during the early DC priming of anti-tumor T cells. A word of caution: small molecule inhibitors that appear to be related may not have the same activities. For example, sorafenib, a multi-kinase inhibitor, targets VEGFR, but it also appears to have immunosuppressive properties, which may be related to its inhibitory effects on MEK signaling.

Apart from impeding VEGFR function, sunitinib has the potential to prevent STAT3 activation, a significant immunosuppressive pathway. Animals with a T cell-specific STAT3-null mutation in the B16 melanoma model exhibited higher overall survival and more tumor-specific T cells than animals of the wild-type. When sunitinib and adoptive T cell transfer were administered to mice in a RENCA renal cancer model, their responses were superior to those of either treatment alone. Sunitinib, however, did not exhibit any further therapeutic effects upon the transfer of T cells deficient in STAT3, indicating that STAT3 is the primary target in this system. In a mouse model of hepatocellular carcinoma, sunitinib-mediated STAT3 inhibition likewise improved the therapeutic benefits of vaccination and adoptive T-cell transfer.

Since JAK2 phosphorylates STAT3 in numerous signaling cascades, using JAK2 inhibitors to reduce STAT3 activation may also be a successful tactic. JAK2 inhibitor-treated tumor-bearing mice showed increased DC maturation and T cell polarization towards a Th1 phenotype, with enhanced IL-2 and IFN-γ production, similar to studies conducted with sunitinib. JAK2 inhibitors reduce PDL-1 expression in tumor cells transcriptionally while enhancing the therapeutic benefits of DC vaccination.

Indoleamine-pyrrole 2,3-dioxygenase (IDO) catalyzes the breakdown of tryptophan, an amino acid necessary for optimal T cell function, into metabolites that are directly toxic to T cells and crucial for immune tolerance. This is another immunosuppressive pathway mediated by tumor associated myeloid cells. It was discovered that imatinib unexpectedly reduced the expression of IDO in myeloid cells. Imatinib promoted tumor destruction in a murine model of gastrointestinal stromal tumors by increasing the ratio of intra-tumoral CD8+ CTLs to Tregs. When imatinib and CTLA4 antibodies were administered simultaneously, the production of IFN-γ by $CD8^+$ T cells was increased more than when either agent was administered alone. Additionally, imatinib may directly inhibit Tregs, reducing both their quantity and ability to suppress. Notably, compared to either monotherapy, the combination of imatinib and a DC vaccine in a BCR-ABL negative lymphoma model resulted in fewer metastases, a decrease in Tregs, and an increase in T cell IFN-γ production. Considering the strong effects of imatinib in this BCR-ABL negative model, more research needs to be done to see if this targeted treatment could be used more widely as a part of combination immunotherapy.

An additional significant element of the tumor microenvironment is inflammatory responses that promote tumor growth. Myeloid cells are essential for these responses because they respond to factors derived from tumors, invade the lesions, and release cytokines that promote tumor growth in a way that is dependent on the PI3K catalytic subunit-γ (p110γ). Therefore, myeloid cell infiltration was reduced by genetic and pharmacologic inhibition of p110γ, which also resulted in a decrease in tumor growth and metastases. Since the p110γ isoform is primarily expressed in immune cells rather than tumor cells, the host appears to be the primary target of these inhibitors. Mutant BRAF is another factor connecting immunoregulation and oncogenic pathways. It is responsible for the secretion of suppressive cytokines from melanoma cells, including VEGF-A and IL-10. Murafenib, an inhibitor of mutant BRAF, increases DC responsiveness by blocking these effects, suggesting that targeted therapies can directly oppose factors that suppress tumor growth.

5.4.7. Challenges for Combining Targeted Therapies and Immunotherapies

While targeted therapies hold great potential to enhance immunotherapy responses, combinatorial approaches are likely to require careful consideration of the timing, dosage, and sequencing of these agents. In this regard, a few targeted treatments that have the ability to stimulate the immune system also exhibit immunosuppressive properties. HSP90 inhibitors, for instance, may improve MHC class I presentation and hence boost CTL-mediated tumor lysis, but they may also reduce certain DC and macrophage functions. Similarly, bortezomib and HDAC inhibitors may prevent some NK cell actions, while the mTOR inhibitor temsirolimus may reduce DCs' capacity to prime tumor-specific T cells.

Can stronger anti-tumor effects be obtained without a commensurate rise in toxicities? This is a second important question for combinatorial therapies. Immunomodulatory drugs like ipilumimab and PD1 antibodies are known to cause inflammatory pathologies as their main side effects. It may be expected that taking medications that influence different stages of the immune response together will increase the risk of these side effects. Pre-clinical research into these toxicities is unquestionably necessary, but it may not fully account for the range of pathology seen in humans. For instance, ipilimumab is known to cause inflammation in the pituitary gland (hypophysitis), a side effect that was not expected from experimental studies in mice. Surprisingly, some pre-clinical studies suggest that specific combination therapies, like 4–1BB agonist antibody and CTLA4 blockade, may lessen rather than increase inflammatory toxicities.

Experimentation will be necessary to determine the best timing and order for using combinations of targeted agents and immunotherapy. However, some insight can be gained by considering which stage of the immune response is most affected by each therapy. Generally speaking, different treatments impact one of four areas of immune activation: dendritic cell presentation and T cell priming, T cell activation and anti-tumor functions, T cell differentiation into memory cells, and antagonism of the tumor microenvironment.

The strategy of targeting therapies that impact dendritic cell priming could involve administering these therapies before any immunotherapies, such as vaccination or adoptive cell transfer, and continuing throughout treatment. This approach may redirect dendritic cell actions towards enhancing T cell effector responses rather than regulatory T cells. For instance, starting sunitinib before tumor vaccination led to better anti-tumor responses compared to administering both concurrently. On the other hand, cycling sunitinib (4 weeks on-2 weeks off) resulted in the accumulation of myeloid-derived suppressor cells and regulatory T cells during the "off" period, possibly due to an unchecked rebound effect of VEGF-A. Pre-treating with monoclonal antibodies like cetuximab or trastuzumab could also be beneficial by improving the uptake of tumor antigens by dendritic cells, leading to their maturation and priming. Conversely, it may be advisable to avoid using agents that hinder dendritic cell function, like HSP90 inhibitors or sorafenib, during this pre-treatment phase to optimize tumor-specific T-cell priming.

Following immunization, targeted treatments that enhance T cell differentiation, such as mTOR inhibitors or GSK3β, may be given to encourage the induction of memory T cells. However, because GSK3β inhibitors may prevent Tscm differentiation into effector T cells and mTOR inhibitors may prevent maximal T cell proliferation, relatively short courses may be given. To sustain effector T cell activation and avoid exhaustion, immunostimulatory agents such as antibodies that block negative checkpoint activation, agonistic costimulatory antibodies, and IAP inhibitors may be administered after T cell priming and continued for a while (possibly intermittently).

Finally, there may be wide-ranging applications for targeted therapies that counteract the immunosuppressive tumor microenvironment, ranging from treatment consolidation to prior tumor vaccination. This group of drugs may include gemcitabine and 5-fluorouracil (5-FU), which both kill MDSCs, cyclophosphamide, which kills Tregs, imatinib, which inhibits IDO, sunitinib, which antagonizes MDSCs and Tregs, and p110γ inhibitors, which stop tumor-promoting inflammation. However, a potential impact on T cell effector function needs to be carefully studied.

A recent Phase I/II clinical trial combining the immune checkpoint blocking antibody ipilimumab with the mutant BRAF inhibitor vemurafenib is testing some of these concepts in patients with metastatic melanoma. The goal of this significant study is to induce a strong immune memory to translate the frequent tumor regressions brought about by vemurafenib into long-lasting clinical responses. The potential of CTLA4 blockade to enhance T cell responses and impede energy production may be enhanced by vemurafenib's capacity to raise CTL recognition of tumor cells and to reduce tumor immunosuppression. This trial will give an initial estimate of overall survival as well as assess the combination therapy's safety and tolerability. The patterns of clinical response will be especially interesting because the two modalities work well together to achieve tumor control.

A Closer Look

Anti-microtubule Agents

Chemicals derived from plants called anti-microtubule agents stop cell division by interfering with the function of microtubules. The crucial cellular structure known as microtubules is made up of two proteins called α- and β-tubulin. Among other things, these are hollow, rod-shaped structures that are necessary for cell division. Given that they are dynamic structures, microtubules are always assembling and disassembling. The two main classes of anti-microtubule agents are vinca alkaloids and taxanes. While both of these drug classes cause microtubule dysfunction, their modes of action are diametrically opposed: vinca alkaloids inhibit microtubule assembly, while taxanes inhibit microtubule disassembly. They can cause the cancer cells to undergo a mitotic catastrophe by doing this. After that, there is a cell cycle arrest, which triggers apoptosis, or planned cell death. These medications can influence blood vessel growth, which is a crucial process used by tumors to proliferate and spread.

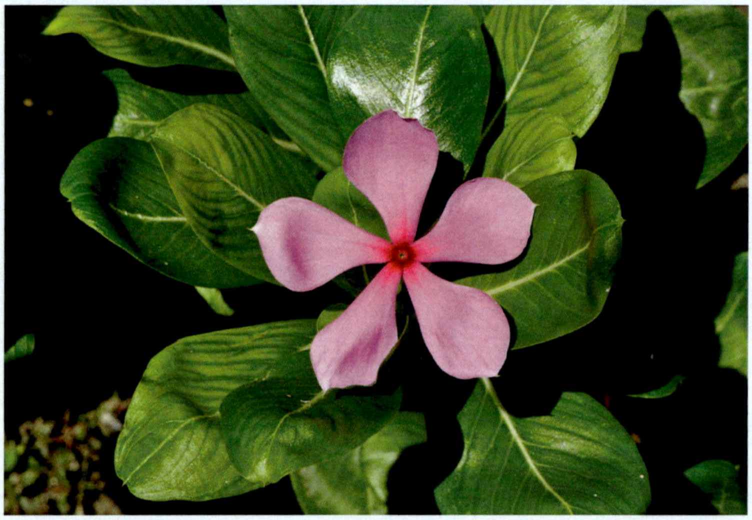

Catharanthus roseus: By Biswarup Gangulyb – Own work, CC BY-SA 3.0, https://commons.wikimedia.org/w/index.php?curid=11072973.

Catharanthus roseus, formerly known as *Vinca rosea*, is the Madagascar periwinkle from which vinca alkaloids are derived. They bind to particular tubulin sites and prevent tubulin from assembling into microtubules. Vincristine and vinblastine are two examples of the natural products that make up the original vinca alkaloids. Vinorelbine, vindesine, and vinflunine are examples of semi-synthetic vinca alkaloids that were created as a result of the success of these medications for the treatment of non-small-cell lung cancer. These medications are cycle-specific. They attach themselves to tubulin molecules in the S-phase and obstruct the normal formation of microtubules needed for the M-phase.

Taxanes are semi-synthetic, natural medications. The Pacific yew, Taxus brevifolia, was the original source of paclitaxel, the first medication in their class. Now, a substance discovered in the bark of another yew tree, Taxus baccata, is used to create this medication and another in the class, docetaxel, semi-synthetically.

Podophyllum peltatum, the American mayapple, and *Sinopodophyllum hexandrum*, the Himalayan mayapple, are the main sources of podophyllotoxin, an anti-tumorous lignan. It inhibits the formation of microtubules by binding to tubulin, a mechanism that is similar to that of vinca alkaloids. It possesses anti-microtubule activity. Teniposide and etoposide, two additional medications with distinct modes of action, are synthesized from podophyllotoxin.

Summary

- Chemotherapy is a distinctively different approach from surgery and radiation therapy to treat cancer. Chemotherapy is used as primary treatment, neoadjuvant, adjuvant treatment, and as palliative.
- Chemotherapy is often used as a neoadjuvant treatment. When chemotherapy is used as neoadjuvant treatment, it is designed to reduce the size and or bulk of the tumor so surgical resection can more easily be performed.
- The development of cytotoxic chemotherapy at the beginning of the twentieth century revolutionized the treatment of cancer, especially the treatment of disseminated diseases such as leukemia.
- The cell cycle is an ordered series of events that involves several sequential phases. The purpose of the cell cycle is for cells to reproduce themselves, to replace dead or injured cells and add new ones during tissue growth.
- Pharmacokinetics is the study of drug absorption, distribution, metabolism and excretion, or the movement of drugs within the body.
- Childhood cancer is very rare; hence the best way to search for better treatments is to conduct multi-institutional trials within a cooperative group, which may be either national or international.
- Chemotherapeutic agents have the same cytotoxic effect on both normal and malignant cells. This cell toxicity is often dose-limiting and restrictive.
- Cytotoxic chemotherapy is extremely toxic and has many unwanted side effects. Some side effects, such as nausea and vomiting and alopecia, are unpleasant but are reversible and not life-threatening.
- Antimicrobial agents are any of a large variety of chemical compounds and physical agents that are used to destroy microorganisms or to prevent their development.
- The modulation of chromosomal supercoiling by topoisomerase-catalyzed strand breakage and rejoining reactions is needed for DNA synthesis, mRNA transcription and cell division.
- By competitively blocking the biosynthesis of tetrahydrofolate, which acts as a carrier of one-carbon fragments and is required for the ultimate synthesis of DNA, RNA and bacterial cell wall proteins, trimethoprim and sulfonamides interfere with folic acid metabolism in the microbial cell.

References

1. Akbari, R., Hakemi Vala, M., & Hashemi, A. (2018). Action mechanism of melittin-derived antimicrobial peptides, MDP1 and MDP2, de novo designed against multidrug resistant bacteria. *Amino Acids, 50*(9), 1231–1243. https://doi.org/10.1007/s00726-018-2594-1.
2. Beaudoin, T., Stone, T. A., & Glibowicka, M. (2018). Activity of a novel antimicrobial peptide against P. aeruginosa biofilms. *Scientific Reports, 8*(1), 14728. https://doi.org/10.1038/s41598-018-33117-6.

3. Boruchov, A. M., et al. (2005). Activating and inhibitory IgG Fc receptors on human DCs mediate opposing functions. *Journal of Clinical Investigation, 115*, 2914–2923. https://doi.org/10.1172/JCI24772.

4. Breidenstein, E. B., de la Fuente-Núñez, C., & Hancock, R. E. (2011). Pseudomonas aeruginosa: All roads lead to resistance. *Trends in Microbiology, 19*, 419–426. https://doi.org/10.1016/j.tim.2011.04.005.

5. Candido, E. S., Cardoso, M. H., & Chan, L. Y. (2019). Short cationic peptide derived from archaea with dual antibacterial properties and anti-infective potential. *ACS Infectious Diseases, 5*(7), 1081–1086. https://doi.org/10.1021/acsinfecdis.9b00060.

6. Cerceo, E., Deitelzweig, S. B., Sherman, B. M., & Amin, A. N. (2016). Multidrug-resistant Gram-negative bacterial infections in the hospital setting: Overview, implications for clinical practice, and emerging treatment options. *Microbial Drug Resistance, 22*, 412–431. https://doi.org/10.1089/mdr.2016.0068.

7. Dechant, M., et al. (2008). Complement-dependent tumor cell lysis triggered by combinations of epidermal growth factor receptor antibodies. *Cancer Research, 68*, 4998–5003. https://doi.org/10.1158/0008-5472.CAN-07-6239.

8. Drenkard, E. (2003). Antimicrobial resistance of Pseudomonas aeruginosa biofilms. *Microbes and Infection, 5*, 1213–1219. https://doi.org/10.1016/j.micinf.2003.09.004.

9. El Solh, A. A., & Alhajhusain, A. (2009). Update on the treatment of Pseudomonas aeruginosa pneumonia. *Antimicrobial Agents and Chemotherapy, 64*, 229–238. https://doi.org/10.1128/AAC.00630-08.

10. Hancock, R. E., & Speert, D. P. (2000). Antibiotic resistance in Pseudomonas aeruginosa: Mechanisms and impact on treatment. *Drug Resistance Updates, 3*, 247–255. https://doi.org/10.1054/drup.2000.0152.

11. Hirsch, E. B., & Tam, V. H. (2010). Impact of multidrug-resistant P. aeruginosa infection on patient outcomes. *Expert Review of Pharmacoeconomics & Outcomes Research, 10*, 441–451. https://doi.org/10.1586/erp.10.49.

12. Hodi, F. S., et al. (2008). Immunologic and clinical effects of antibody blockade of cytotoxic T lymphocyte-associated antigen 4 in previously vaccinated cancer patients. *Proceedings of the National Academy of Sciences of the United States of America, 105*, 3005–3010. https://doi.org/10.1073/pnas.0712232105.

13. Hsu, Y. F., et al. (2010). Complement activation mediates cetuximab inhibition of non-small cell lung cancer tumor growth in vivo. *Molecular Cancer, 9*, 139. https://doi.org/10.1186/1476-4598-9-139.

14. Kawabe, M., et al. (2009). Heat shock protein 90 inhibitor 17-dimethylaminoethylamino-17-demethoxygeldanamycin enhances EphA2+ tumor cell recognition by specific CD8+ T cells. *Cancer Research, 69*, 6995–7003. https://doi.org/10.1158/0008-5472.CAN-08-4680.

15. Ko, J. S., et al. (2009). Sunitinib mediates reversal of myeloid-derived suppressor cell accumulation in renal cell carcinoma patients. *Clinical Cancer Research, 15*, 2148–2157. https://doi.org/10.1158/1078-0432.CCR-08-1332.

16. Lee, H., Pal, S. K., Reckamp, K., Figlin, R. A., & Yu, H. (2011). STAT3: A target to enhance antitumor immune response. *Current Topics in Microbiology and Immunology, 344*, 41–59. https://doi.org/10.1007/82_2010_105.

17. Leffers, N., et al. (2009). Prognostic significance of tumor-infiltrating T-lymphocytes in primary and metastatic lesions of advanced stage ovarian cancer. *Cancer Immunology, Immunotherapy, 58*, 449–459. https://doi.org/10.1007/s00262-008-0589-5.

18. Li, B., et al. (2009). Anti-programmed death-1 synergizes with granulocyte macrophage colony-stimulating factor-secreting tumor cell immunotherapy providing therapeutic benefit to mice with established tumors. *Clinical Cancer Research, 15*, 1623–1634. https://doi.org/10.1158/1078-0432.CCR-08-1646.

19. Lister, P. D., Wolter, D. J., & Hanson, N. D. (2009). Antibacterial-resistant Pseudomonas aeruginosa: Clinical impact and complex regulation of chromosomally encoded resistance mechanisms. *Clinical Microbiology Reviews, 22*, 582–610. https://doi.org/10.1128/CMR.00040-09.

20. Marechal, R., et al. (2010). Putative contribution of CD56 positive cells in cetuximab treatment efficacy in first-line metastatic colorectal cancer patients. *BMC Cancer, 10*, 340. https://doi.org/10.1186/1471-2407-10-340.

21. Miller, R. E., et al. (2002). 4-1BB-specific monoclonal antibody promotes the generation of tumor-specific immune responses by direct activation of CD8 T cells in a CD40-dependent manner. *Journal of Immunology, 169*, 1792–1800. https://doi.org/10.4049/jimmunol.169.4.1792.

22. Mitsui, J., et al. (2010). Two distinct mechanisms of augmented antitumor activity by modulation of immunostimulatory/inhibitory signals. *Clinical Cancer Research, 16*, 2781–2791. https://doi.org/10.1158/1078-0432.CCR-09-2210.

23. Molchanova, N., Wang, H., & Hansen, P. R. (2019). Antimicrobial activity of α-peptide/β-peptoid lysine-based peptidomimetics against colistin-resistant Pseudomonas aeruginosa isolated from cystic fibrosis patients. *Frontiers in Microbiology, 10*, 275. https://doi.org/10.3389/fmicb.2019.00275.

24. O'Brien, S. G., et al. (2003). Imatinib compared with interferon and low-dose cytarabine for newly diagnosed chronic-phase chronic myeloid leukemia. *The New England Journal of Medicine, 348*, 994–1004. https://doi.org/10.1056/NEJMoa022457.

25. Olga, P., Lucia, B., Inès, B., Laura, F. G., Mónica, G. B., Antón, A., María, L., German, B., & Maria, T. (2020). Strategies to combat multidrug-resistant and persistent infectious diseases. *Antibiotics, 9*(65). https://doi.org/10.3390/antibiotics9020065.

26. Park, S. Y., Park, H. J., Moon, S. M., Park, K. H., & Chong, Y. P. (2012). Impact of adequate empirical combination therapy on mortality from bacteremic Pseudomonas aeruginosa pneumonia. *BMC Infectious Diseases, 12*, 308. https://doi.org/10.1186/1471-2334-12-308.

27. Romoli, O., Mukherjee, S., & Mohid, S. A. (2019). Enhanced silkworm cecropin B antimicrobial activity against Pseudomonas aeruginosa from single amino acid variation. *ACS Infectious Diseases, 5*(7), 1200–1213. https://doi.org/10.1021/acsinfecdis.9b00138.

28. Taipale, M., Jarosz, D. F., & Lindquist, S. (2010). HSP90 at the hub of protein homeostasis: Emerging mechanistic insights. *Nature Reviews Molecular Cell Biology, 11*, 515–528. https://doi.org/10.1038/nrm2918.

29. Wang, Y., Wang, X. Y., Subjeck, J. R., Shrikant, P. A., & Kim, H. L. (2011). Temsirolimus, an mTOR inhibitor, enhances anti-tumor effects of heat shock protein cancer vaccines. *British Journal of Cancer, 104*, 643–652. https://doi.org/10.1038/bjc.2011.5.

30. Yasir, M., Dutta, D., & Willcox, M. D. P. (2019). Comparative mode of action of the antimicrobial peptide melimine and its derivative Mel4 against Pseudomonas aeruginosa. *Scientific Reports, 9*(1), 7063. https://doi.org/10.1038/s41598-019-43573-6.

Chapter

6

MEDICINAL CHEMISTRY OF CENTRAL NERVOUS SYSTEM (CNS) DRUGS

Contents

Introduction

Among the first pharmacologic agents to be discovered by early humans were drugs that act on the central nervous system (CNS), and they continue to be the most commonly used class of drugs. Among other things, these include drugs that alleviate pain, suppress nausea, lower fever, and treat a variety of neurologic and psychiatric disorders. Furthermore, many over-the-counter CNS-acting medications are used to elevate mood.

The mechanisms by which different drugs act in the central nervous system are often complicated and not fully understood. However, the field of CNS pharmacology has seen significant advancements in methodology in recent decades. Nowadays, it is feasible to investigate how a medication affects a single neuron or even a single receptor within a synapse. Numerous significant advancements in CNS research have their roots in the data gathered from these kinds of investigations. First, almost all medications that affect the central nervous system (CNS) clearly target particular receptors that alter synaptic transmission. Even some non-receptor-mediated actions, like those of alcohol and general anesthetics, can cause noticeable changes in synaptic transmission. These exceptions to the rule are not universally acknowledged.

Second, medications are among the most useful instruments for researching how the central nervous system functions, from the formation of long-term memory to the mechanism underlying convulsions. In these kinds of studies, both antagonists and agonists that mimic endogenous substances—and are frequently more selective than the latter—are very helpful. Third, some of the most productive theories about the mechanisms underlying disease have come from analyzing the effects of medications with established clinical efficacy. For instance, knowledge of how antipsychotic medications affect dopamine receptors has served as the foundation for significant theories about the pathophysiology of schizophrenia. Research on how different agonists and antagonists affect γ-aminobutyric acid (GABA) receptors has led to new ideas about the pathophysiology of several conditions, such as epilepsy and anxiety.

Orientation and Directional Terms

Term	Definition	Illustration
Serotonin	Serotonin is an inhibitory neurotransmitter. Serotonin helps regulate mood, sleep patterns, sexuality, anxiety, appetite and pain. Diseases associated with serotonin imbalance include seasonal affective disorder, anxiety, depression, fibromyalgia and chronic pain. Medications that regulate serotonin and treat these disorders include selective serotonin reuptake inhibitors (SSRIs) and serotonin-norepinephrine reuptake inhibitors (SNRIs).	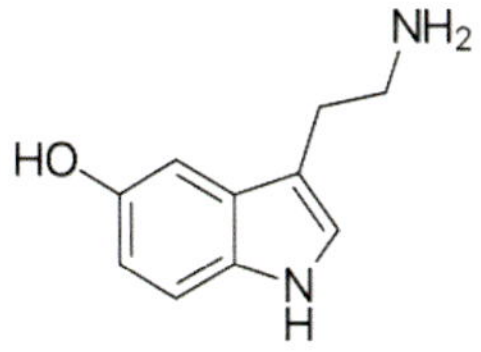
Caffeine	A stimulant present in tea, coffee, cola beverages, analgesic drugs, and agents used to increase alertness. It is also used in to prevent and treat pulmonary complications of premature birth.	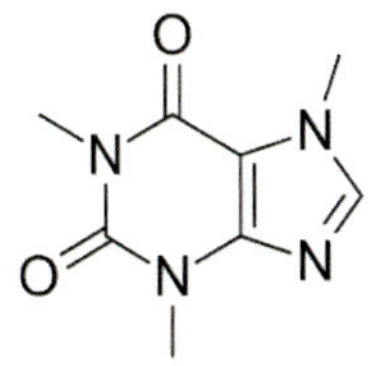
Histamine	Histamine regulates body functions including wakefulness, feeding behavior and motivation. Histamine plays a role in asthma, bronchospasm, mucosal edema and multiple sclerosis.	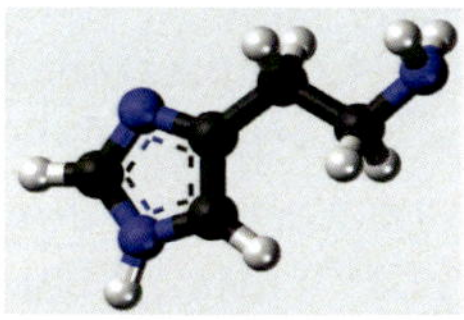
Dopamine	Dopamine plays a role in your body's reward system, which includes feeling pleasure, achieving heightened arousal and learning. Dopamine also helps with focus, concentration, memory, sleep, mood and motivation. Diseases associated with dysfunctions of the dopamine system include Parkinson's disease, schizophrenia, bipolar disease, restless legs syndrome and attention deficit hyperactivity disorder (ADHD). Many highly addictive drugs (cocaine, methamphetamines, amphetamines) act directly on the dopamine system.	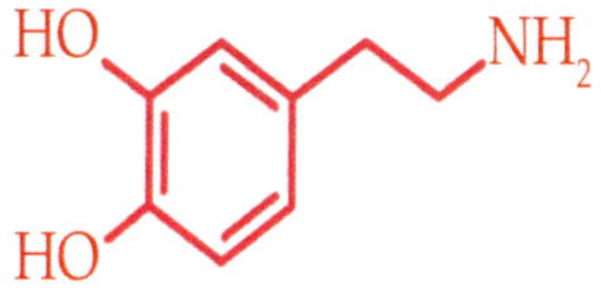
Norepinephrine	Norepinephrine (also called noradrenaline) increases blood pressure and heart rate. It's most widely known for its effects on alertness, arousal, decision-making, attention and focus.	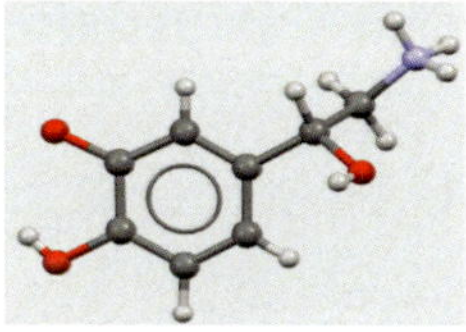

6.1. Organization of the CNS

The two main components of the central nervous system are the brain and spinal cord. The cranium shields the brain, which is housed inside the skull. Lying caudally to the brain, the spinal cord is continuous with it. The vertebrae protect it. The spinal cord extends from the base of the skull, passes through the foramen magnum or begins below it, and ends approximately level with the first or second lumbar vertebra, taking up the upper portions of the vertebral canal.

6.1.1. White and Gray Matter

The neurons and tissue of the central nervous system (CNS) and the peripheral nervous system (PNS) differ from one another under the microscope. Gray and white matter make up the central nervous system. Brain tissue exhibits this macroscopically as well. Axons and oligodendrocytes make up the white matter, whereas neurons and unmyelinated fibers make up the gray matter. Glial cells, also known as CNS supporting cells, are present in both tissues in varying numbers (though the white matter has more of them). Different glial cell types have different roles. For example, Bergmann glia act almost as a scaffolding for neuroblasts to climb during neurogenesis, while microglia are a specialized type of macrophage that are involved in the brain's immune system and the removal of different metabolites from brain tissue. Astrocytes may be involved in the transportation of fuel and other helpful substances from the brain's capillaries to neurons, as well as the clearance of metabolites. Astrocytes will multiply after a CNS injury, resulting in gliosis, a type of neuronal scar tissue devoid of functioning neurons (Figure 6.1).

Within the brain, more white matter forms tracts and commissures, while the cortex, which is made up of neuron bodies that make up gray matter, makes up the cerebrum, midbrain, and hindbrain. In addition to cortical gray matter, subcortical gray matter is composed of numerous distinct nuclei.

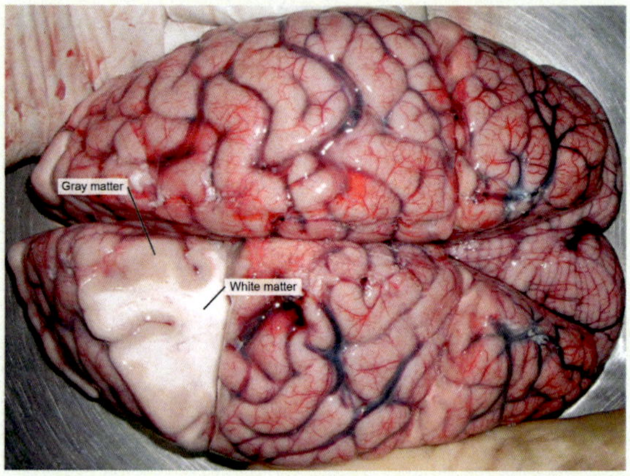

Figure 6.1. *Dissection of a human brain with labels showing the clear division between white and gray matter.*

Source: ByOpenStax-https://cnx.org/contents/FPtK1zmh@8.25:fEI3C8Ot@10/Preface, CCBY4.0, https://commons.wikimedia.org/w/index.php?curid=30147908.

6.1.2. Spinal Cord

The peripheral nervous system projects as spinal nerves (and occasionally segmental nerves) from and to the spinal cord. The spinal cord and the skin, joints, muscles, etc., are connected by nerves. allow the efferent motor and afferent sensory stimuli and signals to be transmitted. This permits the senses to be perceived as well as the voluntary and involuntary movements of muscles.

The brain stem is the source of all 31 spinal nerves, some of which form plexa as they branch out, such as the sacral plexa and brachial plexa. Both sensory and motor signals are carried by each spinal nerve, but they synapse at different locations in the spinal cord: either from the periphery to sensory relay neurons that send the information to the central nervous system (CNS) or from the CNS to motor neurons that send the information out. Information is sent up to the brain from the spinal cord via spinal tracts, the thalamus, and finally the cortex via the last common pathway.

6.1.2.1. Cranial Nerves

Peripheral nerves of the PNS that synapse through intermediaries or ganglia directly on the CNS exist in addition to the spinal cord. These 12 nerves, collectively referred to as cranial nerves, are located in the head and neck area. Information is transmitted to and from the CNS by cranial nerves, which also supply specific muscles (like the trapezius muscle, which is innervated by accessory nerves and some cervical spinal nerves).

The olfactory and optic nerves are two pairs of cranial nerves that are frequently regarded as CNS structures. This is since they directly synapse on CNS neurons rather than first on peripheral ganglia. The olfactory epithelium is important because it expresses CNS tissue in direct contact with the environment, facilitating the administration of some medications.

6.1.3. Brain

Located at the front of the spinal cord is the brain. The majority of the CNS is made up of the brain. When discussing the nervous system as a whole, it is frequently mentioned as the primary structure. The primary brain-based neural system (CNS) unit. Although the spinal cord can process reflexes and perform certain tasks related to spinal locomotion, the brain is the primary nervous system processing unit.

6.1.3.1. Brainstem

The midbrain, the pons, and the medulla make up the brainstem. Given their similar structures and functional characteristics, the medulla and spinal cord can be thought of as an extension of one another. This is where the tracts that travel from the spinal cord to the brain pass through. The medulla nuclei are responsible for breathing and blood pressure regulation. Balance, taste, hearing, and the control of the muscles in the face and neck are all mediated by other nuclei.

The ventral anterior side of the brainstem contains the pons, the next structure rostral to the medulla. Pontine nuclei, one type of pons nuclei, communicate information between the cerebral cortex and the cerebellum by working with it. Nuclei related to taste, breathing, and sleep are located in the dorsal posterior pons. The mesencephalon, also known as the midbrain, is located rostrally and above the pons. Among other nuclei connecting various regions of the motor system are those found in the cerebellum, basal ganglia, and both cerebral hemispheres. In addition, the midbrain houses several components of the visual and auditory systems, including those that regulate automatic eye movements.

Numerous pathways for motor and autonomic control of the face and neck are accessed and exited by the brainstem as a whole through cranial nerves. The tenth cranial nerve mediates autonomic control of the organs. The brainstem plays a major role in this kind of autonomic regulation of the body. These processes may involve the heart, blood vessels, and pupils, among other bodily parts. The reticular formation is a collection of brainstem nuclei that are involved in arousal and alertness.

6.1.3.2. Cerebellum

Behind the pons is the cerebellum. Numerous lobes and dividing fissures make up the cerebellum. Controlling posture and coordinating the movements of various body parts, such as the head, eyes, and limbs, are among its functions. Moreover, it performs actions that have been trained and refined via repetition, and it can adjust to newly acquired motions.

The cerebellum exhibits connections to parts of the cerebral cortex related to language and cognition, despite its prior classification as a motor structure. Medical imaging methods like functional magnetic resonance imaging and Positron emission tomography have demonstrated these relationships.

The cerebellum's body contains more neurons than any other brain structure, including the larger cerebrum. However, because it has fewer distinct neuronal types than other brain structures, it is also better understood. It manages and processes vestibular organ balance information, motor information, and sensory stimuli.

6.1.3.3. Diencephalon

The thalamus and hypothalamus are the two diencephalon structures that are important to note. The thalamus serves as an intermediary between the cerebral hemispheres and incoming pathways from the peripheral nervous system and the optical nerve (although it does not receive input from the olfactory nerve). It was formerly thought of as just a "relay station," but it also sorts the data that is sent to the cerebral hemispheres (neocortex). The thalamus links the cerebellum and basal ganglia to the cerebrum in addition to conducting information sorting from the periphery. The thalamus, like the SCN, is involved in wakefulness and consciousness, just like the previously mentioned reticular system.

Many primal emotions or feelings, including hunger, thirst, and maternal bonding, are controlled by the hypothalamus. This is partially regulated by the pituitary gland's hormone secretion control. The hypothalamus also influences motivation and a host of other behavioral issues.

6.1.3.4. Cerebrum

The majority of the human brain's visual cortex is found in the cerebrum of both cerebral hemispheres. The cerebral hemispheres are composed of several structures, including the hippocampus, amygdala, cortex, and basal ganglia. Together, the hemispheres govern a sizable range of mental processes, including emotion, memory, perception, and motor abilities. In addition, the cerebral hemispheres represent the brain's cognitive capacities.

The corpus callosum and various commissures connect the hemispheres of the brain. The cortex, composed of gray matter, is a crucial part of the cerebral hemispheres as it covers the brain's surface. The cerebral cortex is responsible for planning and executing daily tasks. The hippocampus aids in memory storage, the amygdala facilitates emotional perception and communication, and the basal ganglia coordinate voluntary movements.

6.1.4. Difference from the Peripheral Nervous System

This distinguishes the PNS, which is made up of Schwann cells, axons, and neurons, from the CNS. Similar roles are played by Schwann cells and oligodendrocytes in the PNS and CNS, respectively. Both contribute to the axons' myelin sheaths, which serve as a type of insulation that improves and speeds up the transmission of electrical signals along nerves. Since CNS axons are frequently millimeters or less in length, they do not require the same level of isolation as peripheral nerves. Peripheral nerves, like those leading to the big toe, can reach lengths of more than one meter. Myelination is required to guarantee that signals travel at a fast enough speed.

There are differences in the ways that oligodendrocytes and Schwann cells myelinate nerves. Typically, a Schwann cell myelinates an individual axon, encircling it entirely. Sometimes, particularly in regions with short axons, they may myelinate a large number of axons. Typically, multiple axons are myelinated by oligodendrocytes. They envelop and enclose the axon by projecting thin projections of their cell membrane in this manner.

6.1.5. Functional Divisions of the Nervous System

Although there are differences between anatomical and functional divisions of the nervous system, the nervous system can also be divided based on its functions. The same functions that the PNS and the CNS contribute to are those that can be ascribed to distinct ganglia in the periphery or to distinct areas of the brain (like the cerebral cortex or the hypothalamus). Trying to fit functional differences into anatomical divisions is problematic because a single structure can occasionally serve multiple functions. For instance, the optic nerve transmits signals from the retina that are either processed by the hypothalamus for processing in the cortex of the cerebral brain or utilized for the reflexive responses of smooth muscle tissue.

There are two ways to think about the functional division of the nervous system. The nervous system's primary roles are integration, response, and sensation. Second, the divisions of control over the body that result from the response are primarily defined by the somatic and autonomic domains. Additionally, a section of the peripheral nervous system known as the enteric nervous system is in charge of a particular group of gastrointestinal-related autonomic control functions.

6.1.5.1. Basic Functions

The nervous system is involved in receiving information about the environment around us (sensation) and generating responses to that information (motor responses). The nervous system can be split into areas that control response (motor functions) and sensation (sensory functions). It is necessary to incorporate a third function, though. Integration of sensory data with memories, emotional state, learning (cognition), and other sensations is necessary. An association or integration area is a term used to describe certain areas of the nervous system. Higher cognitive processes like memory, learning, and emotion are combined with sensory perceptions to generate an answer. This process is known as integration.

- **Sensation:** The primary function of the nervous system is to receive information from the environment, known as sensation. This includes inputs about what is happening both outside and inside the body. The sensory functions of the nervous system detect changes from homeostasis or specific events in the environment, which are called stimuli. The most well-known senses are taste, smell, vision, hearing, and balance. Taste and smell rely on chemical substances, vision on light, hearing on sound, and balance on the perception of head position in space. These senses have specialized organs to detect stimuli and are referred to as special senses. In addition to these, there are general senses like touch, pain, and temperature sensed by the skin. Special and general senses provide conscious awareness, known as somatic sensation. Visceral senses, on the other hand, are related to internal stimuli and are not consciously perceived. Both somatic and visceral sensory information is processed by the Peripheral Nervous System and transmitted to the Central Nervous System in an inward direction known as afferent.
- **Integration:** The nervous system processes information received

by sensory structures and communicates it to other parts of the body. In addition to being compared or integrated with other stimuli, memories of prior stimuli, or an individual's state at a specific moment are also considered. This causes a particular response to be generated. A batter is not guaranteed to swing just because they see a baseball pitched to them. It will be necessary to take into account the ball's speed and trajectory. To get a walk to first base, the batter may want to let this pitch pass by if the count is three balls and one strike. Perhaps the batter's team has such a large lead that it would be enjoyable to simply swing away.

- **Response:** The nervous system uses the sensory stimuli as a basis for producing a response. A response that would be immediately apparent would be to move your muscles, like taking your hand away from a hot stove, but the term has other applications. All three types of muscle tissue can contract due to the nervous system. For instance, during exercise, an increase in heart rate affects cardiac muscle, skeletal muscle contracts to move the skeleton, and smooth muscle contracts to move food through the digestive tract. In addition, responses involve the neural regulation of bodily glands, such as the eccrine and merocrine sweat glands in the skin, which produce and secrete sweat to regulate body temperature. As a result, the motor response targets muscles and glands, which activate when prompted to execute the response. This is why they are referred to as effectors. Responses can be classified as either involuntary or unconscious (such as smooth muscle contraction, cardiac muscle regulation, or gland activation) or voluntary or conscious (such as the contraction of skeletal muscle). The somatic nervous system controls voluntary responses, while the autonomic and enteric nervous systems—discussed in the following section—are in charge of involuntary responses. The Central Nervous System produces motor information, which is then transmitted to the Peripheral Nervous System. Additionally, this outward direction is efferent. While they are distinct, afferent and efferent have the same sound. Utilizing the acronym SAME, which stands for Sensory Afferent Motor Efferent, can help you remember their distinctions.

6.1.5.2. Controlling the Body

Most of the time, functional differences in responses allow for the division of the nervous system into two sections. Both voluntary motor responses, also known as somatic responses, and conscious perception, or somatosensation, are governed by the somatic nervous system (SNS). Skeletal muscle contractions are referred to as voluntary motor responses, but they are not always voluntary in the sense that you have to want to perform them. Certain somatic motor responses are reflexive, meaning they frequently occur without the conscious choice to do so. Your friend will startle you and you might scream or jump back if they jump out from behind a corner and yell "Boo!". It is a reflex involving contractions of the skeletal muscles; you may not have wanted to give your friend a reason to make fun of you, but you did not choose to do that. As a person learns motor skills, other motor responses become automatic, or unconscious (also known as "habit learning" or "procedural memory").

Involuntary bodily control is the responsibility of the autonomic nervous system (ANS), which is typically employed to maintain homeostasis (the internal environment's regulation). Autonomic processes receive their sensory input from sensory structures that are attuned to either internal or external environmental stimuli. The motor output includes glandular tissue, cardiac muscle, and smooth muscle. The autonomic nervous system's function is to maintain homeostasis by regulating the body's organ systems. The autonomic nervous system regulates the function of sweat glands, for instance. Sweating aids in the cooling of your body when you're hot. It is a system of homeostasis. But you may also begin to perspire if you're anxious. That is the body's reaction to an emotional state; it is not homeostatic.

Table 6.1. Nervous System-Divisions

	Sensation	**Integration**	**Motor Response**
Somatic	Conscious perception of environmental changes (light, sounds, molecules in food, movement, temperature, touch, etc) through somatic sensory neurons of PNS	Information processed inbrain and spinal cord (CNS)	Voluntary and reflex response via skeletal muscles
Autonomic	Unconscious perception of external or internal changes (light, molecules, organ stretch, etc) through visceral sensory neurons in both CNS and PNS	Information processed in brain (particularly hypothalamus and brainstem) and spinal cord (CNS)	Involuntary movement of cardiac muscle, smooth muscle, glands
Enteric	Unconscious perception of internal changes (molecules, movement, stretch) within the gastrointestinal tract through visceral sensory neurons in gastrointestinal tract	Information processed within the gastrointestinal tract (PNS)	Involuntary movement of smooth muscle and glands of digestive system

Source: https://med.libretexts.org/Bookshelves/Anatomy_and_Physiology/Human_Anatomy_(OERI)/11%3A_Nervous_System_and_Nervous_Tissue/11.02%3A_Organization_and_Functions_of_the_Nervous_System.

The nervous system has another division that deals with functional responses. Your digestive system's glandular tissue and smooth muscle are under the direction of the enteric nervous system (ENS). It is independent of the CNS and makes up a sizable portion of the PNS. However, because the neural structures that comprise the enteric system are a part of the autonomic output that controls digestion, it is occasionally appropriate to think of the enteric system as a component of the autonomic system. Although the two have some differences, there will be a significant amount of overlap for the purposes of this discussion (Table 6.1).

Neurons and glial cells make up nervous tissue. The soma, or cell body, and processes make up a neuron's fundamental structure. Dendrites—which receive information—and axons—which transmit information—are the two categories into which processes fall. The myelin sheath, which is rich in lipids, covers a portion of the axons. Because myelin contains a lot of fat, axons covered in it appear white. Therefore, depending on how the nervous tissue appears in unstained tissue, it can also be categorized as gray matter or white matter.

Depending on where they are located, the cell bodies of neurons group together in areas known as ganglia or nuclei. Additionally, depending on where they are located, neuronal axons have a tendency to bundle up into structures called nerves (fibers) or tracts (columns). Anatomy and physiology allow for the division of the nervous system into distinct sections. The peripheral nervous system (PNS) and central nervous system (CNS) are the two anatomical divisions. The brain and spinal cord make up the central nervous system. Within the CNS, bundles of axons known as tracts are found within the white matter, and localized collections of neuron cell bodies known as nuclei are found within the gray matter. The PNS is composed of nerves, which are bundles of axons, and ganglia, which are collections of neuron cell bodies. When an axon enters the PNS, it can be a component of a nerve; however, when it crosses the CNS, it transforms into a tract.

According to their respective roles, the nervous system can be functionally separated into three regions: those for integration, sensation, and response generation. The central and peripheral anatomy contain all of these functional regions. Another way to categorize the nervous system is according to how it governs the body. Skeletal muscle movement is the outcome of functions carried out by the somatic nervous system (SNS). Somatic refers to any sensory or integrative function that causes skeletal muscle to move. The autonomic nervous system (ANS) is in charge of processes that impact smooth or cardiac muscle or trigger the secretion of glands.

The central and peripheral nervous systems each have different roles in autonomic processes. The sensations involved in triggering somatic responses may also be the ones that lead to autonomic functions. The integrative roles of the somatic and autonomic systems may also overlap. The nervous system's unique division, the enteric nervous system, is in charge of regulating the digestive organs. The enteric nervous system and the autonomic nervous system share certain components. Since the enteric nervous system is the nervous tissue found in the digestive system's organs, it can only be found in the periphery.

6.2. Drugs Acting Upon the Central Nervous System

Every cellular operation is guided by the central nervous system. The spinal cord carries thousands of sensory inputs that the peripheral nervous system processes and forwards to the brain. After processing all of the information, the brain deems 99 % of it irrelevant. Certain regions of the central nervous system fire nerve impulses to organs or tissue in response to sensory data analysis, allowing the body to react appropriately.

Numerous effects on the activity and operation of the central nervous system can be produced by chemical influences. There may be ambiguity in the explanations for the mechanisms of drug action due to our limited understanding of the neurotransmitters and various brain regions. The three known neurotransmitters are: serotonin, which is involved in emotion, pain, sleep, and biological rhythms; acetylcholine, which is involved in memory and learning; and norepinephrine, which is involved in mania, depression, and emotions.

6.2.1. Central Nervous System Stimulants

Drugs classified as stimulants work by stimulating the central nervous system. Cocaine, caffeine, and different amphetamines are examples of psychic stimulants. These medications are intended to lessen weariness and drowsiness while increasing mental alertness. Caffeine over 200 mg, or roughly two cups of coffee, does not, however, improve mental function; instead, it may exacerbate headaches, tremors, anxiety, and irritability. People who drink a lot of coffee develop a psychic dependence on caffeine. A person may have mild withdrawal symptoms, such as headache, agitation, and nervousness, if they stop drinking coffee (Figure 6.2).

In terms of their stimulatory effect, caffeine and the chemically related xanthines theophylline and theobromine decrease in the following order. They might be present in certain over-the-counter medications. Caffeine functions as an antagonist by blocking adenosine receptors. Given that the structure of caffeine and the adenosine group are similar. This implies that both caffeine and adenosine will bind to adenosine receptors. Although it prevents neurotransmitters from being released from presynaptic sites, it synergizes with angiotensin or norepinephrine to enhance their effects. Caffeine's stimulating effects seem to be due to its antagonistic effects on adenosine receptors, which appears to stimulate the release of neurotransmitters.

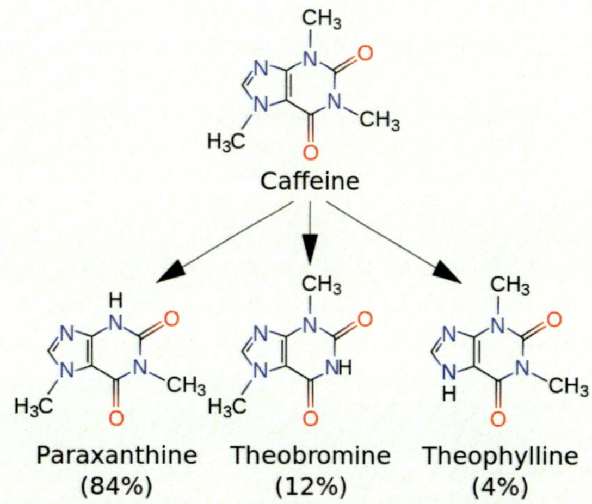

Figure 6.2: *Caffeine and theophylline.*

Source: By Icey – Own work, created in Inkscape, Public Domain, https://commons.wikimedia.org/w/index.php?curid=1073029.

6.2.2. Amphetamines

Excessive norepinephrine release from peripheral nervous system storage sites is what causes amphetamine-induced stimulation. Whether the same process takes place in the central nervous system is unknown. There are two alternative hypotheses regarding their mechanism of action: either they act on serotonin receptor sites or they are broken down more slowly than norepinephrine. Amphetamine in therapeutic doses improves mood, lessens hunger and fatigue, improves concentration, and increases motivation and productivity. They provide powerful, energizing, powerful, self-assured, focused, and more motivated feelings. There is less of a need to eat or sleep (Figure 6.3).

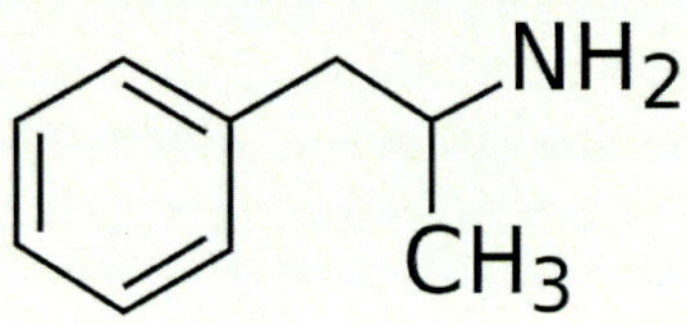

Figure 6.3: *Amphetamines.*

Source: By Wesalius – Own work, Public Domain, https://commons.wikimedia.org/w/index.php?curid=39657831.

Amphetamines are the collective term for levoamphetamine (Benzedrine), dextroamphetamine (Dexedrine), and methamphetamine (Methedrine). The isomers of levoamphetamine and dextroamphetamine are combined to form benzoedrine. Compared to the levo isomer, the dextro isomer has several times the potency. The abuse and misuse of amphetamines is a serious issue. Examples of this include housewives who take diet pills, athletes who want to perform better, truck drivers who drive nonstop from coast to coast, and students who stay up late studying for tests.

6.3. Neurotransmitters and Their Receptors

Neurotransmitters are chemical messengers that travel throughout the body, carrying, enhancing, and balancing signals between target cells and neurons, also referred to as nerve cells. These target cells could be found in other neurons, muscles, or glands. Our brains are constantly producing billions of neurotransmitter molecules to keep our breathing, heartbeat, learning, and levels of concentration under control. They may also have an impact on a range of psychological processes, including joy, fear, fear, and mood. The body and brain contain a variety of neurotransmitters, such as endorphins, epinephrine, norepinephrine, glutamate, serotonin, and dopamine.

6.3.1. How Neurotransmitters Work

Neurons must be able to communicate with one another in order for signals to be transmitted throughout the body. Neurones are not merely linked to one another, though. Each neuron has a synapse, or tiny gap, at the end. For a signal to reach the next cell, it must be able to pass through this gap. This happens via a mechanism called neurotransmission. The synapse, a location where neurons can exchange signals, is where an action potential usually arrives before a neurotransmitter is released from what is referred to as the axon terminal.

Vesicles, which are tiny sacs containing neurotransmitters, are released when an electrical signal reaches the end of a neuron. The neurotransmitters pass through the opening in these sacs and travel toward the nearby cells at the synapse.

These cells have receptors on them where neurotransmitters can attach and cause cellular changes. Upon release, the neurotransmitter attaches to the receptor site on the other neuron across the synaptic gap, either stimulating or inhibiting the receiving neuron, depending on the neurotransmitter.

Neurotransmitters and receptors function as a lock and key combination. A neurotransmitter, which is the key, can only bind to a particular receptor, which is the lock, just as a specific lock can only be opened with the correct key. Changes in the receiving cell are triggered if the neurotransmitter is able to function at the receptor site.

Neurotransmitters can occasionally bind to receptors to send an excitatory electrical signal down the cell. In certain instances, the neurotransmitter has the ability to obstruct the signal and stop the message from getting through (inhibitory).

6.3.1.1. Inactivation of Neurotransmitters

What happens to a neurotransmitter when its function is fulfilled? There are three ways in which a neurotransmitter can cease to function after it has produced the intended result.

- **Degradation**: An enzyme modifies the neurotransmitter's structure to prevent the receptor from recognizing it.
- **Diffusion:** The neurotransmitter drifts away from the receptor
- **Reuptake:** The axon of the neuron that released the neurotransmitter takes up the entire molecule.

6.3.1.2. Criteria for Neurotransmitters

The identification of neurotransmitters themselves can be a challenging task. Although the vesicles containing neurotransmitters are visible to scientists, it is more difficult to determine what substances are stored in the vesicles. As a result, when deciding whether or not to classify a chemical as a neurotransmitter, neuroscientists have established a number of guidelines:

Presence of the chemical within the cell. The chemical is present in the neuron or is either synthesized there.

- *Stimulus-dependent release.* The neuron releases it when stimulated in the right amounts.
- *Action on the postsynaptic cell.* The postsynaptic neuron needs to have receptors that the chemical will bind to, and the presynaptic neuron needs to release the chemical.
- *A mechanism for removal.* Once the chemical has completed its task, there is a specific mechanism in place to remove it from its site of activation.

6.3.2. Classification of Neurotransmitters

Neurotransmitters are essential for daily survival and proper functioning. Although the precise number of neurotransmitters is still unknown, over 60 different chemical messengers have been found. The functions of neurotransmitters can be categorized as follows:

- **Excitatory Neurotransmitters:** These neurotransmitters increase the probability that a neuron will fire an action potential by having excitatory effects on the neuron. The excitatory neurotransmitters norepinephrine and adrenaline are a couple of the main ones.
- **Inhibitory Neurotransmitters:** These neurotransmitters work as inhibitors, meaning they lessen the possibility that a neuron will fire an action potential. Gamma-aminobutyric acid and serotonin are two important inhibitory neurotransmitters (GABA).
- **Modulatory Neurotransmitters:** These neurotransmitters, also known as neuromodulators, have the ability to influence multiple neurons at once. The effects of other chemical messengers are also influenced by these neuromodulators. While synaptic neurotransmitters are rapidly released from axon terminals to affect other receptor neurons, neuromodulators diffuse more widely and have a slower rate of action. Among the neurotransmitters that function as neuromodulators are cannabinoids, acetylcholine,

dopamine, serotonin, and histamine. Depending on the kind of receptors that are present, some neurotransmitters, like acetylcholine and dopamine, can have both excitatory and inhibitory effects.

6.3.3. Actions

Synapses, which are specialized contact sites where neurotransmitters transmit signals, are how neurons communicate with one another. Neurotransmitters may be released into the synaptic cleft in response to an action potential that reaches the presynaptic terminal. Following their binding to receptors on the postsynaptic membrane, these neurotransmitters either stimulate or inhibit the receiving neuron. The receiving neuron may produce its own action potential to carry on information transmission to the following neuron in the network if the total excitatory influences surpass the inhibitory influences. Complex neural networks and information flow are made possible by this process.

6.3.3.1. Modulation

A neurotransmitter can affect a target cell in an excitatory, inhibitory, or modulatory manner. The neurotransmitter's interaction with receptors at the post-synaptic membrane determines the outcome. Trans-membrane ion flow is influenced by neurotransmitters, which can either increase (excitatory) or decrease (inhibitory) the likelihood that the cell they come into contact with will generate an action potential. Type I synapses are those that have receptors that have excitatory effects, whereas Type II synapses have receptors that have inhibitory effects. Because of this, even though synapses differ greatly, they all transmit the same two kinds of messages. The two varieties have distinct looks and are mostly found on various regions of the neurons that are affected by it. All synaptic membranes contain receptors with modulatory properties, and when neurotransmitters bind to these receptors, signaling cascades are triggered that aid in cell function regulation. Numerous outcomes can arise when neurotransmitters bind to receptors that have modulatory effects. For example, by attracting more or fewer receptors to the synaptic membrane, it could lead to a change in the sensitivity to subsequent stimuli.

On the shafts or spines of dendrites, type I (excitatory) synapses are usually found, while type II (inhibitory) synapses are usually found on a cell body. Furthermore, the synaptic vesicles of Type I synapses are spherical, while those of Type II synapses are flattened. In a Type I synapse, the material on the presynaptic and postsynaptic membranes is denser than in a Type II synapse, and the Type I synaptic cleft is wider. Lastly, a Type I synapse has a larger active zone than a Type II synapse.

A neuron is separated into two zones by the locations of its Type I and Type II synapses: the excitatory dendritic tree and the inhibitory cell body. From an inhibitory standpoint, an action potential is triggered by excitation that enters over the dendrites and travels to the axon hillock. Applying inhibition to the cell body near the axon hillock, the source of the action potential, is the best way to stop the message. Imagine excitation triumphing over inhibition as another method to understand excitatory-inhibitory interaction. Reducing the cell body's inhibition is the only way to produce an action potential at the axon hillock if the cell body is normally in an inhibited state. The excitatory message in this "open the gates" strategy is like a racehorse about to sprint down the track, but first the inhibitory starting gate needs to be removed.

6.3.3.2. Neurotransmitter Actions

A neurotransmitter can only directly affect a receptor by activating it, as previously mentioned. As a result, the connections between the neurons that use the transmitter and the chemical makeup of the receptors determine how a neurotransmitter system behaves.

- In the brain and spinal cord, glutamate is used at the vast majority of fast excitatory synapses. The majority of "modifiable" synapses also use it, i.e., able to change its strength in both directions. The primary components of the brain involved in memory storage are believed to be modifiable synapses. Overindulgence in glutamate release can overstimulate the brain, resulting in excitotoxicity, which kills off cells and causes seizures or strokes. Chronic illnesses such as ischemic stroke, epilepsy, amyotrophic lateral sclerosis, Parkinson's disease, Alzheimer's disease, and Huntington's disease have all been linked to excitotoxicity.
- The vast majority of fast inhibitory synapses in almost every region of the brain use GABA. Numerous sedatives and tranquilizers work by amplifying GABA's effects. Consequently, the inhibitory transmitter in the spinal cord is glycine.
- The first neurotransmitter identified in the peripheral and central nervous systems was acetylcholine. It stimulates the somatic nervous system's skeletal muscles and can either excite or inhibit the autonomic nervous system's internal organs. It can be identified by its function as the transmitter at the neuromuscular junction, which joins motor neurons and muscles. The paralytic arrow poison cure works by obstructing the ability of these synapses to transmit information. Although it does so through various receptor types, such as muscarinic and nicotinergic receptors, acetylcholine also functions in a variety of brain regions.
- In the brain, dopamine is involved in many critical processes, such as the control of motor behavior, motivation-related pleasures, and emotional arousal. Dopamine is essential to the reward system; high levels of dopamine have been associated with schizophrenia and low levels with Parkinson's disease.
- The neurotransmitter serotonin is a monoamine. About 90% of it is generated and present in the intestine, with the remaining 10% occurring in neurons of the central nervous system. It controls the following: behavior, temperature, mood, memory and learning, appetite, sleep, muscle contraction, and the operation of the endocrine and cardiovascular systems. Since some depressed patients are observed to have lower concentrations of serotonin metabolites in their brain tissue and cerebrospinal fluid, it is hypothesized to play a part in depression.
- Neurotransmitters classified as catecholamines include norepinephrine. Tyrosine is the

amino acid from which it is synthesized. One of norepinephrine's main functions in the peripheral nervous system is to trigger the release of the stress hormone adrenaline (i.e., from the adrenal glands, such as adrenaline.

- Tyrosine is used to make the neurotransmitter and hormone epinephrine. The adrenal glands release it, and it contributes to the fight-or-flight reaction. Vasoconstrictive effects of epinephrine encourage elevated blood pressure, heart rate, and energy mobilization. Vasoconstriction affects metabolism by encouraging the body to break down glucose that is released into the blood. Airway relaxation, or bronchodilation, is another effect of epinephrine.

6.3.4. Types of Neurotransmitters

Neurotransmitters can be categorized and classed in a variety of ways. They can sometimes be simply separated into peptides, amino acids, and monoamines. Furthermore, neurotransmitters can be divided into six different types:

- **Amino Acids**
    - o **Gamma-aminobutyric acid (GABA):** The primary inhibitory chemical messenger in the body is this naturally occurring amino acid. In addition to helping with vision and motor control, GABA helps control anxiety. Benzodiazepines, which are used to treat anxiety, work by making GABA neurotransmitters more effective, which can heighten emotions of calmness and relaxation.
    - o **Glutamate:** Glutamate, the neurotransmitter that is most prevalent in the nervous system, is involved in cognitive processes like learning and memory. Glutamate overdosage can result in excitotoxicity, which can kill cells. Alzheimer's disease, stroke, and epileptic seizures are among the illnesses and brain injuries linked to this excitotoxicity brought on by glutamate accumulation.
- **Peptides**
    - o **Oxytocin:** In the brain, this potent hormone functions as a neurotransmitter. It plays a part in social recognition, bonding, and sexual reproduction and is produced by the hypothalamus. Pitocin, a synthetic form of oxytocin, is frequently used as a labor and delivery aid. During labor, the uterus contracts due to the effects of both pitocin and oxytocin.
    - o **Endorphins:** These neurotransmitters encourage feelings of euphoria while blocking the transmission of pain signals. The body naturally produces these chemical messengers in response to pain, but other stimuli, like aerobic exercise, can also cause them to be released. An instance of a pleasurable sensation brought on by endorphin production is the "runner's high.".

- **Monoamines**
    - **Epinephrine:** Epinephrine, also referred to as adrenaline, is classified as a neurotransmitter and a hormone. In general, the adrenal system releases the stress hormone epinephrine. But in the brain, it serves as a neurotransmitter.
    - **Norepinephrine:** This naturally occurring substance is a neurotransmitter that is involved in the body's fight-or-flight response and is crucial for alertness. Its function is to assist in preparing the body and mind for action during stressful or dangerous situations. This neurotransmitter's levels are normally highest during stressful situations and lowest during sleep.
    - **Histamine:** This natural substance functions in the brain and spinal cord as a neurotransmitter. It is generated as a byproduct of the immune system's reaction to infections and contributes to allergic reactions.
    - **Dopamine:** Dopamine, sometimes referred to as the "feel-good" neurotransmitter, plays a role in motivation, reward, and addiction. Numerous addictive substance classes raise dopamine levels in the brain. The synchronization of bodily movements is another crucial function of this chemical messenger. Dopamine-producing neurons in the brain are lost in Parkinson's disease, a degenerative condition that impairs motor function and causes tremors.
    - **Serotonin:** Serotonin is a neurotransmitter and hormone that is crucial for controlling mood, appetite, anxiety, sleep patterns, and sexuality. Antidepressant drugs known as selective serotonin reuptake inhibitors (SSRIs) are frequently prescribed to treat anxiety, panic disorder, depression, and panic attacks. By preventing serotonin from being reabsorbed in the brain, SSRIs balance serotonin levels, which can elevate mood and lessen anxiety.
- Purines
    - **Adenosine:** This organic substance functions as a neuromodulator in the brain, suppressing arousal and promoting better sleep.
    - **Adenosine triphosphate (ATP):** ATP is known as the energy currency of life and functions as a neurotransmitter in both the central and peripheral nervous systems. It is involved in autonomic control, sensory transduction, and communication with glial cells. Studies indicate that ATP may be implicated in various neurological issues such as pain, trauma, and neurodegenerative disorders.
- **Gasotransmitters**
    - **Nitricoxide:** This substance has an effect on smooth

muscles, relaxing them to permit blood vessels to widen and improve blood flow to particular body parts.

- **Carbonmonoxide:** When exposed to high concentrations of this colorless, odorless gas, people may experience toxic and possibly fatal effects. But the body can also naturally produce it, and when it does, it functions as a neurotransmitter to help control the body's inflammatory response.

- **Acetylcholine:** In its class, this neurotransmitter is unique. It is the main neurotransmitter linked to motor neurons and is present in both the central and peripheral nervous systems. It affects learning and memory as well as how muscles move (Figure 6.4 and Table 6.2).

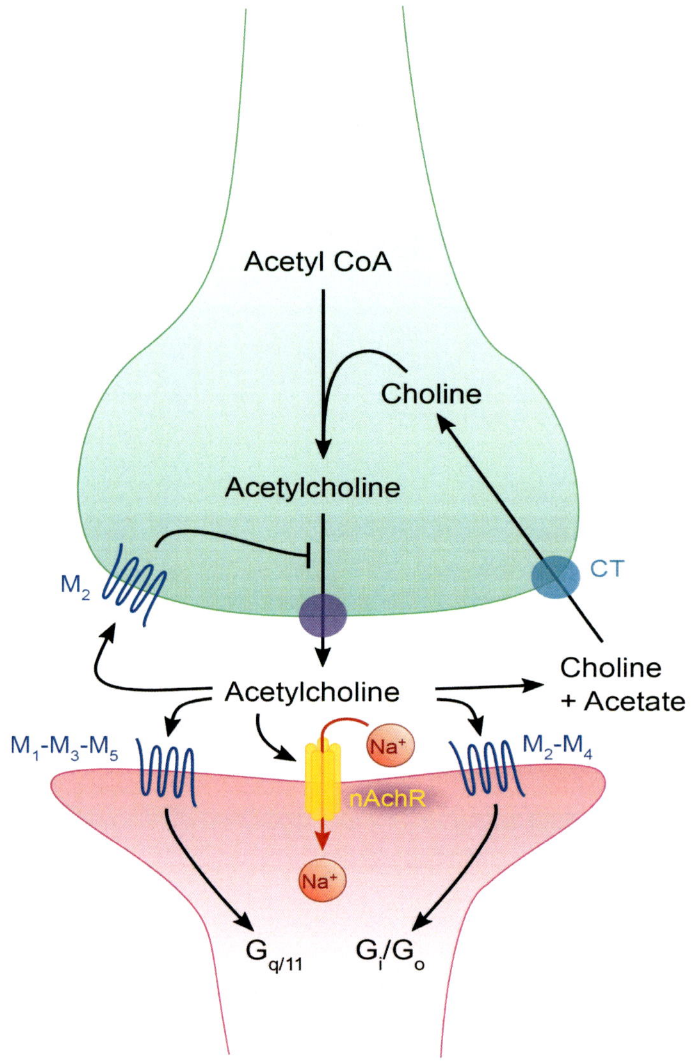

Figure 6.4. *Acetylcholine is cleaved in the synaptic cleft into acetic acid and choline.*

Source: By Pancrat-Ownwork, CCBY-SA3.0, https://commons.wikimedia.org/w/index.php?curid=15253818.

Table 6.2. List of Neurotransmitters, Peptides, and Gaseous Signaling Molecules

Neurotransmitters				
Category	**Name**	**Abbreviation**	**Metabotropic**	**Ionotropic**
Small Tooltip Small molecule: Amino acids (Arg)	Arginine	Arg, R	α_2-Adrenergic receptors, imidazoline receptors	NMDA receptors
Small: Amino acids	Aspartate	Asp, D	–	NMDA receptors
Small: Amino acids	Glutamate	Glu, E	Metabotropic glutamate receptors	NMDA receptors, kainate receptors, AMPARs
Small: Amino acids	Gamma-aminobutyric acid	GABA	$GABA_B$ receptors	$GABA_A$ receptors, $GABA_A$-ρ receptors
Small: Amino acids	Glycine	Gly, G	–	NMDA receptors, glycine receptors
Small: Amino acids	D-serine	Ser, S	–	NMDA receptors
Small: Acetylcholine	Acetylcholine	ACh	Muscarinic acetylcholine receptors	Nicotinic acetylcholine receptors
Small: Monoamine (Phe/Tyr)	Dopamine	DA	Dopamine receptors, trace amine-associated receptor 1	–
Small: Monoamine (Phe/Tyr)	Norepinephrine (noradrenaline)	NE, NAd	Adrenergic receptors	–

Small: Monoamine (Phe/ Tyr)	Epinephrine (adrenaline)	Epi, Ad	Adrenergic receptors	–
Small: Monoamine (Trp)	Serotonin (5-hydroxyt-ryptamine)	5-HT	Serotonin receptors (all except 5-HT_3)	5-HT_3
Small: Monoamine (His)	Histamine	H	Histamine receptors	–
Small: Trace amine (Phe)	Phenethylamine	PEA	Human trace amine-associated receptors: hTAAR1Tooltip human trace amine associated receptor 1, hTAAR2Tooltip human trace amine associated receptor 2	–
Small: Trace amine (Phe)	*N*-methylphen-ethylamine	NMPEA	hTAAR1	–
Small: Trace amine (Phe/Tyr)	Tyramine	TYR	hTAAR1, hTAAR2	–
Small: Trace amine (Phe/Tyr)	octopamine	Oct	hTAAR1	–
Small: Trace amine (Phe/Tyr)	Synephrine	Syn	hTAAR1	–
Small: Trace amine (Trp)	Tryptamine		hTAAR1, various serotonin receptors	–
Small: Trace amine (Trp)	*N*-methyltryptamine	NMT	hTAAR1, various serotonin receptors	–
Lipid	Anandamide	AEA	Cannabinoid receptors	–

Lipid	2-Arachidonoy-lglycerol	2-AG	Cannabinoid receptors	–
Lipid	2-Arachidonyl glyceryl ether	2-AGE	Cannabinoid receptors	–
Lipid	*N*-Arachidonoyl dopamine	NADA	Cannabinoid receptors	TRPV1
Lipid	Virodhamine		Cannabinoid receptors	–
Small: Purine	Adenosine	Ado	Adenosine receptors	–
Small: Purine	Adenosine triphosphate	ATP	P2Y receptors	P2X receptors
Small: Purine	Nicotinamide adenine dinucleotide	β-NAD	P2Y receptors	P2X receptors
		Neuropeptides		
Category	**Name**	**Abbreviation**	**Metabotropic**	**Ionotropic**
Bombesin-like peptides	Bombesin		BBR1–2-3	–
Bombesin-like peptide	Gastrin releasing peptide	GRP	–	–
Bombesin-like peptide	Neuromedin B	NMB	Neuromedin B receptor	–
Bradykinins	Bradykinin		B1, B2	–
Calcitonin/CGRP family	Calcitonin		Calcitonin receptor	–
Calcitonin/CGRP family	Calcitonin gene-related peptide	CGRP	CALCRL	–
Corticotropin-releasing factors	Corticotropin-releasing hormone	CRH	CRHR1	–
Corticotropin-releasing factors	Urocortin		CRHR1	–
Galanins	Galanin		GALR1, GALR2, GALR3	–
Galanins	Galanin-like peptide		GALR1, GALR2, GALR3	–

Gastrins	Gastrin		Cholecystokinin B receptor	–
Gastrins	Cholecystokinin	CCK	Cholecystokinin receptors	–
Granins	Chromogranin A	ChgA	–	–
Melanocortins	Adrenocorticotropic hormone	ACTH	ACTH receptor	–
Melanocortins	Proopiomelanocortin	POMC	Melanocortin 4 receptor	–
Melanocortins	Melanocyte-stimulating hormones	MSH	Melanocortin receptors	–
Neurohypop-hyzeals	Vasopressin	AVP	Vasopressin receptors	–
Neurohypo-phyzeals	Oxytocin	OT	Oxytocin receptor	–
Neurohypo-phyzeals	Neurophysin I		–	–
Neurohypo-phyzeals	Neurophysin II		–	–
Neurohypo-phyzeals	Copeptin		–	–
Neuromedins	Neuromedin U	NmU	NmUR1, NmUR2	–
Neuropeptide B/W	Neuropeptide B	NPB	NPBW1, NPBW2	–
Neuropeptide B/W	Neuropeptide S	NPS	Neuropeptide S receptors	–
Neuropeptide Y	Neuropeptide Y	NY	Neuropeptide Y receptors	–
Neuropeptide Y	Pancreatic polypeptide	PP	–	–
Neuropeptide Y	Peptide YY	PYY	–	–
Opioids	Enkephalins		δ-Opioid receptor	–
Opioids	Dynorphins		κ-Opioid receptor	–
Opioids	Neoendorphins		κ-Opioid receptor	–

Opioids	Endorphins		μ-Opioid receptors	–
Opioids	Endomorphins		μ-Opioid receptors	–
Opioids	Morphine		μ-Opioid receptors	–
Opioids	Nociceptin/orphanin FQ	N/OFQ	Nociceptin receptors	–
Orexins	Orexin A	OX-A	Orexin receptors	–
Orexins	Orexin B	OX-B	Orexin receptors	–
Parathyroid hormone family	Parathyroid hormone-related protein	PTHrP	–	–
RFamides	Kisspeptin	KiSS	GPR54	–
RFamides	Neuropeptide FF	NPFF	NPFF1, NPFF2	–
RFamides	Prolactin-releasing peptide	PrRP	PrRPR	–
RFamides	Pyroglutamylated RFamide peptide	QRFP	GPR103	–
Secretins	Secretin		Secretin receptor	–
Secretins	Motilin		Motilin receptor	–
Secretins	Glucagon		Glucagon receptor	–
Secretins	Glucagon-like peptide-1	GLP-1	Glucagon-like peptide 1 receptor	–
Secretins	Glucagon-like peptide-2	GLP-2	Glucagon-like peptide 2 receptor	–
Secretins	Vasoactive intestinal peptide	VIP	Vasoactive intestinal peptide receptors	–
Secretins	Growth hormone–releasing hormone	GHRH	Growth hormone–releasing hormone receptor	–

Secretins	Pituitary adenylate cyclase-activating peptide	PACAP	ADCYAP1R1	–
Somatostatins	Somatostatin		Somatostatin receptors	–
Tachykinins	Neurokinin A		–	–
Tachykinins	Neurokinin B		–	–
Tachykinins	Substance P		–	–
Tachykinins	Neuropeptide K		–	–
Other	Agouti-related peptide	AgRP	Melanocortin receptor –	
Other	*N*-Acetylasparty-lglutamate	NAAG	Metabotropic glutamate receptor 3 (mGluR3)	–
Other	Cocaine- and amphetamine-regulated transcript	CART	Unknown G_i/G_o-coupled receptor	–
Other	Gonadotropin-releasing hormone	GnRH	GnRHR	–
Other	Thyrotropin-releasing hormone	TRH	TRHR	–
Other	Melanin-concentrating hormone	MCH	MCHR 1,2	–
Gasotransmitters				
Category	**Name**	**Abbreviation**	**Metabotropic**	**Ionotropic**
Gaseous signaling molecule	Nitric oxide	NO	Soluble guanylyl cyclase	–
Gaseous signaling molecule	Carbon monoxide	CO	–	Heme bound to potassium channels
Gaseous signaling molecule	Hydrogen sulfide	H2S	–	–

Source: https://en.wikipedia.org/wiki/Neurotransmitter

6.3.5. Problems with Neurotransmitters

Just like in many other bodily functions, things can go wrong from time to time. Perhaps it should come as no surprise that a system as large and intricate as the human nervous system could experience issues. Among the things that could go wrong are the following:

- Neurons might not manufacture enough of a particular neurotransmitter
- Neurotransmitters may be reabsorbed too quickly
- Too many neurotransmitters may be deactivated by enzymes
- Too much of a particular neurotransmitter may be released

Diseases and medications that alter neurotransmitters can have a variety of negative effects on the body. Deficits in specific neurotransmitters are linked to conditions like Parkinson's, epilepsy, and Alzheimer's. Some neurotransmitters are referred to as "feel-good" chemicals because they have a significant impact on mood and play a vital role in the brain. Dopamine, serotonin, oxytocin, norepinephrine, and endorphins are the five main neurotransmitters.

Because neurotransmitters are known to have an impact on mental health issues, doctors frequently prescribe drugs that alter the body's chemical messengers to treat a range of psychiatric disorders. Dopamine, for instance, has been linked to conditions like schizophrenia and addiction. Depression and OCD are two mood disorders that are influenced by serotonin. Anxiety disorders are associated with dopamine, GABA, serotonin, and norepinephrine levels. Doctors and psychiatrists may prescribe medications, like SSRIs, to help treat anxiety or depression symptoms. Medications can be used in conjunction with other therapeutic treatments, such as cognitive-behavioral therapy, or they can be used alone on occasion.

6.3.6. Drugs That Influence Neurotransmitters

Possibly the most useful use of neurotransmitter function research and discovery has been in the creation of medications that affect chemical transmission. These medications have the ability to alter neurotransmitter effects, which can lessen the symptoms associated with certain illnesses.

- **Agonists vs. Antagonists:** Certain medications, referred to as agonists, work by amplifying the effects of particular neurotransmitters. Other medications, known as antagonists, work to prevent the effects of neurotransmission.
- **Direct vs. Indirect effects:** Depending on whether these neuro-acting medications have an indirect or direct effect, they can be further divided. Because their chemical structures are so similar to those of neurotransmitters, those that have a direct effect function by imitating them. Indirect effects are achieved by means of the synaptic receptors.

Medications used to treat conditions like anxiety and depression, such as benzodiazepines, tricyclic antidepressants, and selective serotonin reuptake inhibitors (SSRIs), can affect neurotransmission.

For instance, SSRIs like Paxil (paroxetine) and Prozac (fluoxetine) increase serotonin levels in the brain by preventing serotonin from being absorbed by nerve cells. Cholinesterase inhibitors, like Aricept (donepezil), work by blocking the enzymes that break down acetylcholine, which can help Alzheimer's patients function more cognitively. Psychoactive substances like cocaine, heroin, and marijuana also have an impact on neurotransmission. Heroin functions as a direct-acting agonist, sufficiently emulating the natural opioids found in the brain to activate the receptors linked to them. One drug that affects dopamine transmission in an indirect manner is cocaine.

Neurotransmitters are essential for neural communication because they affect mood, learning, and involuntary movements, among other things. This system has a great deal of interconnectivity and complexity. Neurotransmitters have specific functions, but illnesses, medications, and even the actions of other chemical messengers can have an impact on them.

6.3.7. Barriers to CNS Drug Delivery

There are several obstacles that prevent drugs from being delivered systemically to the central nervous system (CNS), which helps to explain why many CNS diseases remain untreated despite this fact.

6.3.7.1. Blood-Brain Barrier

The BBB is a distinct membranous barrier that firmly isolates the brain from the bloodstream, as is now widely known. There is a permeability barrier separating the blood inside brain capillaries from the extracellular fluid in brain tissue because the blood capillaries in the central nervous system (CNS) are structurally distinct from the blood capillaries in other tissues. The capillaries found in the brain and spinal cord of vertebrates are lined with a layer of unique endothelial cells that are sealed with tight junctions and lack fenestrations, which prevents solutes from the circulation from moving quickly into other organs. Similar to this barrier, tight epithelium is also present in the skin, bladder, colon, and lung, among other organs. The brain-capillary endothelium is a component of this permeability barrier, which is referred to as the BBB. There are three types of glial cells and ependymal cells that line the cerebral ventricles. Astrocytes regulate the biochemical environment of neurons and provide the structural framework for them. The limbs or foot processes of astrocytes, which extend and abut each other, enclose the capillaries and are closely linked to the blood vessels to form the blood-brain barrier (BBB). The myelin sheath, which envelops axons and is necessary for the rapid transfer of action potentials via salutatory conduction, is formed and maintained by oligodendrocytes. Mononuclear macrophages derived from blood are called microglias. The tight junctions between endothelial cells results in a very high trans-endothelial electrical resistance of 1500–2000 W.cm2 compared to 3–33 W.cm2 of other tissues which reduces the aqueous based para-cellular diffusion that is observed in other organs.

The human brain is thought to contain 650 km of capillaries with a surface area of 12 m^2. Despite this, the capillaries function as an extremely effective barrier that prevents lipid-insoluble substances like polar molecules and small ions from entering the brain. Consequently, many promising drugs lose some of their therapeutic value, and brain diseases have shown to be particularly resistant to treatment. This is a serious issue just in light of the prevalence of brain disorders. Almost all medications used today to treat brain disorders are lipid-soluble and easily pass through the blood-brain barrier when taken orally. Fortunately, because of their limited transport across the blood-brain barrier (BBB), antimicrobial b-lactam antibiotics do not cause such central nervous system (CNS) side effects when administered intravenously or orally. However, when administered intracerebroventricularly, these antibiotics do cause severe convulsions. Furthermore, grepafloxacin, a lipophilic new quinolone antimicrobial agent, is not able to enter the brain despite being widely distributed into various tissues. This prevents the development of central nervous system side effects like headache and dizziness, which are caused by the displacement of g-aminobutyric acid (GABA) from the GABA receptor binding sites.

However, because benzodiazepines are lipophilic and easily cross the blood-brain barrier, they have been used as sedative-hypnotic agents. One example of this is diazepam. Nevertheless, cyclosporin A, an immunosuppressive medication that is more lipophilic than diazepam, has extremely restricted BBB transport. Vinca alkaloids (e.g., vincristine and vinblastine) hardly enter the brain, causing difficulty in the treatment of brain tumors. Levodopa is a hydrophilic medication that is effective in treating Parkinson's disease, but it can easily cross the blood-brain barrier.

Certain areas of the central nervous system lack the expression of classical BBB capillary endothelial cells, but they do have peripheral-like microvessels. These regions are known as the circumventricular organs (CVOs) because they are close to the brain's ventricles. The pineal gland, the organum vasculosum of the lamina terminalis, the subfornical organ, the subcommisaral organ, the area postrema, the median eminence, the neurohypophysis, and the choroid plexus are among the CVOs. Although the capillaries in the CVO brain regions are more permeable to solutes, transport from the abluminal extracellular fluid (ECF) to the brain ECF is hindered by the formation of tight junctions between the tanycytes of other regions and the epithelial cells of the choroid plexus. Given that the choroid plexus is the primary location for the production of cerebrospinal fluid (CSF) and that the CSF and brain ECF are freely exchanged, it may be significant when thinking about the transport of peptide drugs.

An extra enzymatic component exists in the BBB. When solutes pass through the cell membrane, they are exposed to the many degrading enzymes found inside endothelial cells, which are highly metabolically active organelles with high densities of mitochondria. The majority of peptides, including naturally occurring neuropeptides, are recognized by BBB enzymes and are quickly broken down.

Additionally, the blood-brain barrier is strengthened by a significant presence of P-glycoprotein (Pgp), a transporter protein that actively removes various drug molecules from the endothelial cell cytoplasm before they can enter the brain parenchyma.

6.3.7.2. Blood-Cerebrospinal Fluid Barrier

The blood-cerebrospinal fluid barrier (BCB) is the second barrier that a drug administered systemically encounters before entering the central nervous system (CNS). The BCB also carefully controls the flow of blood-borne molecules into the CSF because the CSF can exchange molecules with the brain parenchyma's interstitial fluid. From a physiological perspective, the BCB is located in the choroids plexus epithelium, which is arranged to restrict the entry of molecules and cells into the CSF. At the borders separating the blood from the CSF, the choroid plexus and the arachnoid membrane collaborate. The arachnoid membrane, which is located between the dura and pia on the exterior of the brain, is a double-layered structure formed by the folding of ependymal cells over one another. The subarachnoid space, a component of the double layer, aids in CSF drainage.

Tight junctions stop substances from the blood from passing through the arachnoid membrane. The arachnoid membrane plays a mostly passive role in forming the blood-CSF barrier because it is normally impermeable to hydrophilic substances. The CSF is created by the choroid plexus, which also actively controls the CSF's molecule concentration. The highly vascularized, "cauliflower-like" masses of pia mater tissue that dip into ependymal cell-formed pockets make up the choroid plexus. The choroid plexus predominates in the lateral ventricles located inside the right and left cerebral hemispheres as well as the fourth ventricle, which is located close to the base of the brain.

The choroidal epithelium's cells are altered and possess epithelial traits. These ependymal cells have a lot of mitochondria, basolateral interdigitations, and microvilli on the CSF side. A continuous sheet of ependymal cells, which border the ventricles, encircles the choroid plexus. The choroid plexus's capillaries are fenestrated, non-continuous, and have gaps between the capillary endothelial cells that permit small molecules to flow freely. However, the nearby choroidal epithelial cells form tight junctions that hinder the majority of macromolecules from efficiently entering the CSF from the blood. However, these epithelial-like cells have shown a low resistance as compared the cerebral endothelial cells, approximately 200 $W.cm^2$, between blood and CSF.

Furthermore, an active organic acid transporter system in the choroids plexus that can propel CSF-borne organic acids into the bloodstream strengthens the BCB. Consequently, the CSF actively removes a range of therapeutic organic acids that would otherwise diffuse into the brain parenchyma, including the antibiotic penicillin, the anti-neoplastic agent methotrexate, and the antiviral drug zidovudine. Moreover, there are frequently significant differences in the composition of the CSF and the brain parenchyma's interstitial fluid, which may indicate the existence of the so-called CSF-brain barrier. The unbreakable diffusion distances needed for the CSF and the brain interstitial fluid to equilibrate are the cause of this barrier. Consequently, a drug's ability to enter the CSF does not ensure that it will enter the brain.

6.3.7.3. Blood-Tumor Barrier

Delivering drugs intracranially is even more difficult when the target is a brain tumor. Clinical implications arise from the BBB's presence in the microvasculature of CNS tumors. For instance, intracranial metastases frequently continue to grow even in response to chemotherapeutic agents delivered through the cardiovascular system for primary and secondary systemic tumors. A range of physiological barriers common to all solid tumors impede drug delivery via the cardiovascular system in CNS malignancies where the BBB is severely compromised. A heterogeneous distribution of microvasculature throughout the tumor interstitial compromises drug delivery to neoplastic cells in a solid tumor, resulting in spatially inconsistent drug delivery.

Moreover, when a tumor gets bigger, its vascular surface area shrinks, which lessens the amount of blood-borne molecules that can pass through it. The high interstitial tumor pressure and accompanying peri-tumoral edema cause an increase in hydrostatic pressure in the normal brain parenchyma next to the tumor, and at the same time, intra-capillary distance increases, increasing the diffusional requirement for drug delivery to neoplastic cells. Consequently, extra-tumoral interstitial drug concentrations may be abnormally low due to the cerebral microvasculature in these tumor-adjacent normal brain regions being even less drug-permeable than normal brain endothelium. Brain tumors can also cause localized, nonhomogeneous disruptions to the blood-brain barrier.

In conclusion, the delivery of drugs to the CNS via the cardiovascular system is often precluded by a variety of formidable barriers including the BBB, the BCB, and the BTB.

6.4. Medicinal Chemistry of Drugs for Neurological Disorders

Conditions affecting the brain, spinal cord, and the body's nerves as a whole are referred to as neurological disorders. These encompass a broad spectrum of illnesses, including cerebral aneurysms, Bell's palsy, Alzheimer's disease, attention deficit hyperactivity disorder (ADHD), brain tumors, traumatic brain injuries, carpal tunnel syndrome, diabetic neuropathy, epilepsy, and essential tremor. These also include conditions that affect movement, such as muscular dystrophy (progressive muscle weakness), Parkinson's disease, migraine, multiple sclerosis, myasthenia gravis, and amyotrophic lateral sclerosis (ALS). There are known to be over 600 neurological conditions that affect people.

A number of neurological disorders, including drug-induced movement disorders such as tremors, neuroleptic malignant syndrome (NMS), serotonin syndrome (serotonin excess), permanent cerebellar syndrome, tardive dyskinesia, and other tardive syndromes, are brought on by medication side effects.

The neurological condition being treated will determine how it is treated. Every medication therapy is tailored to treat a particular illness. Drug therapy, for instance, might involve the administration of drugs via pumps or implanted devices (like spinal cord and deep brain stimulators). Certain treatments are as simple as physical therapy or brain surgery.

Thankfully, there is a wide range of medical professionals who treat neurological conditions. These professionals include neurologists, neurosurgeons, psychiatrists, vascular surgeons, radiologists, primary care physicians, nurse practitioners, physical and occupational therapists, to mention a few.

These are a few of the drugs that are frequently prescribed to treat neurological conditions.

6.4.1. Anticonvulsants

According to CDC estimates, 3.4 million Americans suffer from epilepsy, or seizures. Among the most often prescribed drugs for neurological conditions are anticonvulsants, which include levetiracetam (Keppra), topiramate (Topamax), lamotrigine (Lamictal), oxcarbazepine (Trileptal), and divalproex sodium (Depakote). These medications may cause nausea, vomiting, double vision, headaches, drowsiness, and liver damage as adverse effects. The side effects of more recent anticonvulsants, such as pregabalin (Lyrica) and gabapentin (Neurontin), are lower. They are used to treat nerve pain, including postherpetic neuralgia and diabetic neuropathy.

6.4.2. Parkinson's Disease Medications

Patients with Parkinson's disease may experience improved function when taking medications like levodopa and carbidopa. The brain can access more dopamine as a result of these drugs. Other neurological drugs such as dopamine agonists such as ropinirole (Requip), rotigotine (Neupro), and pramipexole (Mirapex) are used to treat symptoms such as muscular rigidity in Parkinson's patients.

Be aware that extrapyramidal symptoms are a possible side effect of some antipsychotic medications. At high dosages, there is an increased chance of experiencing these symptoms, which can mimic those of Parkinson's disease. Your physician may choose to switch to a different medication, reduce the dosage of the causing agent (an antipsychotic), or treat specific symptoms with anti-Parkinson's medication to treat Parkinsonian symptoms. Such a side effect is less common in patients treated with more recent atypical antipsychotics such as clozapine, quetiapine, and olanzapine.

6.4.3. Medications Used to Treat Dementia

Alzheimer's disease, dementia with Lewy bodies, and Parkinson's dementia are treated with neurological drugs known as cholinesterase inhibitors, which include donepezil (Aricept), galantamine (Razadyne), and rivastigmine (Exelon). These medications can cause headaches, nausea, diarrhea, and insomnia as side effects.

6.4.4. Antidepressants

Antidepressant medications, such as monoamine oxidase inhibitors, tricyclic antidepressants, and selective serotonin reuptake inhibitors (SSRIs), are frequently prescribed for neurological conditions. One in eight Americans, or roughly 13% of the population, is estimated by the CDC to be taking an antidepressant.

6.4.5. Beta Blockers

Propranolol and other beta blockers are used to treat high blood pressure. Nevertheless, patients with illnesses affecting the nervous system, such as essential tremors and migraine headaches, may also be prescribed this medication.

6.4.6. Thrombolytics

This class of drugs, also known as blood thinners, is intended to break up blood clots that are obstructing blood flow to the brain, legs, heart, or lungs. A few examples are streptokinase, urokinase, prourokinase, Tenecteplase, anistreplase, alteplase (t-PA), and reteplase. Notably, taking certain drugs may raise your risk of blood clots. For instance, women who use oral contraceptives and hormone replacement therapy have increased rates of blood clots, stroke, and cerebrovascular disease. Modifications in lifestyle such as diet, exercise, stopping smoking, and weight loss can help reduce this risk.

Conditions affecting the peripheral nerves and central nervous system can be effectively treated with a wide range of medications. Give your doctors a thorough medical history that includes all of the medications you have tried in the past and how you responded to them to get the most out of any neurological treatments. Additionally, provide your medical professionals with an exhaustive list of all the medications you are currently taking, including prescription, over-the-counter, dietary, and herbal supplements. By doing this, you can prevent drug interactions between your prescriptions.

A Closer Look

Everyday Connection: How Much of Your Brain Do You Use?

Is it true that people only utilize 10% of their brains? Perhaps you have seen a website advertisement promising to reveal the key to unleashing your mind's full potential, as though 90% of your brain was lying around waiting to be used. Never click on an advertisement of that kind. It's untrue.

Measuring brain activity during task performance is a simple approach to determine an individual's brain usage. Functional magnetic resonance imaging (fMRI), which can produce and present a three-dimensional map of the brain's most active regions, is an example of this type of measurement. Because it measures changes in the tissue over time in response to an experimental condition or event, this procedure differs from standard magnetic resonance imaging.

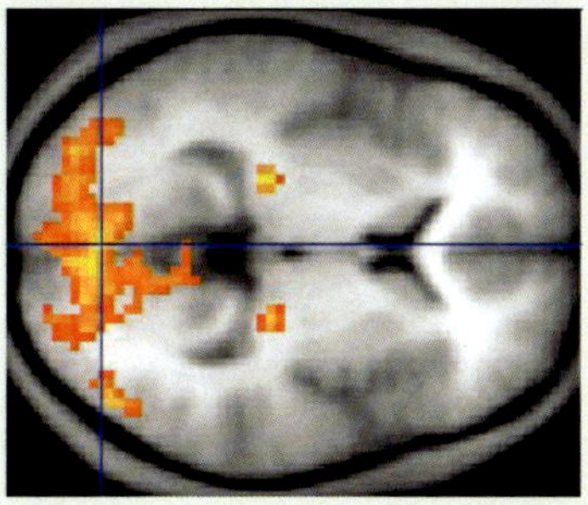

Figure 6.5. *Functional Magnetic Resonance Imaging (fMRI) of the brain.*

Source: By OpenStax, licensedunderCCBY4.0, https://med.libretexts.org/Bookshelves/Anatomy_and_Physiology/Human_Anatomy_(OERI)/11%3A_Nervous_System_and_Nervous_Tissue/11.02%3A_Organization_and_Functions_of_the_Nervous_System.

The fundamental premise is that increased blood flow will occur in active nervous tissue. Brain activity can be measured across the board by asking the subject to complete a visual task. Imagine conducting an experiment where the participant is instructed to gaze at a screen featuring a black dot in the center, known as a fixation point. A faceless picture is displayed on the screen, offset from the center. The person being interviewed must examine the photo and determine what it is. If the person in the photo is someone they know, they are instructed to press a button. In the event that the photo featured a well-known person, the subject would press the button; alternatively, if it featured an unidentified stranger, the subject would not.

The sensory areas involved in vision would be active in this task, as would integrating areas, motor areas involved in eye movement, and motor areas involved in finger-pressing the button. These regions are dispersed throughout the brain, and fMRI scans would reveal activity in more than 10% of the brain (some research indicates that, depending on blood flow to the tissue, approximately 80% of the brain uses energy during specific tasks like the one mentioned above). Not all of the tasks that the brain is capable of performing are included in this task. The body is largely motionless inside the MRI machine, there is no language response, and the autonomic processes that would be going on in the background are not taken into account.

Summary

- The CNS consists of two major structures: the brain and spinal cord. The brain is encased in the skull, and protected by the cranium. The spinal cord is continuous with the brain and lies caudally to the brain. It is protected by the vertebrae.
- Microscopically, there are differences between the neurons and tissue of the CNS and the peripheral nervous system (PNS). The CNS is composed of white and gray matter. This can also be seen macroscopically on brain tissue. The white matter consists of axons and oligodendrocytes, while the gray matter consists of neurons and unmyelinated fibers
- From and to the spinal cord are projections of the peripheral nervous system in the form of spinal nerves (sometimes segmental nerves). The nerves connect the spinal cord to skin, joints, muscles etc., and allow for the transmission of efferent motor as well as afferent sensory signals and stimuli.
- Stimulants are drugs that exert their action through excitation of the central nervous system. Psychic stimulants include caffeine, cocaine, and various amphetamines. These drugs are used to enhance mental alertness and reduce drowsiness and fatigue.
- The stimulation caused by amphetamines is caused by excessive release of norepinephrine from storage sites in the peripheral nervous system. It is not known whether the same action occurs in the central nervous system.
- Neurotransmitters are chemical messengers that carry, boost, and balance signals between neurons (also known as nerve cells) and target cells throughout the body. These target cells may be in glands, muscles, or other neurons.
- There are many different ways to classify and categorize neurotransmitters. In some instances, they are simply divided into monoamines, amino acids, and peptides.
- Neurological disorders are conditions that affect the brain, spinal cord (central nervous system), and the nerves distributed throughout the body. They include a wide range of conditions such as attention deficit hyperactivity disorder (ADHD), Alzheimer's disease, Bell's palsy, brain tumors, traumatic brain injuries, carpal tunnel syndrome, cerebral aneurysms, diabetic neuropathy, epilepsy, and essential tremor.
- Drugs used to treat Parkinson's disease, such as carbidopa and levodopa, can help patients with this condition function better. These medications increase the amount of dopamine available to the brain.
- Neurological medications called cholinesterase inhibitors, such as donepezil (Aricept), galantamine (Razadyne), and rivastigmine (Exelon), are used to treat Alzheimer's disease, dementia with Lewy bodies, and Parkinson's dementia. Adverse effects of these drugs include nausea, diarrhea, headache, and insomnia.
- Beta blockers such as propranolol are used to treat high blood pressure. However, this medication is also prescribed to treat patients with medical conditions affecting the nervous system, for example, essential tremors and migraine headaches.

References

1. Albert, P. R., Vahid-Ansari, F., & Luckhart, C. (2014). Serotonin-prefrontal cortical circuitry in anxiety and depression phenotypes: Pivotal role of pre- and post-synaptic 5-HT1A receptor expression. *Frontiers in Behavioral Neuroscience, 8*, 199. https://doi.org/10.3389/fnbeh.2014.00199.

2. Arias-Carrión, O., Stamelou, M., Murillo-Rodríguez, E., Menéndez-González, M., & Pöppel, E. (2010). Dopaminergic reward system: A short integrative review. *International Archives of Medicine, 3*, 24. https://doi.org/10.1186/1755-7682-3-24.

3. Benarroch, E. E. (2010). Adenosine triphosphate: A multifaceted chemical signal in the nervous system. *Neurology, 2010 Feb 16;74(7):601-7.*

4. Berg, K. A., & Clarke, W. P. (2018). Making sense of pharmacology: Inverse agonism and functional selectivity. *International Journal of Neuropsychopharmacology, 21*(10), 962–977. https://doi.org/10.1093/ijnp/pyy071.

5. Boto, T., & Tomchik, S. M. (2019). The excitatory, the inhibitory, and the modulatory: Mapping chemical neurotransmission in the brain. *Neuron, 101*(5), 763–765. https://doi.org/10.1016/j.neuron.2019.02.021.

6. Ghose, A. K., Herbertz, T., Hudkins, R. L., et al. (2012). Knowledge-based, central nervous system (CNS) lead selection and lead optimization for CNS drug discovery. *ACS Chemical Neuroscience, 3*(1), 50–68. https://doi.org/10.1021/cn200100h.

7. Hanafy, K. A., Oh, J., & Otterbein, L. E. (2013). Carbon monoxide and the brain: Time to rethink the dogma. *Current Pharmaceutical Design, 19*(15), 2771–2775. https://doi.org/10.2174/1381612811319150013.

8. Herculano-Houzel, S. (2009). The human brain in numbers: A linearly scaled-up primate brain. *Frontiers in Human Neuroscience, 3*, 31. https://doi.org/10.3389/neuro.09.031.2009.

9. Hitchcock, S. A., & Pennington, L. D. (2006). Structure-brain exposure relationships. *Journal of Medicinal Chemistry, 49*(26), 7559–7583. https://doi.org/10.1021/jm060642i.

10. Kayalioglu, G. (2009). The vertebral column and spinal meninges. In *The Spinal Cord* (pp. 17–36). Elsevier. https://doi.org/10.1016/B978-0-12-374247-6.50007-9.

11. Kihara, T., & Shimohama, S. (2004). Alzheimer's disease and acetylcholine receptors. *Acta Neurobiologiae Experimentalis, 64*(1), 99–106. Retrieved April 16, 2022, from https://pubmed.ncbi.nlm.nih.gov/15190684/ (accessed on 22 May 2024).

12. Lee, M. S., Johansen, L., Zhang, Y., et al. (2007). The novel combination of chlorpromazine and pentamidine exerts synergistic anti-proliferative effects through dual mitotic action. *Cancer Research, 67*(23), 11359–11367. https://doi.org/10.1158/0008-5472.CAN-07-2235.

13. Magon, N., & Kalra, S. (2011). The orgasmic history of oxytocin: Love, lust, and labor. *Indian Journal of Endocrinology and Metabolism, 15*, S156–S161. https://doi.org/10.4103/2230-8210.84851.

14. Moini, J., & Piran, P. (2020). Meninges and ventricles. In *Functional and Clinical Neuroanatomy* (pp. 95–129). Elsevier. https://doi.org/10.1016/B978-0-12-817424-1.00004-5.

15. Mullard, A. (2011). Could pharma open its drug freezers? *Nature Reviews Drug Discovery, 10*(6), 399–400. https://doi.org/10.1038/nrd3473.

16. Mullard, A. (2012). 2011 FDA drug approvals. *Nature Reviews Drug Discovery, 11*(2), 91–94. https://doi.org/10.1038/nrd3657.

17. Nagappan, P. G., Chen, H., & Wang, D. Y. (2020). Neuroregeneration and plasticity: A review of the physiological mechanisms for achieving functional recovery post-injury. *Military Medical Research, 7*(1), 30. https://doi.org/10.1186/s40779-020-00259-3.

18. Nielsen, J. A., Zielinski, B. A., Ferguson, M. A., Lainhart, J. E., & Anderson, J. S. (2013). An evaluation of the left-brain vs. right-brain hypothesis with resting state functional connectivity magnetic resonance imaging. *PLOS ONE, 8*(8), e71275. https://doi.org/10.1371/journal.pone.0071275.

19. Nuutinen, S., & Panula, P. (2010). Histamine in neurotransmission and brain diseases. *Advances in Experimental Medicine and Biology, 709*, 95–107. https://doi.org/10.1007/978-1-4419-8056-4_10.

20. Oprea, T. I., Davis, A. M., Teague, S. J., et al. (2001). Is there a difference between leads and drugs? A historical perspective. *Journal of Chemical Information and Computer Sciences, 41*(5), 1308–1315. https://doi.org/10.1021/ci010366a.

21. Pajouhesh, H., & Lenz, G. R. (2005). Medicinal chemical properties of successful central nervous system drugs. *NeuroRx, 2*(4), 541–553. https://doi.org/10.1602/neurorx.2.4.541.

22. Palmer, A. M., & Alavijeh, M. S. (2012). Translational CNS medicines research. *Drug Discovery Today, 17*(19–20), 1068–1078. https://doi.org/10.1016/j.drudis.2012.05.001.

23. Paul, S. M., Mytelka, D. S., Dunwiddie, C. T., et al. (2010). How to improve R&D productivity: The pharmaceutical industry's grand challenge. *Nature Reviews Drug Discovery, 9*(3), 203–214. https://doi.org/10.1038/nrd3078.

24. Perry, M., Stansfeld, P. J., Leaney, J., et al. (2006). Drug binding interactions in the inner cavity of hERG channels: Molecular insights from structure-activity relationships of clofilium and ibutilide analogs. *Molecular Pharmacology, 69*(2), 509–519. https://doi.org/10.1124/mol.105.016741.

25. Purves, D., Augustine, G. J., Fitzpatrick, D., et al. (2001). What defines a neurotransmitter? In *Neuroscience* (2nd ed.). Sunderland, MA: Sinauer Associates.

26. Sheffler, Z. M., Reddy, V., & Pillarisetty, L. S. (2020). Physiology, neurotransmitters. In *StatPearls*. StatPearls Publishing. Retrieved December 23, 2020, from https://www.ncbi.nlm.nih.gov/books/NBK539894/ (accessed on 22 May 2024).

27. Sprouse-Blum, A. S., Smith, G., Sugai, D., & Parsa, F. D. (2010). Understanding endorphins and their importance in pain management. *Hawaii Medical Journal, 69*(3), 70–71.

28. Tank, A. W., & Leewong, D. (2015). Peripheral and central effects of circulating catecholamines. *Comprehensive Physiology, 5*(1), 1–15. https://doi.org/10.1002/cphy.c140007.

29. Valenzuela, C. F., Puglia, M. P., & Zucca, S. (2011). Focus on: Neurotransmitter systems. *Alcohol Research & Health, 34*(1), 106–120.

30. Veber, D. F., Johnson, S. R., Cheng, H. Y., et al. (2002). Molecular properties that influence the oral bioavailability of drug candidates. *Journal of Medicinal Chemistry, 45*(12), 2615–2623. https://doi.org/10.1021/jm020017n.

31. Wang, R., & Reddy, P. H. (2017). Role of glutamate and NMDA receptors in Alzheimer's disease. *Journal of Alzheimer's Disease, 57*(4), 1041–1048. https://doi.org/10.3233/JAD-160763.

Chapter 7

DRUG METABOLISM AND TOXICOLOGY

Contents

Introduction

The metabolic breakdown of drugs by living things, typically facilitated by specialized enzymatic systems, is known as drug metabolism. More broadly speaking, the metabolic pathways that alter the chemical structure of substances that are outside of an organism's natural biochemistry, like drugs and poisons, are referred to as xenobiotic metabolism. These pathways are a type of biotransformation thought to have an ancient origin and are found in all major groups of organisms. These processes frequently work to detoxify harmful substances (though occasionally the metabolic intermediates of xenobiotics can also have harmful effects on their own). Pharmacokinetics is the study of drug metabolism. Pharmacology and medicine both heavily rely on the metabolism of pharmaceutical drugs. For instance, a drug's pharmacologic action's duration and potency are dictated by its rate of metabolism. Medication metabolism also influences multidrug resistance in infectious diseases and in cancer chemotherapy. Dangerous drug interactions are frequently caused by certain drugs acting as substrates or inhibitors of xenobiotic metabolism-related enzymes. These pathways are also crucial to environmental science, since microorganisms' xenobiotic metabolism dictates whether a pollutant will persist in the environment or be broken down during bioremediation. Due to their potential to cause herbicide and pesticide resistance, the xenobiotic metabolism enzymes, in particular the glutathione S-transferases, are also significant in agriculture. Three phases make up drug metabolism. Enzymes like cytochrome P450 oxidases add polar or reactive groups to xenobiotics during phase I. In phase II reactions, these altered compounds are subsequently conjugated to polar compounds. Glutathione S-transferases and other transferase enzymes catalyze these reactions. Phase III is the last stage where the conjugated xenobiotics might undergo additional processing before being recognized by efflux transporters and pumped out of the cells. Drug metabolism frequently changes lipophilic substances into more easily excreted hydrophilic products.

Orientation and Directional Terms

Term	Definition	Illustration
Biochemical conversion	It is the process where microorganisms break down the biomass to produce useful end products.	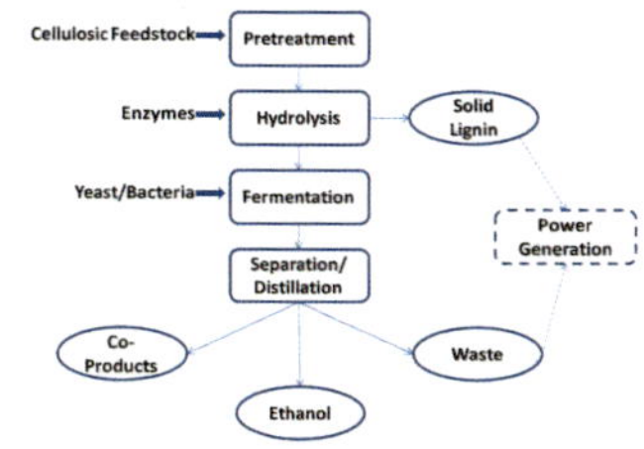
Enzymatic systems	There are several enzyme systems that catalyze reactions to neutralize free radicals and reactive oxygen species. These enzymes include: superoxide dismutase. glutathione peroxidize.	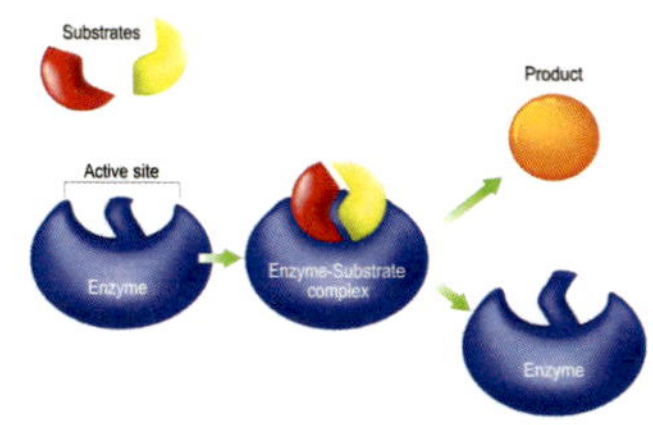
Cytochrome	Cytochrome contains a heme prosthetic group embedded within a porphyrin ring. Porphyrin rings are comprised of four pyrrole structures.	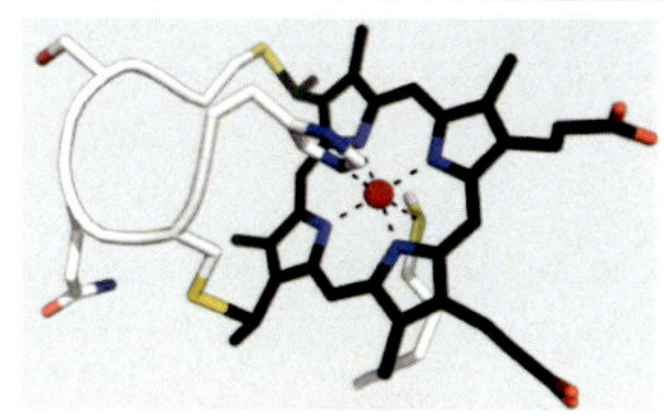
Biotransformation	A metabolic process that takes place mainly in the liver and helps to facilitate the excretion of both exogenous and endogenous substances.	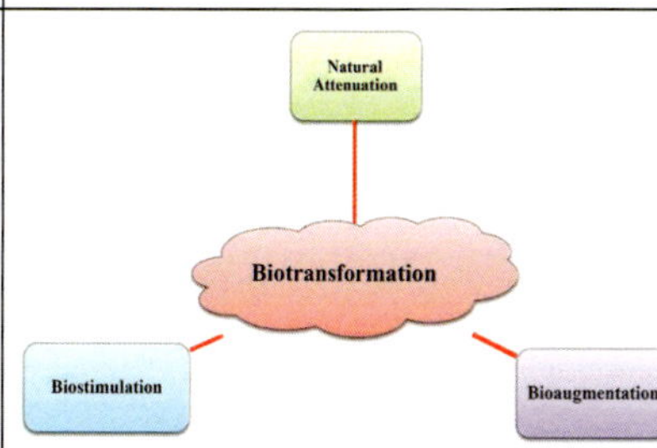
Bioinorganic chemistry	Bioinorganic chemistry is an important field that helps scientists to analyze the relationship between different metals, inorganic substances, and organisms.	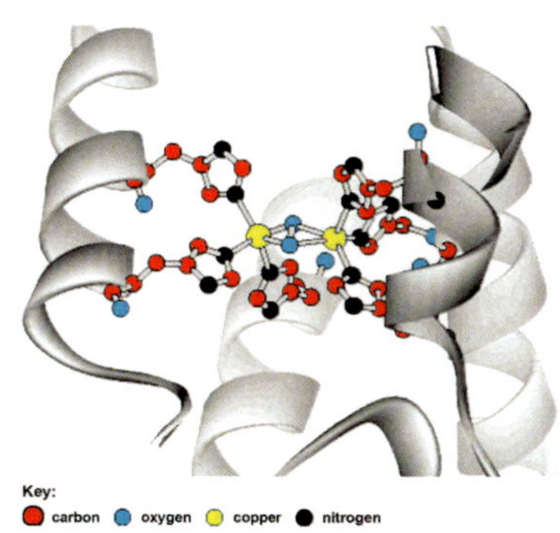

7.1. Drug Metabolism

Humans need medicines to treat illnesses, but they are also foreign substances to the body. Therefore, the body makes an effort to eliminate them as soon as possible. It is ideal for medications to leave the body as soon as possible after they start to act as a drug. The longer a medication is in the body, the more adverse effects it causes. The human body naturally gets rid of these foreign substances, or medications. The drug metabolism process primarily facilitates this. The biochemical conversion of one chemical form to another, usually carried out by specialized enzymatic systems, is known as drug metabolism. It frequently entails the transformation of lipophilic chemical substances—drugs—into highly polar derivatives that the body can eliminate with ease (Figure 7.1).

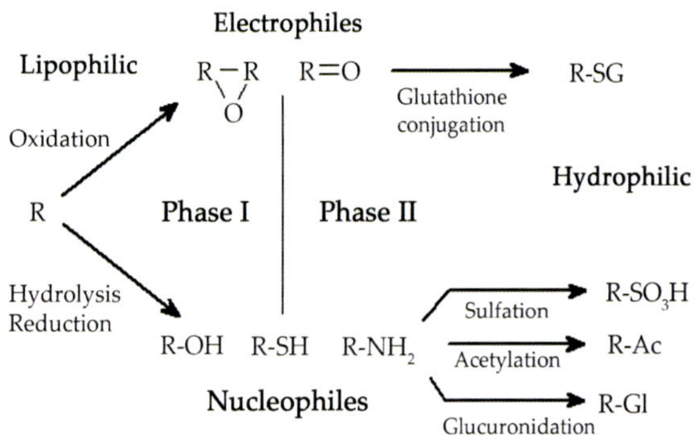

Figure 7.1. *General pathway of drug metabolism.*

Source: By TimVickers – Own work, Public Domain, https://commons.wikimedia.org/w/index.php?curid=4549628.

Lipid soluble substances build up in the body and cause toxic reactions because they are passively reabsorption into the bloodstream from the renal tubules. The body has an arsenal in the form of a metabolic system to prevent the same. This system converts drugs that are lipophilic, water-insoluble, and nonpolar into metabolites that are more polar, water-soluble, and readily excretable from the body. Drug metabolism is therefore appropriately and fittingly referred to as a detoxification process. For a drug to take effect, some of the metabolites are necessary. Prodrugs are being designed with this phenomenon in mind. Reactive metabolites (RM), which are harmful to the human body, can also be produced by the same metabolic process. This process, known as drug bioactivation, is dependent on certain structural characteristics of the compounds in question. There are efforts underway to prevent the production of these reactive metabolites.

7.1.1. Metabolic Organs

Drug metabolism is a fascinating and intricate process that requires a deep understanding of chemistry. The smooth endoplasmic reticulum of the liver cell serves as the main location for drug metabolism. This is a result of the abundance of various types of enzymes in large quantities. Hepatic metabolism is the name given to the drug metabolism that takes place in the liver. Every biological tissue in the body has the capacity to metabolize drugs, except for the liver. Extrahepatic metabolism is the term for the drug metabolism process that takes place in organs other than the liver. The placenta, kidney, lungs, skin, adrenal glands, and gastrointestinal tract epithelial cells are among the other sites. These sites do, however, only have a small part in this process. The majority of drugs (roughly 70%) go through metabolism, which is facilitated by the enzymes found in the locations listed above.

7.1.2. Chemistry of Drug Metabolism

Enzymes are essential for the conversion of one chemical species to another during the chemical process of drug metabolism. The cytochrome P450 family of enzymes is the main group connected to these metabolic processes. These enzymes' structural characteristics and functional capabilities make up the bioinorganic components of drug metabolism.

7.1.2.1. Bioinorganic Chemistry of Drug Metabolism

The cytochrome P450 (CYP) enzymes, also known as microsomal mixed function oxidases, are membrane-bound proteins found in the smooth endoplasmic reticulum of the liver and other tissues.

$$\text{CYP} + \underset{\text{Substrate/Drug}}{\text{Sub-H}} + O_2 + H^+ \xrightarrow{\text{NADPH} \rightarrow \text{NADP}^+} \underset{\text{Oxidised Substrate/Drug}}{\text{Sub-OH}} + H_2O$$

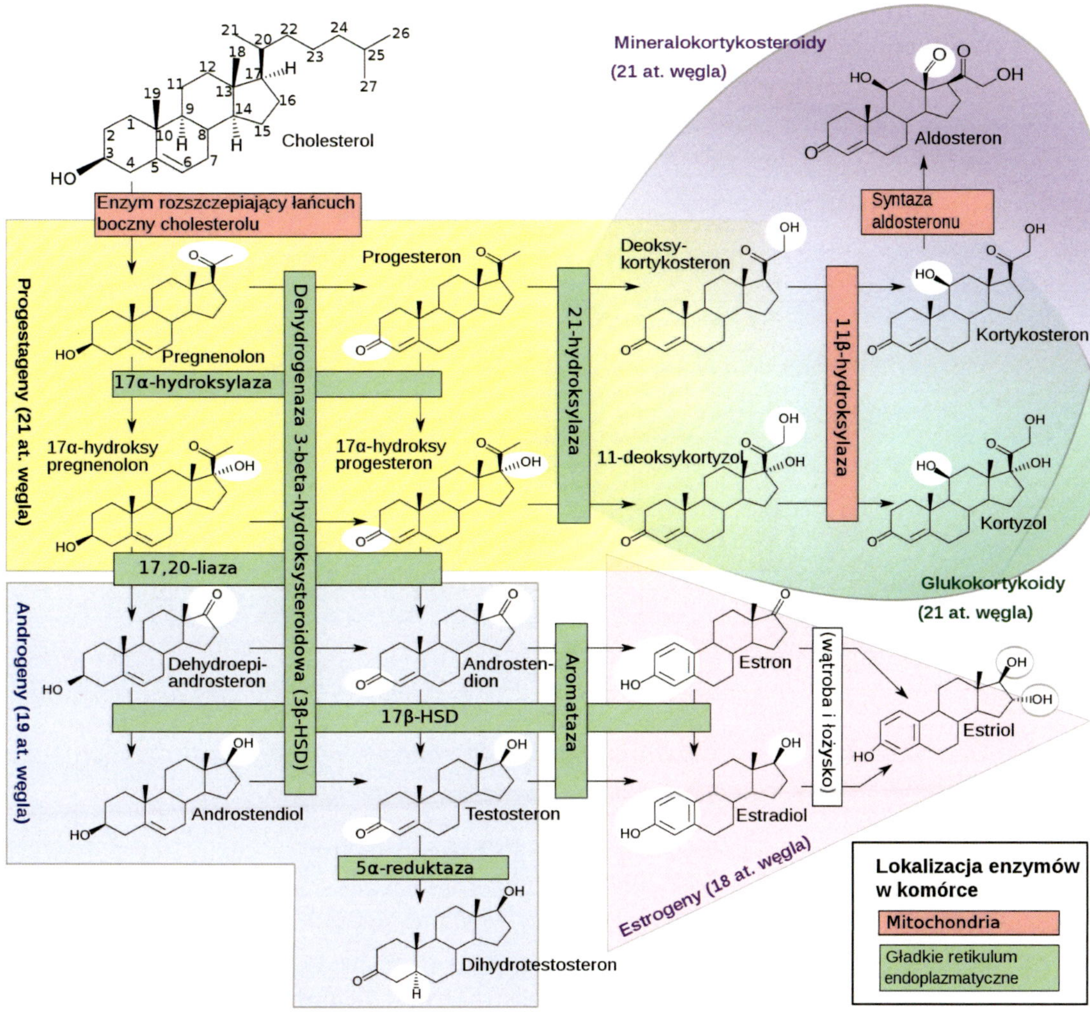

Figure 7.2. *The catalytic cycle of CYP450, leading to the oxidation of substrate.*

Source: By David Richfield (Slashme) and Mikael Häggström. Derived from previous version by Hoffmeier and Settersr. In external use, this diagram may be cited as:(2014). "Diagram of the pathways of human steroidogenesis". WikiJournal of Medicine 1 (1). DOI:10.15347/wjm/2014.005. ISSN 20018762. – Häggström M, Richfield D (2014). "Diagram of the pathways of human steroidogenesis". WikiJournal of Medicine 1 (1). DOI:10.15347/wjm/2014.005. ISSN 20024436., CC0, https://commons.wikimedia.org/w/index.php?curid=4494399.

They play a crucial role in Phase I drug biotransformation. These enzymes contain a heme prosthetic group, consisting of an iron-porphyrin unit. The heme center within these enzymes is responsible for oxidizing hydrophobic compounds into more hydrophilic or polar metabolites for elimination from the body. CYP450 enzymes are named for their ability to bind carbon monoxide with high affinity in the reduced state, resulting in a distinctive UV absorbance at 450 nm. These enzymes facilitate the transfer of oxygen atoms to substrates, converting them into oxidized products and water.

The comprehensive process of CYP metabolism has been explicated in the catalytic cycle depicted in Figure 7.2. Based on the amino-acid sequence, the more than 300 distinct CYP enzymes have been divided into a number of families and subfamilies. Of these, eighteen CYP families—mostly those of CYP1, CYP2, and CYP3—have been found in mammals. Figure 7.3 shows the percentage contribution of each CYP isoform to drug metabolism (Table 7.1).

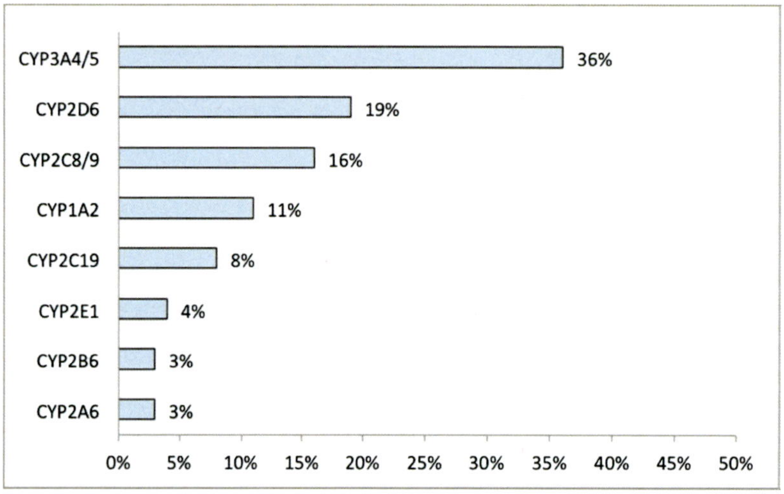

Figure 7.3. *The percentage contribution of various CYP isoforms in antifungal drug metabolism.*

Source: *By en: User: Ibrmrn3000 – This file was derived from: Proportion of drugs metabolized by different CYPs.png, CC0, https://commons.wikimedia.org/w/index.php?curid=54978591.*

With regard to the heme prosthetic group of CYP450, the iron atom can exist in Fe^{2+} (reduced) or Fe^{3+} (oxidized) states. These enzymes use one Fe-S (cysteine) covalent bond and ionic interactions to bind the heme prosthetic group to a polypeptide chain made up of several amino acids. The oxidation reactions carried out by CYP450 enzymes are caused by the active species of these enzymes, Cpd I. Figure illustrates the heteroatom oxidation process that Cpd I catalyzes schematically. 7 points. The binding of the substrate to the enzyme's active site is the initial step. As a result, a reactant complex is formed, and oxygen is then transferred from Cpd I to the substrate's heteroatom. This results in the product complex, where the oxygen atom is still attached to the heme-iron but the transfer of oxygen to the heteroatom is nearly complete. The next step involves the product containing the oxidized heteroatom exiting the enzyme's active site (Figure 7.4).

Table 7.1. Most Common Cytochrome P450 (CYP450) Enzymes in Humans

Enzyme	Upper Limit of Normal Percentage of Total Hepatic CYP450 (%)
CYP3A4	37
CYP3A5	1
CYP2C9	29
CYP1A2	16.3
CYP2A6	14
CYP2B6	5.3
CYP2D6	4.3
CYP2C19	3.8

Note: As this is a range, values do not completely sum to 100%.

Source: Fatunde, O. A., Brown, S. A. The Role of CYP450 drug metabolism in precision cardio-oncology. International Journal of Molecular Sciences. 2020; 21(2):604. https://doi.org/10.3390/ijms21020604.

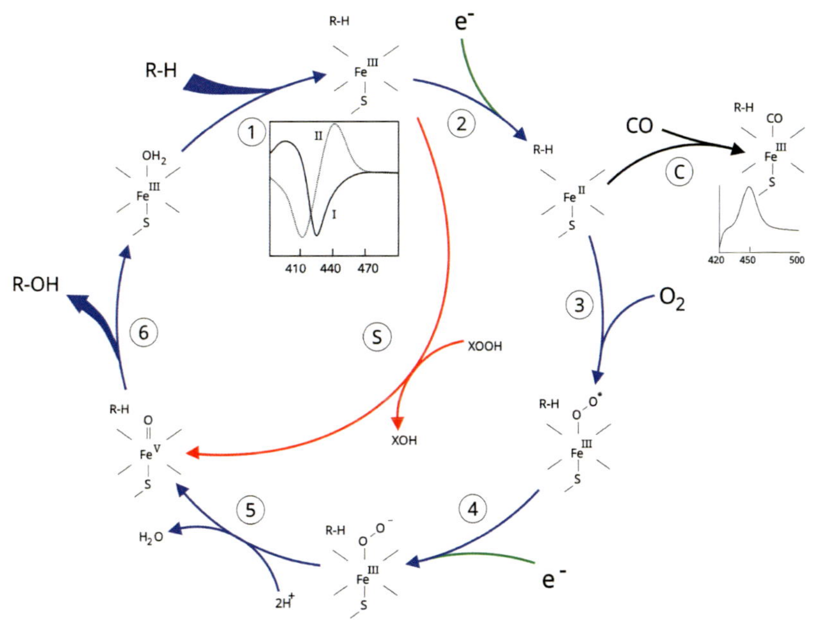

Figure 7.4. *The most important portion of the catalytic cycle of CYP450, leading to heteroatom oxidation of substrate.*

Source: By Slashme at English Wikipedia when using this image in external works, it may be cited as follows: Richfield, David. "Medical gallery of David Richfield 2014". Wikiversity Journal of Medicine 1 (2). doi:10.15347/wjm/2014.009. ISSN 2001–8762. – M.Sc. Thesis, David Richfield (User:Slashme), Public Domain, https://commons.wikimedia.org/w/index.php?curid=4325740.

Studies have been done on additional drug metabolism reaction mechanisms that resemble heteroatom oxidation. Mechanistic information about the bioinorganic chemistry occurring inside the cytochrome active site cavity is provided by computational chemistry techniques. Quantum mechanical (QM) and quantum mechanical/ molecular mechanical (QM/MM) techniques are among these techniques. To clarify the mechanism, the computational studies make use of the active species Cpd I and theoretical techniques. Shaik and colleagues, for instance, have covered the processes of CH hydroxylation, N-oxidation, S-oxidation, olefin epoxidation, and Ndealkylation in a variety of substrates. Fig. 7.5 illustrates the CH hydroxylation reaction mechanism. Creating the ferric-alcohol complex first requires Cpd I to abstract hydrogen from the alkane (RH). Radical rebound then occurs on the iron-hydroxo intermediate. After that, this lets go of the alcohol and returns the body to its resting state (i.e., the water complex), as illustrated in Figure. 7.5.

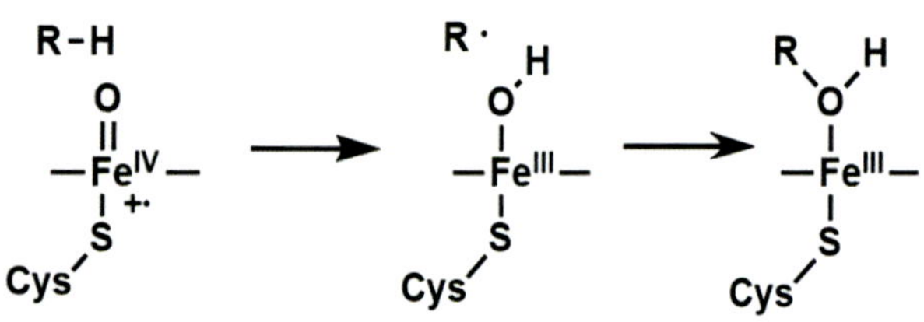

Figure 7.5. *The mechanism for CH hydroxylation.*

Source: By Pwnsey – Own work, CC BY-SA 4.0, https://commons.wikimedia.org/w/index.php?curid=38850591.

Through the application of the QM/MM method, Thiel and colleagues have reinforced the mechanistic details even further and established the foundation for a number of metabolic reactions that are catalyzed by various CYP isoforms in the body. Visser and Shaik clarified a novel proton shuttle mechanism for benzene's CH hydroxylation.

7.1.2.2. Bioorganic Chemistry of Drug Metabolism

Understanding the different kinds of drug metabolism reactions is crucial to comprehending the idea of drug metabolism. As was previously mentioned, drug metabolism can result in a variety of outcomes, including detoxification or bioactivation. Phase I (functionalization) and Phase II (conjugation) reactions are the two main categories into which the detoxification reactions can be separated. The reactions could happen (i) in a sequential fashion, (ii) on their own, or (iii) all at once.

- **Detoxification Reactions: Phase I Reactions:** These processes, which include oxidation, reduction, hydrolysis, cyclization, and decyclization, are referred to as nonsynthetic reactions. These reactions occur in the liver and are primarily carried out by mixed function oxidases, which typically involve CYP450. A polar group is either created in these reactions or, if it already exists, is revealed. Phase II reactions follow these reactions. The majority of Phase I products go through Phase II reactions rather than being immediately eliminated. The following are some examples of different Phase I reactions:
  - o **Oxidation:** This reaction is the most frequent one, increasing the hydrophilicty of the substrates by adding a polar functional group, like –OH. Oxidation reactions have been categorized in accordance with the possibility of this reaction happening at multiple locations in drugs.

    Oxidation at the carbon center: This includes aliphatic

groups, aromatic rings, and olefinic centers. A number of significant medications are being metabolized by this process, including the analgesics acetanilide, phenylbutazone, valproic acid, carbamazepine, and minoxidil (which is an antihypertensive).

Reactions on C–N, C–S, and C–O systems are involved in oxidation at carbon–heteroatom systems. N-dealkylation, oxidative deamination, N-oxide formation, and N-hydroxylation are the oxidation reactions that occur on C–N systems. Ndealkylation takes place in substrates where the nitrogen atom is directly connected to an alkyl group. Methamphetamine, an antidepressant, is one example of a substance that is converted to amphetamine through Ndealkylation. Oxidative deamination is the process by which amphetamine is further broken down into phenylacetone and ammonia.

In C–S systems, S-dealkylation, S-oxidation, and desulfuration are possible reactions. The process of S-dealkylation is carried out through α-carbon hydroxylation, e.g., 6 methylmercaptopurine. Through the process of desulfuration, the barbiturate medication thiopental is changed into pentobarbital. This process results in the cleavage of the C=S bond and the formation of a C=O product. Substrates containing a sulfide unit (-S-) exhibit the S-oxidation reaction. Methymazole (antithyroid), cimetidine (antihistaminic), ranitidine (antihistaminic), chlorpromazine (antipsychotic), and other medications are examples of medications that undergo S-oxidation. Anti-diabetic medications in the thiazolidinedione class, including pioglitazone and rosiglitazone, also experience the Soxidation reaction. Theoretical chemistry has been utilized to clarify the mechanistic aspects of S-oxidation. Other significant oxidation processes at the carbon center include oxidative aromatization, oxidative dehalogenation, and o-dealkylation. Medication like the analgesic phenacetin and the antitussive codeine are metabolized by O-dealkylation. Oxidative dehalogenation is the process by which halothane, a general anesthetic, is metabolized.

- **Reduction:** Amino and hydroxyl, two polar functional groups produced by the reduction reactions, may go through additional metabolic processes. Many functional groups, like carbonyl and hydroxyl, may be the subject of these reactions.

  Ketones and aliphatic and aromatic aldehydes can undergo the reduction reaction. Drugs that go through this metabolic process include naltrexone (which treats alcohol dependence), methadone (an analgesic), and chloral hydrate (a sedative and hypnotic). This metabolic process is carried out by N-containing compounds containing nitro, azo, or N-oxide. Nitrazepam, a hypnotic and anxiolytic, and prontosil, an antibiotic that fights bacteria, are two examples of drugs that are reduced to their corresponding amines. Drugs containing halogen atoms can be reduced by substituting them with Hatom, e.g., halothane.

o **Hydrolysis:** The substrate undergoes a significant chemical change during these reactions. After being hydrolyzed, esters yield alcohols and carboxylic acids. Esters are typically administered as prodrugs, which are changed into active forms, e.g., by hydrolysis, and aspirin (antipyretic, analgesic). Compared to esters, drug molecules with amide functionality hydrolyze more slowly. Amidases catalyze these reactions. It rarely happens in primary amides, but it does happen in secondary and tertiary amides, e.g., procainamide (an antiarrhythmic drug) (Figure 7.6).

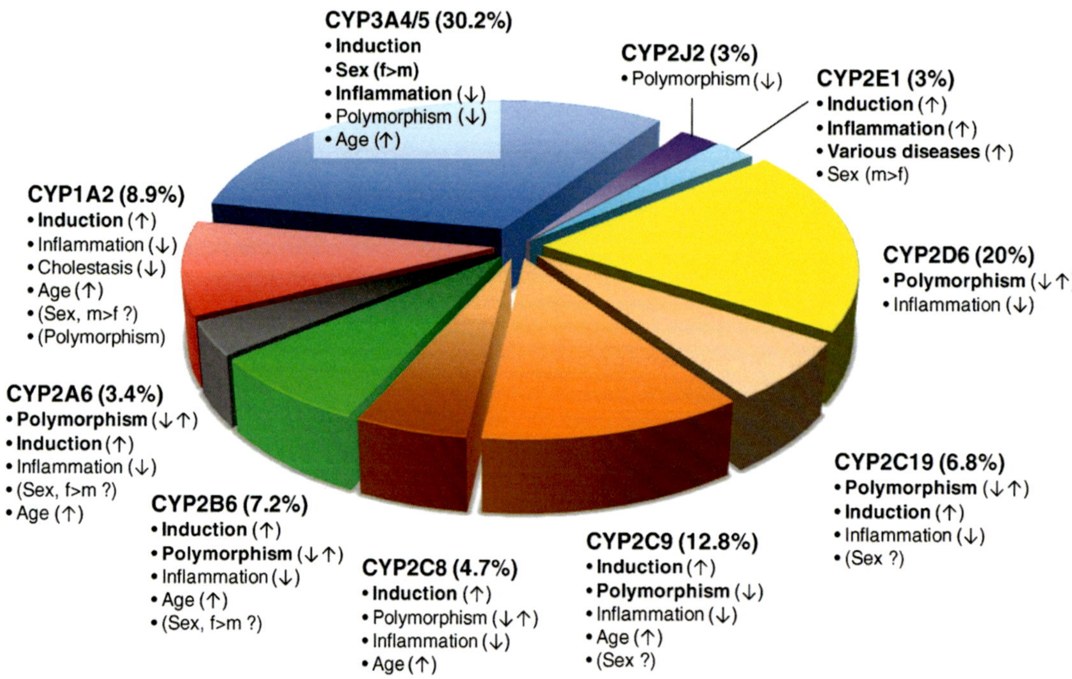

Figure 7.6. *The pie chart depicts the various P450 isoforms, the percentage of clinically used drugs metabolized by the isoform and factors inducing or inhibiting the respective P450 enzyme, thereby influencing variability. The most important factors influencing variability are in bold, with a vertical arrow indicating increased activity (↑), decreased activity (↓)* or both (↑↓). *Biologic sex (female (f) or male (m)) and rarely polymorphism (CYP1A2) can be of controversial significance. In total, 248 CYP-related drug metabolism pathways were analyzed (excluding chemicals and endogenous substrates).*

Source: *Fatunde OA, Brown S-A. The Role of CYP450 drug metabolism in precision cardio-oncology. International Journal of Molecular Sciences. 2020; 21(2):604. https://doi.org/10.3390/ijms21020604.*

- **Detoxification Reactions: Phase II Reactions:** Phase II reactions occur after Phase I reactions and typically involve the metabolites produced in Phase I. During Phase II reactions, molecules like glucuronic acid, glutathione, sulfate, and glycine are added to the Phase I metabolites. These reactions are essential for drug detoxification and are referred to as conjugation reactions because they involve combining the metabolites with large and polar moieties. Transferase enzymes, including UDP-glucoronsyltransferases, sulfotransferases, and glutathione transferases, catalyze these reactions. While these enzymes form a superfamily similar to CYPs, they metabolize fewer drugs (Figure 7.7).

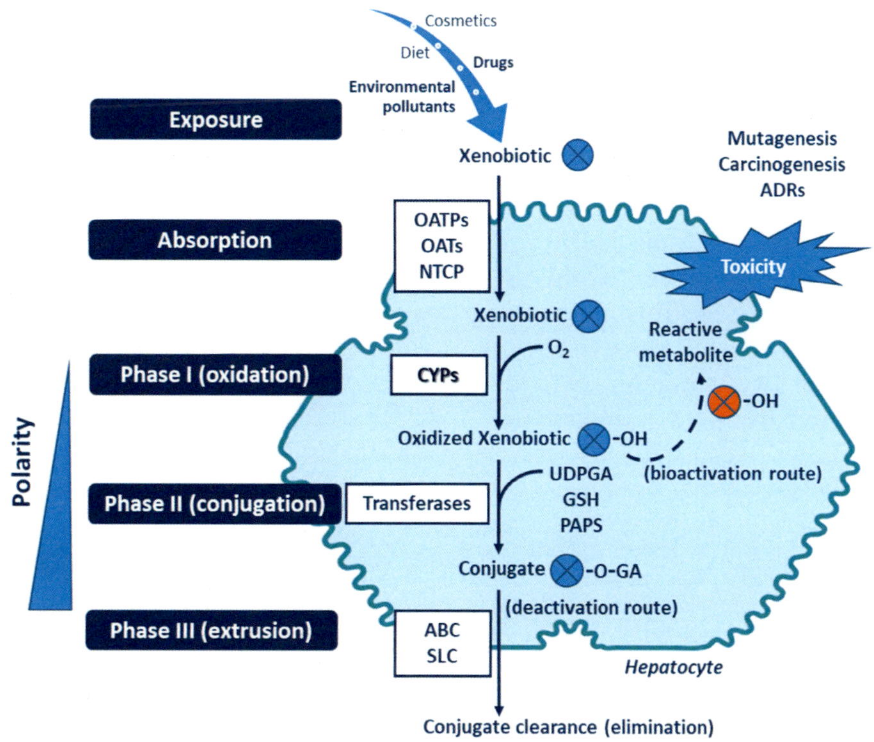

Figure 7.7. *Xenobiotic metabolism in the hepatocyte and the central role of CYPs in biotransformation. Besides hydroxylation, exemplified here, CYPs catalyze a variety of other biotransformation reactions (e.g., epoxidation, dealkylation, oxygenation, dehydrogenation, dehalogenation, among others). Non-CYP mediated metabolism may also occur in Phase I via flavin-containing monooxygenases (FMOs), NAD(P) H:quinone oxidoreductases (NQOs), amine oxidases, alcohol dehydrogenases, esterases and peroxidases. ABC: ATP binding cassette (e.g., multidrug resistance protein family—MRP); GA: glucuronic acid; GSH: glutathione; NTCP: sodium taurocholate cotransporting polypeptide; OAT: organic anion transporters; OATP: organic anion transporting polypeptides; OH: hydroxyl; PAPS: phosphoadenosine-phosphosulfate; SLC: solute carrier transporters; UDPGA: uridine diphosphate-glucuronic acid. Transferases: glutathione S-transferases (GST), methyltransferases, glycine N-acyltransferase (GLYAT), N-acetyltransferases (NAT), sulfotransferases (SULT), UDP-glucuronosyltransferases (UGT).*

Source: *Esteves F, Rueff J, Kranendonk M. The central role of cytochrome P450 in xenobiotic metabolism—A brief review on a fascinating enzyme family. Journal of Xenobiotics. 2021; 11(3):94–114. https://doi.org/10.3390/jox11030007.*

Thus, we have listed both Phase I and II reactions, and the functional groups on which different reactions take place in the body. We have covered the detoxification pathways of drug metabolism; however, we still have to understand the toxic effects of drug metabolism via bioactivation process.

7.1.3. Bioactivation Reactions: Chemistry of Reactive Metabolites and Adverse Drug Effects

In certain cases, the drug metabolism process can result in the production of Reactive Metabolites (RM), which can cause additional toxicity. There are several types of toxicity, including immune-mediated adverse drug reactions (ADRs) and genotoxicity. Adverse drug reactions pose significant challenges to both clinical drug development and drug therapy. Since the liver is in charge of the majority of metabolic reactions, it is the organ most frequently impacted by adverse drug reactions. Because these RMs have a chemically reactive group that produces ADRs, they are specifically referred to as Chemically Reactive Metabolites (CRMs).

7.1.3.1. Structural Alerts

The structural alerts are composed of multiple functional groups related to CRM generation. The following structural warnings are well-known: arylacetic acids; quinones, quinone-methide; nitroaromatics; epoxides, furan, thiophene, anilines, and anilides; hydrazines; thiophenes; terminal alkenes; etc.

But the kind and intensity of negative reactions might not always be indicated by the mere existence of these substructures that could form CRMs. Because they have a higher benefit-to-risk ratio than other drugs on the market, many of them have one structural alert or another. e.g., sulphonamides of aniline as anti-infective agents. Sometimes there is so much clearance that the toxic effects are not noticed. For instance, glucoronidation and sulphation of phenolic OH groups eliminate raloxifene (a medication used to treat osteoporosis), reducing the quantity of quinone and quinone-methide reactive metabolites that are produced. Early on in the drug discovery process, structural alerts have been effectively applied. One example of this is the ocular pain reliever bromofenac, which included aniline, arylacetic acid, and a bromophenyl ring as structural alerts. The carboxylic acid is a structural alert that has drawn everyone's attention. The majority of non-steroidal anti-inflammatory drugs (NSAIDs), including diclofenac and aspirin., have a carboxylate function, and result in a variety of adverse drug reactions. Consequently, it's critical to comprehend the significance of a number of functional groups that could otherwise trigger harmful bodily reactions.

7.1.3.2. Structure–Toxicity Relationship

To identify some functional groups as the structural alerts, a number of techniques can be applied. Utilizing DEREK software is one methodology. The Deductive Estimation of Risk from Existing Knowledge computer program, or DEREK for short, is intended to help toxicologists and chemists anticipate potential toxicological risk regions for novel compounds by analyzing their molecular structures. Various alerts that describe structural features or toxicophores linked to toxicity are used as part of the prediction process of this knowledge-based expert system to identify different structural alerts. The occurrence of bioactivation and additional toxicity in a drug candidate, however, cannot be predicted using any of the currently available in silico tools. Drug candidates' metabolic changes can be predicted by computational tools like Meta Site. By using a ranking derived from the site of metabolism predictions, a computational procedure provides the structure of the metabolites formed. To assist chemists in narrowing down their compound design to lessen CYP-mediated metabolism, it forecasts "hot spots" within the molecule. The molecular moieties that aid in directing the molecule within the cytochrome cavity to place the catalytic center close to the site of metabolism are also highlighted. Still, it is unable to forecast a drug candidate's bioactivation pathway. A thorough understanding of structural alerts would help with efficient drug design, as it is difficult to predict the bioactivation pathways of potential drug candidates. This would ensure that a successful drug candidate lacks any structural alerts that were present in a toxic predecessor. A "structure–toxicity" relationship is the term used to describe this kind of partnership (Table 7.2).

Table 7.2. Toxicity data

Toxicity Data for Compounds Considered in This Study		
Name	CAS Number	log(IGC_{50}^{-1})
Haloalcohols		
2-Chloroethanol *	107–07–3	-1.42
2,2,2-Trichloroethanol *	115–20–8	-0.46
1-Chloro-2-propanol *	127–00–4	-1.49
1-Bromo-2-propanol *	19686–73–8	-1.19
6-Chloro-1-hexanol *	2009–83–8	-0.27
8-Chloro-1-octanol ^	23144–52–7	0.49
3-Bromo-2,2-dimethyl-1-propanol *	40894–00–6	-0.46
6-Bromo-1-hexanol ^	4286–55–9	0.01
8-Bromo-1-octanol ^	50816–19–8	1.04
2-Bromoethanol ^	540–51–2	-0.85
3-Chloro-1-propanol *	627–30–5	-1.40
2,2,2-Tribromoethanol *	75–80–9	0.11
4-Chloro-1-butanol ^	928–51–8	-0.76
1,3-Dichloro-2-propanol *	96–23–1	-0.79
3-Chloro-1,2-propanediol *	96–24–2	-1.63
Halonitriles		
Chloroacetonitrile *	107–14–2	0.85
2-Chloropropionitrile ^	1617–17–01	-0.86
2-Bromopropionitrile *	19481–82–4	0.63
7-Bromoheptanonitrile ^	20965–27–9	0.51
7-Chloroheptanonitrile ^	22819–91–6	0.29
3-Bromopropionitrile ^	2417–90–5	-0.50
Dibromoacetonitrile *	3252–43–5	2.40
4-Bromobutyronitrile *	N/A	-0.47

5-Bromovaleronitrile ^	5414–21–1	-0.21
3-Chloropropionitrile *	542–76–7	-1.00
4-Chlorobutyronitrile *	628–20–6	-0.93
Bromoesters		
Ethyl-5-bromovalerate ^	14660–52–7	0.22
5-Bromopentylacetate *	15848–22–3	0.29
Ethyl-6-bromohexanoate ^	25542–62–5	0.59
Ethyl-4-bromobutyrate *	2969–81–5	-0.03
Ethyl-2-bromopropionate *	535–11–5	1.06
Ethyl-3-bromopropionate *	539–74–2	0.13
Methyl-5-bromovalerate *	5454–83–1	-0.08
Ethyl-2-bromoisobutyrate *	600–00–0	0.15
Ethyl-2-bromovalerate *	615–83–8	0.70
Ethyl-2-bromohexanoate *	615–96–3	0.86
DL-methyl-2-bromobutyrate *	69043–96–5	1.02
Diones		
2,5-Hexanedione *	110–13–4	-1.40
2,4-Pentanedione *	123–54–6	-0.27
2,4-Octanedione *	14090–87–0	0.13
2,3-Hexanedione *	3848–24–6	-0.21
2,3-Butanedione *	431–03–8	-0.23
3,4-Hexanedione *	4437–51–8	-0.01
2,3-Pentanedione *	600–14–6	-0.16
2,4-Nonanedione *	6175–23–1	0.51
3,5-Heptanedione *	724–54–6	-0.38
2,3-Heptanedione ^	96–04–8	0.04
Alkanones		
Acetone *	67–64–1	-2.20
2-Butanone*	79–93–1	-1.75
2-Pentanone ^	107–87–9	-1.22
2-Decanone *	693–54–9	0.58
2-Undecanone *	112–12–9	1.50
2-Tridecanone ^	593–08–8	2.12
Alkanals		
Butyraldehyde *	123–72–8	-0.38
Valeraldehyde *	110–62–3	-0.02

Heptaldehyde *	111–71–7	0.00
Octylaldehyde ^	124–13–0	0.45
Undecylaldehyde *	112–44–7	1.69
Dodecylaldehyde ^	112–54–9	1.76
Alkenals		
2-Butenal *	123–73–9	0.70
2-Pentenal ^	1576–87–0	0.66
2-Hexenal *	6728–26–3	0.76
2-Heptenal *	18829–55–5	1.05
2-Octenal ^	2548–87–0	1.20
2-Nonenal ^	18829–56–6	1.60
2-Decenal ^	3913–81–3	1.85

Source: Toropov, A. A., Duchowicz, P., Castro, E. A. Structure–Toxicity Relationships for Aliphatic Compounds Based on Correlation Weighting of Local Graph Invariants. International Journal of Molecular Sciences. 2003; 4(5), 272–283. https://doi.org/10.3390/i4050272

7.1.3.3. Consequences of Reactive Metabolite Formation

Reactive metabolites (RMs) produced by CYP-mediated metabolism typically cause an enzyme to become inactive, which can either be irreversible or reversible. Mechanism-based inactivation or inhibition (MBI) of CYPs refers to the irreversible inactivation or inhibition of an enzyme. The mechanism that prevents enzyme inactivation makes the name appropriate. Depending on the mechanism, there are two possible categories for this inactivation:

i. Coordination results in the formation of a metabolic-intermediate complex (MIC) between reactive species and heme-iron. Various metabolic transformations, including N-dealkylation and N-hydroxylation, cause the aliphatic and aromatic amines (tamoxifen, an anticancer drug; nortriptyline, an antidepressant) to produce reactive nitroso (R-N=O) intermediate. Conversely, medications containing 1,3-benzdioxole moiety result in the production of reactive carbene intermediate. Both intermediates are nucleophilic and form a coordination bond with heme-iron. The metabolic-intermediate complex (MIC), which results from this coordination, is what stops CYP activity.

ii. Covalent modification of reactive species with heme or amino acid residues: medications that produce reactive epoxide intermediate can cause mechanism-based inhibition of CYPs. These medications include thiophene, furan, olefin, and phenyl groups. Through the creation of a covalent bond as a result of nucleophilic active site residues opening the epoxide ring, CYP activity is inhibited. Additionally, quinone-imine and quinone-methide are reactive species that can form covalent bonds and cause MBI. A few medications, including the HIV protease inhibitor L-754,394, form a reactive epoxide intermediate.

The other medication is paracetamol, whose quinone-imine metabolite (N-acetyl p-benzoquinoneimine; NAPQI) is reactive and lowers GSH levels by binding covalently to liver macromolecules. This causes the body to develop hepatic necrosis. Drug-drug interactions (DDIs), which may be harmful to the body, are a result of this CYP inactivation. For instance, hypertensive patients receiving simvastatin, a calcium-channel blocker, and a strong CYP3A4 inactivator, mibefradil, have an increased incidence of myopathy (muscular weakness) and rhabdomyolysis (breakdown products of damaged skeletal muscles released in blood stream). The mechanism underlying DDI in this case is the inactivation of the CYP-catalyzed metabolism process of simvastatin by mibefradil, which in turn causes an increase in statin plasma levels and ultimately results in death. Mibefradil was later taken off the market due to these deadly effects.

CYP3A4 is known to be involved in the metabolism of tadalafil, a medication used to treat erectile dysfunction, and it also inhibits CYP3A4. The 1,3-benzodioxole group is thought to be the cause of the inhibitory effects. This group is thought to produce the corresponding carbene intermediate after metabolism and then coordinate with the heme iron, as was previously discussed. As such, when used over an extended period of time, it may have negative effects on patients. Similarly, paroxetine, an antidepressant medication, forms a coordination bond with heme-iron by producing a reactive carbene intermediate, which functions as a strong inhibitor of CYP2D6. In a drug-discovery paradigm, mechanism-based inactivation of major human CYP enzymes by novel compounds is routinely evaluated because enzyme inactivation can result in potential DDIs. Up until now, we've talked about the fundamentals of drug metabolism, its bioinorganic and organic chemistry, detoxification, and its bioactivation pathways. Determining the variables influencing this process is crucial because the rate of metabolism of any drug determines its pharmacological action's duration, biological half-life, toxicity, and intensity.

7.2. Drug Metabolism: Approaches, Function and Education

The metabolism of both endogenous and exogenous substances is included in drug metabolism. Most medications lose their pharmacological effects and are eliminated from the body during metabolism. Dust, food, toxins, and air pollutants are just a few of the foreign particles to which the human body is exposed. We refer to these foreign particles as xenobiotics as a group. Xeno refers to something that is foreign to us and not typically found in our bodies. The body possesses a mechanism to alter foreign particles upon their entry and facilitate their expulsion from the body. Metabolism is the term for this process. Drugs are considered foreign particles, hence they are also considered xenobiotics. Biotransformation is another term for the drug metabolism process. Normally, metabolism reduces the pharmacological effect, but occasionally it generates active or toxic metabolites. Prodrugs are substances that go through a metabolic process to have a pharmacological effect. Certain medications are broken down into hazardous, mutagenic, or carcinogenic metabolites. The primary site of metabolism in the body is the liver. First-pass effects are caused by certain medications that are metabolized before entering the bloodstream. The kidney, skin, gastrointestinal tract (GIT), and other organs are also involved in drug metabolism.

Most medications are classified as xenobiotics, or chemicals that the body does not naturally produce. Through a variety of bodily processes, xenobiotics are detoxified, lowering their toxicity and making them more easily excreted. These procedures, also referred to as metabolic biotransformation or drug metabolism, enable the chemical conversion of pharmaceuticals into their metabolites. There are three types of metabolites that result from the metabolism of drugs: inactive, toxic, and active metabolites. Biochemically active substances with therapeutic effects are known as active metabolites, while biochemically inert substances have neither toxic nor therapeutic effects. Similar to active metabolites in terms of biochemistry, toxic metabolites can cause a variety of negative consequences.

A low concentration of active metabolites is found in the systemic circulation as a result of drug metabolism, which takes place at a particular site in the body. First-pass metabolism is the term given to this phenomenon, which restricts the bioavailability of drugs. Enzymes that catalyze metabolism are present all over the body, but first-pass metabolism mostly takes place in the liver. It is essential to comprehend these changes in chemical activity to choose the best pharmacological intervention for each patient. Any healthcare professional who regularly administers medication to patients should be interested in this topic.

7.2.1. Function

Drug excretion from the body is mainly carried out by the kidneys; however, lipophilic drugs are easily absorbed back into the bloodstream by passing through the renal tubules' cell membrane. Therefore, before the drug can be excreted, lipophilic drugs must first be metabolized in the liver. Phase I (modification), Phase II (conjugation), and occasionally Phase III (additional modification and excretion) are the different reactions that can occur during drug metabolism. Phase I modifications include oxidation, reduction, hydrolysis, cyclization/decyclization, and addition or subtraction of oxygen from more polar molecules to change the chemical structure of lipophilic drugs. This process can occasionally turn an inactive prodrug into a medication that is metabolically active. Most metabolites produced by oxidation still have some degree of pharmacological activity. Phase I modification, for instance, changes the popular anxiolytic medication diazepam into desmethyldiazepam and oxazepam. The physiological and psychological effects of diazepam and its metabolites are comparable. The majority of phase I reactions are catalyzed by the cytochrome P450 system, also referred to as microsomal mixed function oxidase.

A drug molecule couples with another molecule in a conjugation reaction during phase II modifications. Conjugation typically makes the compound water soluble and pharmacologically inert, facilitating easy excretion. Methylation, acetylation, sulphation, glucuronidation, and glutathione or glycine conjugation are examples of conjugation mechanisms. These processes can take place in the kidney, liver, lungs, intestines, and other organ systems, among other places. Oxazepam is an example of phase II metabolism; it conjugates with glucuronide, a different molecule. Without undergoing any additional chemical changes, the medication becomes physiologically inactive and is eliminated.

Phase II metabolism, during which conjugates and metabolites are eliminated from the cells, may also be followed by phase III metabolism. Phase I and II process enzymatic catalysis is a crucial component of drug metabolism. For drugs to be efficiently metabolized, liver enzyme composition and concentration are essential. The two enzymes that are most frequently utilized in medicine are cytochrome P450 and monoamine oxidase. These two enzymes are in charge of breaking down numerous xenobiotic and biogenic substances. Monoamine oxidase, as its name implies, catalyzes the breakdown of monoamines, including dopamine and serotonin. Antidepressants called monoamine oxidase inhibitors (MAOI) raise dopamine and serotonin levels in the brain. The family of heme-containing isoenzymes known as the cytochrome P450 system is mainly found in the liver and gastrointestinal tract and is in charge of breaking down a wide range of medications and substances, including steroids and lipids. Amphetamines and opioids are among the many psychoactive substances that cytochrome P450 catalyzes the metabolism of.

7.2.2. Issues of Concern

Drug plasma concentrations can be impacted by drug metabolism, which needs to be taken into account. Drug interactions should worry prescribers because they can have a detrimental effect on the patient's health. For instance, imatinib's plasma concentrations may decrease if rifampin is taken concurrently with imatinib because rifampin can activate CYP3A4 and metabolize imatinib considerably more quickly. As a result, the anticancer effect of imatinib may be diminished. Similarly, imatinib's plasma concentrations rise when omeprazole is taken concurrently with imatinib to treat gastroesophageal reflux disease (GERD). This happens because imatinib is metabolized by CYP3A4, which is strongly inhibited by omeprazole. Imatinib builds up as a result of CYP3A4 inhibition, which can be toxic. Another element that influences drug metabolism is aging. Age-related slowing of drug metabolism increases the risk of side effects in elderly patients. The patient's age should be taken into consideration by prescribers when writing prescriptions. Patients may respond differently to different medications due to genetic polymorphism in the enzymes that break down drugs.

7.2.3. Clinical Significance

The prescriber must take into account the manner and timing of a drug's excretion from the body when implementing any pharmacological intervention. First-order kinetics, which states that the clearance rate is dependent on the drug's plasma concentration, is typically the basis for drug clearance. In other words, the drug's concentration and the elimination rate are related. This type of clearance's rate is chemical-specific and frequently expressed as a half-life. This is the amount of time it takes for the body to flush out half of the medication. Because cocaine, for instance, has a half-life of roughly one hour, the body retains only roughly 62.5 % of the initial dose after four hours. Certain medications, however, are eliminated at a steady rate regardless of plasma concentrations. For instance, ethanol is eliminated from the body at a steady rate of roughly 15 mL/hour regardless of its bloodstream concentration. When enzyme binding sites are saturated at low concentrations, a phenomenon known as zero-order kinetics takes place. Because many medications require clinically significant drug concentration monitoring, kinetics are of interest to the medical community. Comprehending pharmacokinetics, particularly drug excretion, enables healthcare professionals to modify patient-specific treatment plans. A steady-state plasma concentration where drug metabolism and elimination happen at the same time is the goal of therapy.

Numerous factors can impact the highly variable process of metabolism. Depot binding, or the coupling of drug molecules to inactive sites in the body so that the drug is no longer accessible for metabolism, is a major perturber of drug metabolism. This may have an impact on how long pharmacological agents that are prone to depot binding remain active. Tetrahydrocannabinol (THC), the primary psychoactive ingredient in marijuana, is one famous example. Because THC is so lipid-soluble, it binds to users' adipose tissue in the depot. Weeks after the patient's last usage, THC metabolites can be found in their urine due to this interaction, which significantly slows down the drug's metabolism. Enzyme induction is a further factor in drug metabolism. The same chemical is used repeatedly to induce enzymes. As a result of the drug's continuous presence, the body adjusts by producing more of the enzymes needed for the drug's metabolism. This leads to pharmacological tolerance, which is one of the reasons why patients require higher and higher dosages of some medications to achieve the same results.

One good example would be opioids. Long-term opioid analgesic prescription holders observe a gradual decrease in the efficacy of their medication. Notably, induction raises the rate at which all medications processed by the enzyme are metabolized; prolonged use of amphetamines, for instance, results in elevated CYP2D6 concentrations. Because this enzyme is also necessary for the metabolism of some opioids, including oxycodone, a doctor prescribing oxycodone to a patient who uses amphetamines would need to prescribe a higher dose to achieve the intended result. On the other hand, some medications cause an enzyme-inhibiting effect that increases a patient's susceptibility to other medications that are metabolized by those enzymes. Monoamine oxidase inhibition caused by some antidepressants is a well-known example. These substances block the enzyme in the brain that breaks down "pleasure" chemicals, which has psychotherapeutic effects. But when people taking other medications while taking an MAOI, it can lead to abnormally high concentrations of these neurochemicals, which can cause issues. Cocaine, which increases serotonin, dopamine, and norepinephrine concentrations, will have a far more potent effect on a patient taking an MAOI. Numerous physiological issues, such as tachycardia, hypertension, and serotonin syndrome, can result from this interaction.

In addition to 'competing' for the same binding sites on enzymes, drugs that share parts of their metabolic pathways can also reduce the efficiency of enzyme metabolism. The same cytochrome P450 family member, for example, metabolizes alcohol and some sedatives.

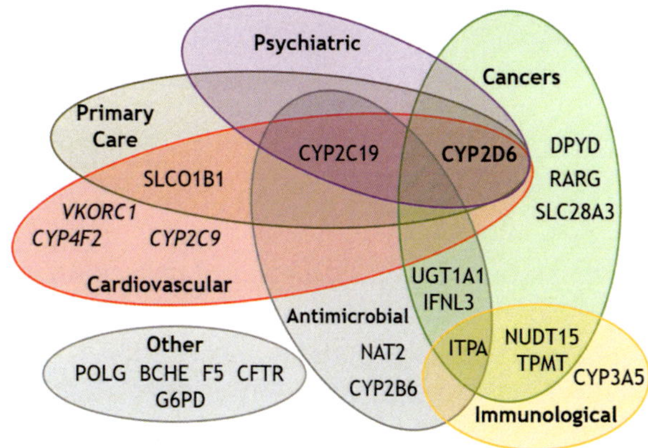

Figure 7.8. *Venn Diagram showing recognized (non-HLA) pharmacogenes according to their association with drugs used in different therapeutic areas. CYP2D6 overlaps with four distinct therapeutic areas. BCHE: Butyrylcholinesterase. CFTR: Cystic fibrosis transmembrane conductance regulator. CYP2B6, CYP2C9, CYP2C19, CYP3A5, CYP4F2: Members of cytochrome P450 superfamily. DPYD: Dihydropyrimidine dehydrogenase. F5: Factor 5. G6PD: Glucose-6-phosphate dehydrogenase. IFNL3: Interferon lambda 3. ITPA: Inosine triphosphate pyrophosphohydrolase. NAT2: N-Acetyltransferase 2. NUDT15: Nudix hydrolase 15. POLG: DNA polymerase subunit γ. RARG: Retinoic acid receptor γ. SLCO1B1: Solute carrier organic anion transporter family member 1B1. SLC28A3: Solute carrier family 28 member 3. TPMT: Thiopurine S-methyltransferase. UGT1A1: UDP-glucuronosyltransferases. VKORC1: Vitamin K epoxide reductase complex.*

Source: Taylor C, Crosby I, Yip V, Maguire P, Pirmohamed M, Turner RM. A review of the important role of CYP2D6 in pharmacogenomics. Genes. 2020; 11(11):1295. https://doi.org/10.3390/genes11111295.

Enzymes that can degrade these substances are few in number. Because most of the required enzymes would be filled with alcohol molecules if pentobarbital were given to a patient who was also metabolizing alcohol, the drug would not be completely metabolized; this is one reason alcohol and other sedative or hypnotic drugs can work in concert when given together (Figure 7.8).

7.2.4. Enhancing Healthcare Team Outcomes

A critical clinical concern for the interdisciplinary healthcare team is drug metabolism. Toavoid clinically significant drug interactions that could have an impact on patients' health, pharmacists and clinicians must collaborate. Nurses keep an eye out for any indications of a hazardous accumulation of metabolites or active medications in a hospital setting. This is particularly important in cases of hepatic or renal insufficiency. Pharmacists dose and oversee the administration of medications, including warfarin, aminoglycoside antibiotics, and fluoroquinolones, by keeping an eye on the drugs' serum levels and renal function. The best chance for achieving the best possible patient care is to use an interprofessional approach to drug dosing and administration in light of the effects of drug metabolism on patients, whether through impaired metabolism, drug-drug interactions, enzymatic induction, or other factors. With fewer unfavorable events, the interprofessional care approach produces better therapeutic outcomes.

7.2.5. Nursing, Allied Health, and Interprofessional Team Interventions

Monitoring and interprofessional interventions are essential for successful results. According to research, interprofessional interventions work best when teams are willing and able to work together, communicate, share decision-making, coordinate care, and integrate their competencies. An efficient method of managing medication through interventions and monitoring is through interprofessional team interventions. As previously stated, different people react differently to medications. Patients may therefore be more vulnerable to unfavorable outcomes if the right precautions are not done. When a patient is not taking their medication as prescribed by a physician or is taking it improperly, teams need to keep an eye on things and take appropriate action. Patient safety should always be the main priority. Adverse event reporting is essential for interprofessional team monitoring. In order for clinical teams to perform interventions and monitoring effectively, they should also receive training.

Topics including standardizing medication dispensing, preventing adverse events by identifying medication errors, and improving team communication can all be covered in training. The goal of Continuing Medication Credits ought to include both monitoring and intervention. An essential component of providing healthcare is communication. Interprofessional teams need to keep developing new strategies for guiding patients through the healthcare continuum. Effective interprofessional education also fosters collaboration, interdisciplinary awareness, respect, and acceptance of the roles that various disciplines play in healthcare delivery. But one must also take the difficulties into account. Every discipline has a distinct methodology and culture. They differ in terms of professional language, qualifications, accountability, and routines as well as rules and regulations. This makes it challenging to standardize on any interventions or drug monitoring. But acknowledging these difficulties is the first step towards making a change. These issues can be resolved, and professionals in all fields—nurses, pharmacists, and doctors—will receive the necessary training to enable them to monitor medication for better health outcomes at any point during the course of treatment.

7.2.6. Drug Metabolism and Drug Design

In the design and development of new drugs, understanding drug metabolism is crucial. A few non-reactive groups that thwart drug metabolism are added if the new drug is rapidly metabolized by the body. For instance, the anti-diabetic medication tolbutamide (Figure 7.9) has a shorter half-life of 2.5 hours. Its methyl group is changed into a carboxyl group during the metabolic process. Drug metabolism has a substantial impact on a drug's pharmacokinetic, pharmacodynamic, and safety. Chlorpropamide, when the methyl group is substituted with a chlorine atom, achieves a longer half-life (12–15 hours) than tolbutamide. Prodrugs are pharmaceuticals that are given in inactive forms. A prodrug is a medication that has had its chemical makeup altered to address issues with excretion, metabolism, absorption, and administration. Liquid functional groups found in prodrugs are readily metabolized by the body. For instance, carbamate, phosphate, and ester. Oral bioavailability is enhanced by masking of polar functional. As an illustration, prodrugs of chloramphenicol and ampicillin are chloramphenicol palmitate and bacampicillin, respectively.

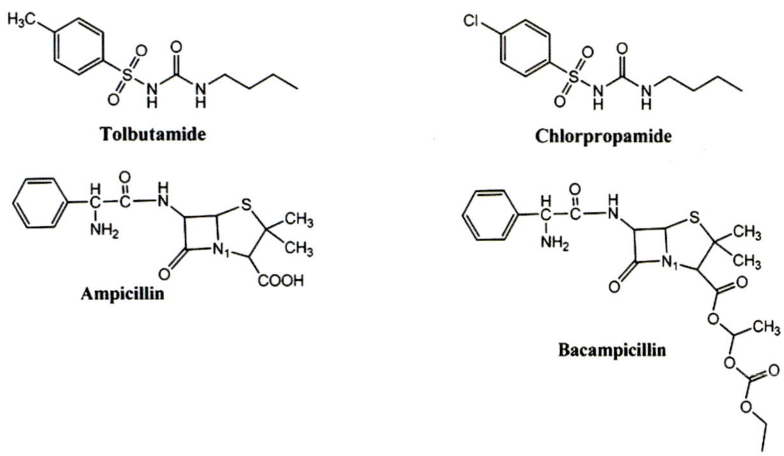

Figure 7.9. *Drug metabolism and drug design.*

Source: ul Amin Mohsin, N., Farrukh, M., Shahzadi, S., & Irfan, M. (2024). Drug metabolism: Phase I and phase II metabolic pathways. IntechOpen. doi: 10.5772/intechopen.112854.

7.2.6.1. In Silico Pharmacokinetic Studies

Poor pharmacokinetic properties account for about 40% of new drug failures in clinical trials. SwissADME, ADMETlab, and pkCSM web tools are now used to assess the pharmacokinetic properties of new compounds. Using online software, 3D structures of compounds are created, and calculations are made for their pharmacokinetic characteristics, or ADMET (absorption, distribution, metabolism, excretion, and toxicity). The oral activity of drug molecules depends on several properties, which can be predicted, including GI absorption, BBB permeation, P-gp substrate, cytochrome P450 enzyme inhibition/induction, and skin permeation. Understanding the behavior of drug molecules in the human body is aided by the prediction of pharmacokinetic properties. The expensive experimental approach is lessened with the aid of in silico predictions. The Lipinski Rule of Five also predicts the drug-likeness of novel molecules. This rule states that drug molecules with more than five hydrogen bond donors, more than ten hydrogen bond acceptors, more than five logP, and more than 500 Daltons in molecular weight have a lower probability of being orally active. Drug molecules absorb poorly when they have a high lipophilicity. Compounds with large weights are also less likely to be absorbed by the GIT. Eighty % of medications have a molecular weight of less than 450. Additionally demonstrating good oral bioavailability are molecules with polar surface areas less than 140°A and fewer rotatable bonds than 10. Pharmacological compounds that adhere to the RO5 have a higher chance of being approved for sale and a lower likelihood of failing clinical trials.

7.2.7. Improving PK and PD Properties

7.2.7.1. Metabolic Soft Spot

After being administered into the body, drugs must reach the site(s) of action to produce their desired pharmacological effects. However, if drugs show inferior PK properties, e.g., due to their high clearance, brief half-life ($t_{1/2}$), and poor bioavailability after oral dosage, their PD effects are probably going to be less than ideal. Studies on the metabolism of human and animal tissue in vitro (e.g., liver) preparations and/or in vivo metabolism research in animals are helpful methods to pinpoint the main drug metabolism pathways (also known as "soft spots").

It is well known that, when these groups are not sterically inhibited and are subject to P450 mediated metabolism, the benzylic C–H bond, the allylic methyl, and the O–, N–, and S–methyl groups are the most preferred metabolic soft spots. The intrinsic reactivity of the substrate sites that are accessible to the ferryl oxidizing species in the P450-substrate complex plays a major role in determining the chemo- and regiospecificity of substrate oxidation as well as the rate of metabolism due to the nature of the enzyme-catalyzed hydroxylation reactions. Therefore, in metabolizing enzyme systems, the propensity to be metabolic soft spots will depend on the intrinsic reactivity of the functional groups and the substrate specificity of the specific molecule bearing this particular functional group (soft spot). Using bioisosteres to replace the identified soft spots is a common strategy to address the metabolic soft spot issue. Bioisosteres are substituents or groups that share similar molecular structures, are similar chemically or physically, and may produce biological properties that are somewhat similar. For instance, a fluorine or chlorine atom, or a -CF3 group, could be utilized in place of a benzylic methyl group in certain situations where it is determined to be a metabolic soft spot.

One strategy to reduce intrinsic clearance in structure-metabolism relationship studies is to block a metabolic soft spot. This may result in a lower total clearance and, if the volume of distribution remains unchanged, a longer half-life for modified molecules. As an instance, zileuton is a 5-lipoxygenase (5-LO) inhibitor used to treat human asthma on a maintenance basis. In cynomolgus monkeys, Zileuton demonstrated half-lives of 0 point 4 hours, and in humans, 2.4 hours. Glucuronidation at the N-hydroxyurea moiety to produce metabolite is the main metabolism pathway for zileuton in cynomolgus monkeys and humans (and the excretion of urine afterward. According to studies on the structure-activity relationship (SAR), the N-hydroxyurea portion is a pharmacophore that is necessary for activity. Only the linker and benzothiophene sections of zileuton could therefore be the target of structural modification to reduce glucuronidation.

Compound 4, which was produced by removing the methyl group from zileuton's linkage group, increased the intrinsic clearance (Clint) in cynomolgus monkey liver microsomes by six times, while also causing a two-fold decrease in half-life and a four-fold increase in plasma clearance in cynomolgus monkeys living in vivo. The glucuronidation at the N-hydroxyurea portion may have been lowered by the steric hindrance of the nearby methyl group from the zileuton linker. According to SAR studies on the linker portion, compounds containing an acetylene linkage generally exhibited longer half-lives, lower plasma clearances, and lower rates of glucuronidation in cynomolgus monkey liver microsomes in vivo. The glucuronidation rate could be considerably lowered by substituting a basic thiophene ring for the benzothiophene portion, according to SAR studies on that portion. And lastly, ABT-761, a second generation 5-LO inhibitor, was found to have a single furan ring and an acetylene linker. In cynomolgus monkey and human liver microsomes, the rate of glucuronidation was >12-fold and >29-fold lower, respectively, than zileuton. In cynomolgus monkeys and humans, ABT-761 demonstrated, respectively, >40- and >29-fold longer half-lives than zileuton. Thus, compared to zileuton at the same dosage, ABT-761 demonstrated a markedly higher level of efficacy. ABT-761 only needs to be taken once daily in humans due to its enhanced potency and PK properties, while zileuton requires multiple daily doses. This work showed that it is possible to enhance the PK characteristics of a new chemical entity (NCE) without compromising or improving upon its pharmacological activity by blocking a metabolism soft spot (Figure 7.10).

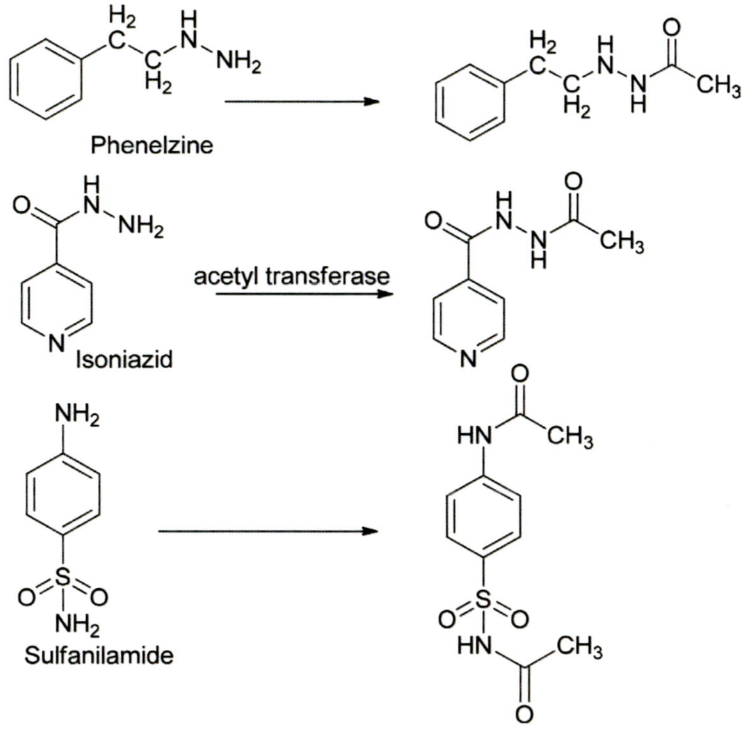

Figure 7.10. *Acetylation of drug molecules having amino group.*

Source: Ul Amin Mohsin, N., Farrukh, M., Shahzadi, S., & Irfan, M. (2024). Drug metabolism: Phase I and phase II metabolic pathways. IntechOpen. doi: 10.5772/intechopen.112854

Studies on 4-(3,4,5-trimethoxybenzoyl)-2-phenylthiazole SMART-H have examined 4-substituted methoxybenzoyl-aryl-thiozoles as novel anti-cancer agents, was found to be a lead that exhibited strong inhibitory effects on tubulin polymerization and cancer cell proliferation. In contrast, SMART-H demonstrated significant metabolic instability in liver microsomes from humans, dogs, rats, and mice, with in vitro half-lives varying from less than five to thirty minutes. The reduction of the ketone functional group was the primary metabolism pathway, according to SMART-H metabolite profiling in human liver microsomes. O-demethylation of SMART-H methoxy groups was the second most common metabolic pathway. As a result, the ketone and methoxy groups of SMART-H were identified as metabolically sensitive areas. In the case of SMART-173A and SMART-176A, the ketone group was substituted with an oxime group and a hydrazide group. In human liver microsomes, SMART-173A and SMART-176A showed a 3- and 2-fold, respectively, increase in metabolic stability. SMART-173A demonstrated a partial retention of anticancer activity against four prostate tumor cell lines, with an average IC50 value of 143 nmol/L (as opposed to that of SMART-H with an IC50 of 44 nmol/L). Conversely, SMART-176A demonstrated a significant loss of anticancer activity, with an average IC50 value of 1250 nmol/L. After removing SMART-H's most labile ketone functional group, SMART-329 increased the metabolic stability by 2-fold. On the other hand, SMART-329 lost all anticancer activity, indicating that the ketone functional group is essential for anticancer action. Upon substituting fluorine atoms for the second soft spot (consisting of three methoxy groups) in SMART-H, SMART-213. There was no anticancer activity and only a slight change in metabolic stability. This implies that the methoxy groups may be involved in the anticancer action as well. It is therefore plausible that structural alteration on or near a lead compound's metabolic soft spots could have a deleterious effect on biological activity.

7.2.7.2. Metabolic Switching and Deuterium Replacement

A large number of small molecule medications are processed by the body's cytochrome P450 (CYP) enzymes. CYPs are a class of enzymes that primarily reside in the endoplasmic reticulum of hepatocytes. They are responsible for a variety of oxidative and reductive biotransformations, such as halocarbon dehalogenation, carbon hydroxylation, bond oxidation, heteroatom oxidation, and hydrocarbon desaturation. When a drug is biotransformed into a metabolite by CYP-catalyzed biotransformation, it first binds to the enzyme's active site and then catalytically turns it into a metabolite via a process known as the P450 catalytic cycle. Although the relationship between the structure and metabolism of drugs involving CYPs is complicated and poorly understood, it is widely acknowledged that the main CYP enzymes that are involved in drug metabolism, such as, e.g., CYP3A, which favors lipophilic substrates and has a large active site. Although substrates rarely interact with CYP through hydrogen bonding or ionic interactions, the binding and orientation of a substrate are frequently dictated by the hydrophobic and steric interactions of the substrate with the specific amino acids at the active site of a CYP enzyme.

The primary determinant of these steric and hydrophobic interactions is lipophilicity (e.g., logP) and the substrates' steric structures. A particular metabolite will then be produced by oxidizing a substrate C-H bond to a C-OH bond through further catalytic turnover. Using a substituent, such as an, e.g., is a common way to block or slow down a molecule's metabolism at a particular site (e.g., a bioisostere, a bulky group, a halogen, or a deuterium atom) to swap out the H-atom in the molecule's C-H bond or to move a bulky group into a nearby location to lessen or prevent the oxidizing species of the iron-bound P450 enzyme from being accessible. The intrinsic reactivity of the molecule's sites that are accessible to the iron-bound oxidizing species in the CYP's active site determines the precise metabolism site in the substrate where the structural modification takes place once the molecule is bound within the active site. Because of the characteristics of active site(s) of CYP enzymes (e.g., blocking the soft spot (also known as the metabolically labile site)) of a lead molecule with one of the aforementioned substituents may alter the binding and orientation of the newly synthesized molecule, changing the original metabolism site to a different C-H bond and leading to the formation of other metabolite(s) to a greater extent than that of the lead compound (CYP 3A4) with a large space binding pocket.

Because CYP enzymes may have multiple binding sites, it is also possible that the blockage of a soft spot of a lead molecule *via* structural modification may cause the binding of the new molecule to the alternative binding site of the metabolizing enzyme, resulting in metabolism on a different site of new molecule. This metabolic switching phenomenon is not uncommon. For example, 7-ethoxycoumarin (Marchitti, Brocker, Stagos & Vasiliou, 2008) was extensively metabolized to 7-hydroxycoumarin (Meyer & Zanger, 1997) with a minor metabolite 6-hydroxy-7-ethoxycoumarin (Nebert & Dalton, 2006) through a CYP1A1-mediated oxidations in rat. Mechanistically, the C-H bond at the α-carbon of the ethoxy group of 7-ethoxycoumarin (Marchitti, Brocker, Stagos & Vasiliou, 2008) is initially oxidized to give an unstable hemiacetal intermediate, which subsequently loses an acetaldehyde to give the metabolite 7-hydroxycoumarin (Meyer & Zanger, 1997). [D2]-7-Ethoxycoumarin (Patilea-Vrana, Anoshchenko & Unadkat, 2019), resulting from the replacement of two hydrogen atoms with deuterium atoms at the α-carbon of the ethoxy group of 7-ethoxycoumarin (Marchitti, Brocker, Stagos & Vasiliou, 2008), showed a 2-fold reduction of the formation of 7-hydroxycoumarin (Meyer & Zanger, 1997) in rat liver microsomes. However, [D2]-7-ethoxycoumarin (Patilea-Vrana, Anoshchenko & Unadkat, 2019) showed a 5-fold increase in the formation of 6-hydroxy-[D2]-7-ethoxycoumarinin in rat liver microsomes, resulting in almost no change of total metabolic stability, compared to 7-ethoxycoumarin (Marchitti, Brocker, Stagos & Vasiliou, 2008). This result suggests that the oxidation of the C-H bond at the α-carbon of the ethoxy group of 7-ethoxycoumarin (Marchitti, Brocker, Stagos & Vasiliou, 2008) was switched to the oxidation of the C-H bond at 6 position of [D2]-7-ethoxycoumarin (Patilea-Vrana, Anoshchenko & Unadkat, 2019). Thus, addressing the metabolically labile sites (or soft spots) of a lead molecule is a systematic SAR process, where multiple factors, including lipophilicity, stereochemistry, and intrinsic reactivity should be considered in the drug design process.

7.2.7.2.1. Source

The "isotope effect" is a technique used in the design of new bioactive molecules to block a metabolic soft spot or change the metabolism's path by substituting deuterium atoms for hydrogen atoms. The deuterated molecule may have decreased metabolism on the carbon atom where the deuterium atom is attached because the carbon-deuterium bond is more difficult to break than the carbon-hydrogen bond. This could potentially lower the in vitro and in vivo clearance or change the metabolism. The search for novel CNS-penetrant and mGlu3-selective negative allosteric modulators served as an example of this. Regarding SAR research, compound 16 was found to be a lead possessing strong biological activity. Compound 16 was found to be metabolically unstable in liver microsomes of both humans and rats, with a calculated hepatic clearance of 18.9 mL/min/kg for humans and 54.01 mL/min/kg for rats. The primary O-demethylation pathway (soft spot) for 16 was CYP-mediated. The extremely shallow allosteric ligand SAR meant that traditional electronic or steric perturbations could not resolve this soft spot issue. Nevertheless, by substituting the deuterium atoms for the hydrogen atoms in the -OCH3 group of 16. Rats' computed hepatic clearance fell from 54.1 mL/min/kg for compound 16 to 35.9 mL/min/kg for compound 17. Rats' plasma clearance likewise dropped following IV dosing, going from 5.2 mL/min/kg for 16 to 2.9 mL/min/kg for 17. The potential metabolic switching for 17 may be the cause of the observed decreased deuterium effect. By replacing the deuterium, a novel compound was found, necessitating additional in vitro and in vivo biological testing.

Tetrabenazine is the subject of another example, where the deuterated form of the drug is a novel formulation with significantly better safety characteristics. Tetrabenazine, a medication that is sold to treat chorea linked to Huntington's disease, undergoes a lot of metabolism to produce an active metabolite 19, which is subsequently processed to produce the active metabolites 20 and 21 through the polymorphic CYP2D6 enzyme. However, the observed clinical adverse effects, e.g., sedation, somnolence, fatigue and insomnia might be associated with not only the high C_{max} of the drug itself but also with the variable levels of active metabolites in patients due to CYP2D6 polymorphism. As a result, finding a dose that lowers chorea while still being well tolerated requires individualized and gradual dosage titration over a number of weeks. SD-809 is a deuterated tetrabenazine product manufactured by Auspex Pharmaceuticals that aims to modify the O-demethylation reaction. Compared to tetrabenazine, SD-809 demonstrated a slightly higher C_{max}, a longer half-life, and a higher exposure. Patients may be able to take SD-809 at a much lower dose in comparison to tetrabenazine to achieve a similar exposure with a lower Cmax. It can be concluded that SD-809 offers a better safety profile if the reported side effects in humans linked to tetrabenazine administration are caused by C_{max}. Auspex Pharmaceuticals released a news release on December 16, 2014, stating that SD-809 demonstrated strong efficacy and safety results in its phase 3 clinical registration trial studies. On April 3, 2017, the FDA authorized SD-809, also known as Austedo, to treat chorea linked to Huntington's disease. In fact, the first deuterated product to receive FDA approval for human use is SD-809 (Austedo).

7.2.7.3. Prodrugs or Active Metabolites as New Drug Candidates

Prodrugs are a class of pharmaceuticals that are administered in an inactive state and are converted to an active state in vivo by chemical or enzymatic means. This is a conventional approach to chemically alter pharmacologically active compounds to address issues related to the site-selective delivery, metabolism, excretion, absorption barrier, and route of administration. Prodrugs frequently contain functional groups that are readily broken down by the body's enzymes or chemicals, such as esters, amides, phosphates, carbonates, or carbamates. Prodrugs are frequently used to increase the oral bioavailability of active molecules by masking their polar or ionizable functional groups. Tenofovir, for instance, is a nucleotide inhibitor of reverse transcriptase, an essential viral enzyme in HIV-1 infections. Tenofovir's low oral bioavailability in humans (less than 5%) was caused by the phosphonic acid group's high hydrophilicity, which restricted its use as a medication. With an oral bioavailability of 39% in humans, the prodrug tenofovir disoproxil was found through SAR studies on bis-carbonate esters of tenofovir. Mechanistically, tenofovir disoproxil is first hydrolyzed to the intermediate 24 by chemical or enzymatic means (carboxyesterases), and then the formaldehyde and CO_2 spontaneously evaporate to produce the monoester intermediate 25. The ultimate hydrolysis of the monoester intermediate 25 to the active medication tenofovir 26 is most likely carried out by phosphodiesterases (Figure 7.11).

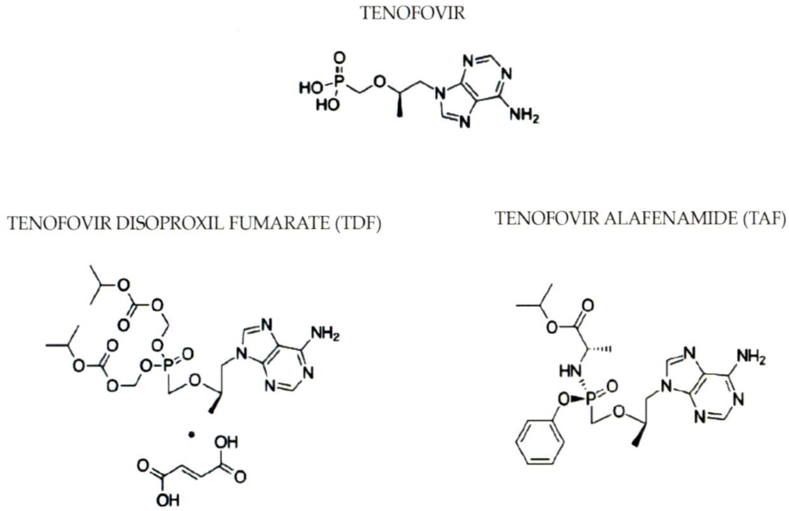

Figure 7.11. *Chemical structures of tenofovir, tenofovir disoproxil fumarate (TDF) and tenofovir alafenamide (TAF).*

Source: Zanella I, Zizioli D, Castelli F, Quiros-Roldan E. Tenofovir, another inexpensive, well-Known and widely available old drug repurposed for SARS-COV-2 Infection. Pharmaceuticals. 2021; 14(5):454. https://doi.org/10.3390/ph14050454.

Drugs are eliminated from the body through metabolism and/or excretion in their intact form after being administered. The latter procedure, which is outside the purview of this work, occasionally entails active transport. The majority of the time, metabolism sites are erratic, and metabolites may exhibit no pharmacological activity at all, activity that is less than, equal to, or greater than the parent molecules' activity. Active metabolites are typically defined as those that possess comparable or superior pharmacological activity. In the following ways, the transformation of drugs into active metabolites differs from the transformation of prodrugs into active drugs. Both pharmaceuticals and their active metabolites are pharmacologically active when it comes to this conversion process. Drugs are metabolized (biotransformed) by enzymes, and the sites of metabolism are unpredictable. Nonetheless, there are specific methods for converting pharmacologically inactive prodrugs into active medications, including enzymatic and chemical processes. The variability of metabolite formation during drug metabolism presents a potential avenue for the identification of active metabolites as novel compounds (NCEs) or novel structural templates for additional drug discovery optimization. A drug molecule's lack of PK–PD correlation or in vivo efficacy–in vitro potency correlation may be a sign of the presence of active metabolites. As an illustration, losartan is used to treat hypertension in humans as an angiotensin II receptor antagonist. To produce the metabolite EXP3174, losartan's alcohol functional group is oxidized to a carboxylic acid group in the body. One of the main metabolites that are circulating in humans is EXP3174. According to in vitro research, EXP3174's IC50 against the angiotensin II receptor is 0.2 nmol/L, while losartan's is 4 nmol/L. It was estimated that the active metabolite EXP3174 may have contributed approximately 14 times the activity of in vitro–in vivo losartan itself by taking into account the in vitro potency, plasma exposure, and the free fraction in plasma. This suggests that more in vitro and in vivo studies on EXP3174 are necessary (Figure 7.12).

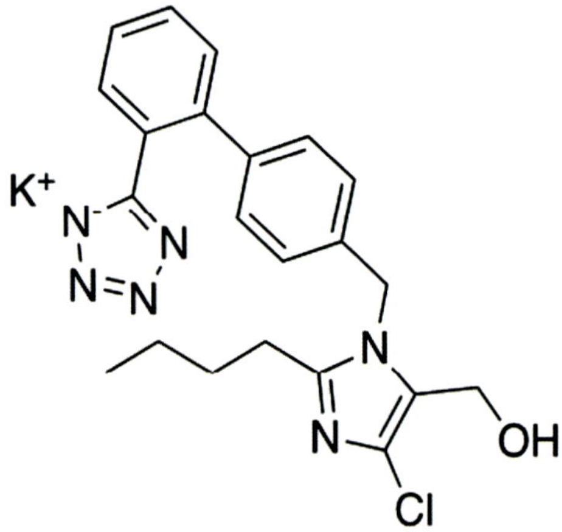

Figure 7.12. *Losartan potassium*

Source: *Foley L, Toney J, Barlow JW, O'Connor M, Fitzgerald-Hughes D, Ramtoola Z. Investigation of the physical, chemical and microbiological stability of losartan potassium 5 mg/ml extemporaneous oral liquid suspension. Molecules. 2021; 26(2):301. https://doi.org/10.3390/molecules26020301.*

In some cases, active metabolites have been developed as new drugs. For example, amitriptyline is a widely used drug for treatment of mental disorders, including depression and anxiety. Amitriptyline is metabolized by CYP2D6, 3A4 and 2C19 to a demethylated metabolite. This metabolite is a more potent and selective norepinephrine reuptake inhibitor with K_i of 4.4 nmol/L, compared to 22.4 nmol/L for amitriptyline, against norepinephrine transporter. Consequently, metabolite underwent development and eventually became a marketed drug, nortriptyline.

7.3. Drug Toxicology

Toxicology is the study of how drugs and chemicals in the environment cause unintended effects, while pharmacology is the scientific field that investigates how drugs change biological systems in an effort to promote health and treat disease. When taken as a whole, these fields cover the molecular underpinnings of drug action, how drugs affect cells, organs, and organisms, how genetic variations affect drug action, and drug discovery. The term "toxicity" describes a substance's potential for poisoning or harm. According to pharmacology, drug toxicity happens when a patient has an excessive amount of a prescription medication in their system, which can have harmful effects. Formally speaking, drug toxicity is defined as a wide range of negative consequences that can result from using drugs at either therapeutic or non-therapeutic dosages.

7.3.1. Causes of Drug Toxicity

Overdosing on medication can lead to drug toxicity, where an excessive amount of the drug accumulates in the body, either due to taking more than the prescribed dosage or the dosage being too high. Some medications can also cause adverse reactions, resulting in harmful side effects even at normal doses. The line between an effective and toxic dose can be thin, as what may be therapeutic for one person could be poisonous for another. Medications with a long half-life can also build up in the bloodstream over time, contributing to toxicity. Factors like age, kidney function, and hydration levels can impact how quickly the body can eliminate a drug, necessitating regular monitoring, such as with lithium levels in the blood.

7.3.2. Mechanisms of Drug Toxicity and Relevance to Pharmaceutical Development

It has been estimated that the average cost of developing a profitable drug is greater than US $1 point7 billion. The cost of pharmaceutical development has been rising for many years. The number of newly approved medications each year, however, is represented by a comparatively flat graph. The challenge of target validation in the face of progressively complex disease domains and the growth of regulatory obstacles are a couple of the causes of the issue. A new drug's development process is thought to take into account an average of 10,000–25,000 different chemicals. A major problem 25 years ago was poor human pharmacokinetics; today, what are the main causes of lead compound attrition?

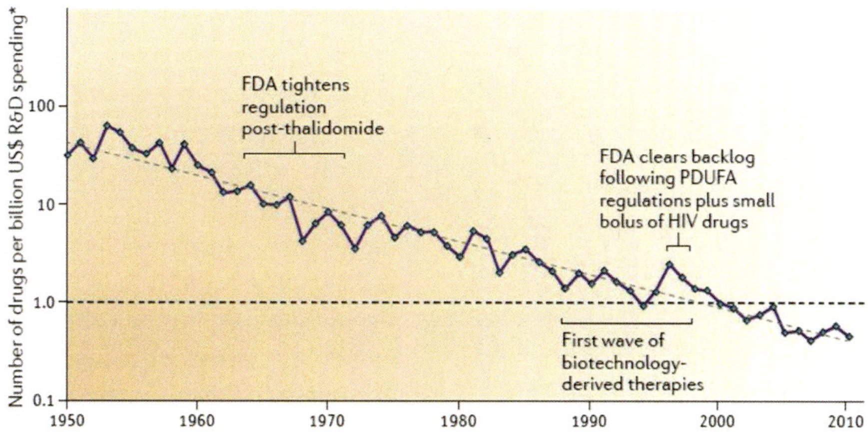

Figure 7.13. *Number of new drugs approved by the U.S.*

Source: Yildirim, O., Gottwald, M., Schüler, P., & Michel, M. C. (2016). Opportunities and challenges for drug development: Public–private partnerships, adaptive designs and big data. Front. Pharmacol. 7, 461. doi: 10.3389/fphar.2016.00461.

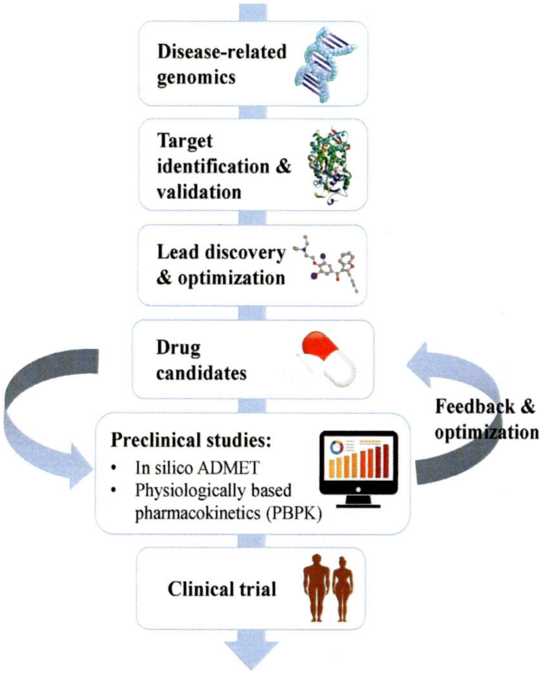

Figure 7.14. *Safety issues at different stages of drug discovery and development.*

Source: Wu, F., Zhou, Y., Li, L., Shen, X., Chen, G., Wang, X., Liang, X., Tan, M., & Huang, Z. (2020). Computational approaches in preclinical studies on drug discovery and development. Front. Chem. 8, 726. doi: 10.3389/fchem.2020.00726

Progress in the comprehension of human cytochrome P450 (P450) and other enzymes, understanding of transporters, and creation of predictive in vitro assays have all contributed to the resolution of this aspect. Toxicological concerns have, however, risen as metabolic problems have decreased. Combined, pre-clinical toxicity (in animals) and adverse events (in humans) represent about one-third of attrition cases. If one excludes the "non-scientific" issues (e.g., If the latter are commercial or financial), the percentage is even higher (Figure 7.13).

The real problem lies in the time and money wasted on compounds that have toxicity problems and must be withdrawn from development. The drug discovery and development process involves several stages where toxicity and safety assessments are conducted. The loss could amount to hundreds of millions of dollars and years of research if substances with toxicity problems are not abandoned until very late. Therefore, in the process of developing new drugs, early decisions are crucial, and they need to be made correctly (Figure 7.14).

7.3.2.1. Contexts of Drug Toxicity

Using the Paracelsus axiom, all compounds are safe at very low doses and toxic at high doses. Here, toxicity and adverse events at doses that are pertinent to patients taking a medication are what we are thinking about, not unintentional drug overdoses. How one approaches the problem of avoiding toxicity or creating substitute compounds that won't have this liability will depend on the context of toxicity. Hepatic and cardiovascular toxicity are the most often reported issues.

On-target, or mechanism-based, toxicity is the first type of toxicity. In other words, the drug's interaction with the same target that results in the intended pharmacological response is what causes the toxicity. Instead of focusing on competitive inhibition, the idea is that the drug's biological response to binding to its target is what causes both the toxic and effective effects. This kind of toxicity is challenging to manage in theory because it manifests in all classes of compounds created to treat the illness. It might be required to alter the disease's target. But statins provide an example of an alternative tactic. Because they block the liver's 3-hydroxy-3-methylglutaryl CoA (HMG CoA) reductase, all statins result in hypercholesterolemia, i.e., the objective. The inhibition of HMGCoA reductase in muscle and potentially other tissues is another reason why statins have negative effects. Protein geranylgeranylation is suppressed. Thankfully, different transport proteins can regulate the distribution of statins across tissues, and while on-target toxicity is a concern, it can be managed through inter-tissue distribution.

Drug toxicity can occur in different contexts. One context is hypersensitivity and immune responses, where drugs can trigger allergic reactions by interacting with proteins in the body and inducing antibody production. For example, penicillins are known to cause allergic reactions due to their ability to bind to proteins and initiate immune responses. Another context is off-target toxicity, where drugs interact with unintended targets in the body, leading to harmful effects. For instance, terfenadine can bind not only to the H1 receptor for antihistaminic effects but also to the hERG channel, causing arrhythmias. To address this issue, it is important to screen and develop drug candidates with lower IC50 and Kd values to minimize off-target interactions.

Bioactivation is the fourth context in which drugs can be toxic. Many medications are transformed into reactive products, which are frequently referred to as "metabolites." These substances alter the proteins they interact with and in some way produce toxicity, though the exact mechanisms are unknown (see infra).

According to one theory, significant regulatory or other proteins undergo modification and lose their functionality. An additional possibility that connects to the second context of toxicity is that the altered proteins trigger immunological responses. According to a review of medications at Bristol-Myers Squibb, "metabolism" was a factor in 28% of the cases where drug candidates were shelved from development.

Idiosyncratic reactions represent the fifth context of toxicity. Idiosyncratic refers to "individual," and these are uncommon, poorly understood events that occur in $1/10^3$ to $1/10^4$ of the population. The fact that so few, if any, animal models are highly predictive makes such responses extremely problematic. Even in extensive clinical trials, it is challenging to identify such adverse events due to their low incidence. However, even a $1/10^4$ incidence can result in hundreds of issues with commonly used medications for which millions of prescriptions may be written.

The context of toxicity has bearing on how difficult it is to predict safety problems.

7.3.2.2. Theories Regarding Mechanisms of Idiosyncratic Reactions

Many researchers have reviewed this subject (Table 7.3). To account for all drugs for which idiosyncrasies have been reported, at least five theories have been put forth, and they might not be mutually exclusive. Polymorphisms or uncommon alleles of metabolism-related enzymes are the first theory. (The term "rare alleles" refers to instances of less than 1–2 percent, so the term "polymorphism" might not be appropriate in this case. The idea is that sensitivity results from a drug's lack of metabolism, which includes a lack of detoxication. For example, a person may be the ~1% of the (Caucasian) population that has a high likelihood of activating a drug (e.g., the extremely quick metabolizers in the P450 2D6 group) and may also lack an enzyme necessary to detoxicate the product, such as glutathione transferase. Consequently, multiplying two polymorphisms at the 1 percent level would result in an incidence of $1/10^4$. Although there are no reliable examples to support any observed idiosyncratic reactions, this scenario is plausible.

The second, which has already been discussed, is the happened theory. The idea is that while some people will activate a medication more than others to produce a hapten, only a small percentage of people will exhibit this response due to differences in immune systems. There is some evidence in the cases of tienilic acid and hydralazine, which cause hepatitis and produce anti-P450 antibodies in humans when activated by human P450s and bound covalently to P450s. The shortcoming is that it hasn't been able to establish whether these incidents are merely coincidental but unconnected or whether they are the cause of the hepatotoxicity. The inflammation model is another name for the third theory. The idea is that while many people experience bioactivation and other events, only some people become more sensitive to inflammation or other predisposing episodes. This phenomenon may be shown in rats given lipopolysaccharide treatments to induce oxidative stress. It's debatable, though, exactly how representative this is as a model for human peculiarities.

Table 7.3. Listing of Published Proposals for Potential Risk Factors of Idiosyncratic Drug Induced Liver Injury (iDILI) with Focus on Cytochrome P450, Drug Dose, Metabolic Drug Parameters and Drug Lipophilicity

Proposed Risk Factors	Comments	Year	First Author
• Cytochrome P450 (CYP) • CYP isoforms	• **Proposal:** Described as classic view, drugs implicated in iDILI are mainly metabolized by CYP. **Comment:** In retrospect, correct assumption but not based on facts or iDILI cases assessed for causality like by RUCAM although this method was quoted. • **Proposal:** Officially proposed, most hepatotoxic drugs are oxidatively metabolized by the CYP system. **Comment:** This sentence statement was not based on any iDILI case assessed for causality by a robust diagnostic algorithm like RUCAM. • **Proposal:** In general, CYP 2C9 and CYP 2 C19 pathways appeared more toxic than CYP 3A and CYP 2D6. Data were retrieved from various databases. **Comment:** Conclusions remain vague because iDILI cases were likely not assessed for causality by RUCAM. • **Proposal:** Being a substrate of CYP enzymes is one of two important predictors of iDILI, having a higher, dose-independent likelihood of causing iDILI based on the adjusted OR (odds ratio) of 5.04 with 95% confidence interval (CI) of 2.34–10.9, p <0.0001. Concomitantly, drugs functioning as CYP inhibitor or inducer had no statistically significant effect on OR. **Comment:** Metabolism data on CYP enzymes for 254 orally administered drugs were collected from the US Liver Toxicity Knowledge Base Benchmark Dataset, but quality details of the used iDILI cases were not provided, lacking especially information whether RUCAM was used for causality assessment or not. Therefore, these data may be considered as preliminary, applicable also to data on CYP isoforms: drugs metabolized by CYP 1A2, CYP 2C8/2C9 and CYP 3A5 are classified having a higher likelihood of causing iDILI as compared with CYP 2D6, CYP 2C19, CYP 3A4, CYP 2B6, and CYP 2E1. Presented were also data of 11 clinical iDILI cases derived from the LiverTox database with causality assessment confirmed by physicians or health care professionals. Many of the assumed iDILI cases of this database were not real iDILI and became a matter of dispute. Other iDILI were derived from Liver Toxicity Biomarker Study, lacking details on causality assessment and biomarkers used. • **Proposal:** As opposed to the proposals made above, recent reports provided clarity on the relationship between drugs implicated in iDILI: Among 36 drugs causing iDILI in published cases assessed for causality using RUCAM, 22 drugs (61.1%) were metabolized through CYP, whereas for the remaining 14 drugs (38.9%) pathways not involving CYPs were responsible for the drug metabolism. As a result, CYP is involved in the majority of drugs implicated in iDILI. Among 619 RUCAM based published iDILI cases caused by drugs metabolized by CYPs, 49.6% of the cases were due to drugs metabolized by CYP 3A4/5, with 24.6% cases by CYP 2C9, 13.2% cases by CYP 2E1, 7.3% cases by CYP 2C19, 3,5% cases by CYP 1A2, and 1.8% cases by CYP 2D6. **Comment:** For the first time, the percentage contribution of CYP and CYP isoform was determined in iDILI cases assessed for causality by RUCAM.	2009 2009 2010 2014 2020	Tarantino, US FDA see, Lammert, Yu, Teschke

• Recommended daily drug dose (RDDD)	• **Proposal:** A relationship was assumed between recommended, not necessarily used, daily drug doses of oral medications with iDILI. The US study cohort retrieved the cases and the used drugs including their recommended daily doses from two publicly available pharmaceutical databases. The drugs were categorized into dosage groups of 10 mg or less, 11 to 49 mg and 50 mg or greater based on daily recommended doses, which originally may show a broad range not allowing for inclusion in a precise dosage group. With atorvastatin as an example for a problematic dosage group attribution, the recommended daily dose was described as ranging between 10 and 80 mg. Among US prescription medicines, a statistically significant relationship was observed between recommended daily drug dose and reported frequency of hepatic adverse events like liver failure, liver transplantation and death caused by iDILI. **Comment:** The proposed daily drug dose dependency of iDILI was not based on the actually used daily dosage but on drugs with a broad dosage range as recommended by the manufacturers. Problematic was also the selection of iDILI cases likely not assessed for causality using RUCAM. Therefore, problems of dosages and iDILI cases limit the validity of published conclusions, classifying the data at best as preliminary. • **Proposal:** High recommended daily drug doses of ≥100 mg daily were assumed as risk factors of iDILI, based on an OR of 6.92 and a 95% CI (3.10–15.63). Data were retrieved from several sources of likely variable, not further described quality. For instance, iDILI cases were used included in the LiverTox database, which is known for presenting many iDILI cases without confirmed causality, causing iDILI cases being non-iDILI cases. Apart from high doses, lipophilicity of the drugs was considered to contribute to the risk of liver injury. **Comment:** The vague quality of the used iDILI cases substantially limits the published conclusions. • **Proposal:** A high daily drug dose, as recommended by the manufacturers but not necessarily as used dose, was considered as one of two important predictors of iDILI. **Comment:** Data were taken from the US Liver Toxicity Knowledge Base Benchmark Dataset, containing iDILI cases likely not assessed for causality using RUCAM. Recommended doses were not necessarily doses actually used. Overall data of insufficient quality caused fragile conclusions. • **Proposal:** A higher recommended daily drug dose was considered as risk factor for iDILI. Basic data were derived from the World Health Organization's Anatomical Therapeutic Chemical classification system and the Micromedex Drugdex® compendium. **Comment:** The quality of the data retrieved from other sources remained unclear, Data were based on recommended but not on actually used drugs and iDILI cases were obviously not assessed for causality using RUCAM. These confounders limit the conclusions as published.	2008 2013 2014 2015	Lammert, Chen, Yu, Weng
• Used daily drug dose (UDDD)	• Proposals: Published in 1999, drugs given at a daily dose of 10 mg or less were rarely or if ever associated with a high incidence of idiosyncratic drug reactions (iDRs), mentioned in the context of published data on the lupus syndrome induced by hydralazine and the increase in mortality with vesnarinone, both conditions that have nothing to do with iDILI. Published 2007, it was claimed as an empirical observation that that iDRs are rare with drugs given at a dose of 10 mg daily or less, whereby iDILI is not mentioned. In 2019, if a drug is given at a total daily dose of 10 mg/day or less, it is unlikely to be associated with a significant incidence of iDILI, considered as an empirical cutoff. The problem with this cutoff remains because it is not based on an iDILI case study. **Comment:** Only in 2019, a drug threshold was attributed to iDILI but without providing new evidence.	1999 2007 2019 2008	Uetrecht, Uetrecht, Uetrecht, Lammert

	• **Proposal:** Swedish cohort: included were 598 iDILI cases, 9% belonged to the ≤10 mg/day group, 14.3% to the 11–49 mg/day group and 77% of cases were caused by medications given at doses ≥50 mg/day. Cases were retrieved from the Swedish Drug Reaction Advisory Committee (SADRAC) and assessed for causality using RUCAM and all included cases had a causality grading of at least possible. **Comment:** The percentage contribution of cases with a possible causality grading was not mentioned, in other studies using iDILI cases of SADAC up to 48% of the cases had a possible causality grading. Therefore, the present data should be taken with caution, because it remains unclear how many cases had the preferred causality gradings of highly probable or probable. It is also unclear how many real liver injury cases were included with alanine aminotransferase (ALT) values of >5 x ULN (upper limit of normal) and whether cases with ALT values of 2 – 5 x ULN were excluded from the study cohort as not real DILI cases.		
• Cumulative drug dose (CDD)	• **Proposal:** There are no valid data proposing that cumulative drug doses could be risk factors of iDILI. **Comment:** This is a major shortcoming in previous risk factor studies on iDILI. However, for a few drugs implicated in iDILI sufficient data were presented for used daily doses and duration of intake, allowing now for calculation of the cumulative drug doses, see below. They ranged from 575 mg to 12,000 mg and provided no trend and no realistic threshold that could be used in the context of risk management In addition, case data were retrieved from the Swedish Hepatic ADR Dataset, known for its problems of correct iDILI definition. • **Proposal:** The potential role of cumulative drug doses for iDILI remained unanswered. **Comment:** However, based on published data of used daily drug doses in 6 patients with length of treatment, cumulative doses were now calculated as shown below and provided cumulative doses from 3200 mg to 60,000 mg. Interestingly, the 60,000 mg was used by patient 6, who recovered. Overall, a valid trend was not found.	2008 2013	Lammert, Chen
• Hepatic drug metabolism (HDM)	• **Proposal:** Oral medications with significant hepatic metabolism are at higher risks for hepatic adverse events. Compared to drugs with <50% hepatic metabolism, drugs with ≥50% hepatic metabolism had a significantly higher frequency of liver failure (28% vs. 9%), fatal DILI (23% vs. 4%). **Comment:** Cases of iDILI and drug characteristics were retrieved from a number of databases with variable quality, and there were no strict inclusion criteria of cases and no causality assessment such as RUCAM. Cases with ALT values above 3 x ULN rather than above 5 x ULN were used, a problematic approach due to inclusion of iDILI cases that were not real liver injury cases. • **Proposal:** Liver metabolism ≥50% was found to be predictive of fatal iDILI lacking synergistic effects with any other risk factor. The study was based on data of the WHO Anatomical Therapeutic Chemical classification system and the Micromedex Drugdex® compendium. **Comment:** The main problem was the obvious lack of a rigorous causality assessment method applied to iDILI cases, which makes this methodological shortcoming the published claims not well evidenced.	2010 2015 2017	Lammert, Weng, McEuen

	• **Proposal:** A hepatic metabolism ≥50% provided for ORs (95%CI): 1.90 (1.18–3.5), classified under the term "consensus" as risk factor for iDILI, although it was admitted that the extent of metabolism is not a strong predictor for iDILI risk. Data were retrieved from various databases including the US LiverTox database despite its known limitations. **Comment:** It was correctly mentioned by the authors as one of several limitations that not all of the datasets considered the causality assessment (e.g., RUCAM score), which they found essential in future studies to characterize iDILI, as reports suggested that some hepatotoxicity recorded in the literature is vague. The authors described other limitations with respect to the used databases.		
• Drug lipophilicity (DL)	• **Proposal:** High lipophilicity per se is not a significant risk factor for iDILI, opposing to the title of the publication: High lipophilicity and high daily dose of oral medications are associated with significant risk for drug-induced liver injury. **Comment:** In fact, lipophilicity alone is not a significant risk factor for iDILI, only if combined with high daily doses. For lipophilicity an OR of 1.83 was calculated, a value that was not statistically significant. • **Proposal:** High drug lipophilicity is not associated with a higher likelihood of causing iDILI. **Comment:** It was correctly mentioned by the authors that data for drug lipophilicity were derived from 254 orally administered drugs collected from the Liver Toxicity Knowledge Base Benchmark Dataset. However, quality details of the used iDILI cases were not provided, lacking especially information whether RUCAM was used for causality assessment or not. Therefore, these data may be considered as provisional. • **Proposal:** According to the published conclusions, it seems that lipophilicity does not play a significant role in predicting a liver risk by an oral drug. **Comment:** These negative results were based on databases and 975 oral medications. • **Proposal:** For lipophilicity as a potential risk factor for iDILI, a consensus among the authors was reached regarding the low OR (95% CI) of 1.55 (109–2.22). For analysis, databases were used including the problematic US LiverTox database, and not all of the iDILI cases were assessed for causality using RUCAM. **Comment:** Results concerning lipophilicity as risk factor of iDILI remain fragile.	2013 2014 2015 2017	Chen, Yu, Weng, McEuen

Source: Teschke, R., Danan, G. Idiosyncratic drug induced liver injury, cytochrome P450, metabolic risk factors and lipophilicity: Highlights and controversies. International Journal of Molecular Sciences. 2021; 22(7), 3441. https://doi.org/10.3390/ijms22073441.

The danger hypothesis is the fourth (theory). Here, the damaged tissue sends out warning signals, e.g., it is not the medication or its metabolites but rather lipid oxidation products and cytokines that cause a toxic reaction. There is no concrete proof that this is a mechanism underlying clinical medication idiosyncracies, but as Uetrecht has noted, if an immunological response is involved, this hypothesis is not incompatible with the hapten theory. The model of pharmacological intervention is the fifth theory. According to this model, medications trigger immune reactions through reversible protein binding, i.e., without a covalent connection. Sulfamethoxazole, an arylamine that is prone to producing reactive metabolites, served as one of the foundations for this proposal. There is some evidence that the peptide-like compound ximelegatran may function in this way.

A Closer Look

Permeability Barriers and Detoxification

One of the main features of xenobiotic toxic stress is that the precise substances to which an organism is exposed will be highly variable and may vary over time. The primary obstacle encountered by xenobiotic detoxification systems is their need to eliminate the seemingly infinite quantity of xenobiotic substances from the intricate blend of chemicals involved in regular metabolic processes. An elegant combination of low-specificity enzymatic systems and physical barriers has been developed as a solution to this issue. Cell membranes serve as hydrophobic permeability barriers that regulate access to the internal environment in all living things. These cell membranes prevent the diffusion of polar compounds, and transport proteins that choose particular substrates from the extracellular mixture facilitate the uptake of beneficial molecules. Because most hydrophilic molecules are not recognized by any particular transporter, they are unable to enter cells due to this selective uptake. However, because hydrophobic compounds cannot be controlled to diffuse across these barriers, organisms cannot use membrane barriers to block the entry of lipid-soluble xenobiotics.

On the other hand, because of the permeability barrier, organisms have evolved detoxification mechanisms that take advantage of the hydrophobicity shared by membrane-permeable xenobiotics. Because of their extremely broad substrate specificities, which enable them to metabolize nearly any non-polar compound, these systems thereby resolve the specificity issue. Because they are polar and typically contain one or more charged groups, useful metabolites are disregarded. Since these species are derived from normal cellular constituents and typically share their polar characteristics, they cannot be used to detoxify the reactive by-products of normal metabolism. Nevertheless, because these substances are scarce, certain enzymes are able to identify and eliminate them. Some examples of these particular detoxification systems are the antioxidant systems that get rid of reactive oxygen species and the glyoxalase system that gets rid of the reactive aldehyde methylglyoxal.

Summary

- Drug metabolism is the metabolic breakdown of drugs by living organisms, usually through specialized enzymatic systems.
- The metabolism of pharmaceutical drugs is an important aspect of pharmacology and medicine. For example, the rate of metabolism determines the duration and intensity of the pharmacologic action of a drug.
- Medicines are required for humans to cure diseases but at the same time, they are foreign objects to the body. Hence, the human body tries to excrete them at the earliest. It is highly desirable that the medicines get eliminated from the human body immediately after showing their drug action
- The chemistry of drug metabolism needs an elaborate understanding – it is a fascinating and a complicated process. The primary site of drug metabolism is the smooth endoplasmic reticulum of the liver cell.
- The drug metabolism process can lead to the generation of Reactive Metabolites (RM) in some instances, which further lead to toxicity. The toxicity may vary from genotoxicity to immune-mediated Adverse Drug Reactions (ADRs).
- Drug metabolism comprises the metabolism of endogenous and exogenous substances. During metabolism most drugs lose the pharmacological activity and are excreted from the body.
- Drugs that share elements of their metabolic pathways can also 'compete' for the same binding sites on enzymes, decreasing their metabolism's efficiency. For instance, alcohol and certain sedatives are metabolized by the same member of the cytochrome P450 family.
- Drug metabolism is an essential clinical concern for the interprofessional healthcare team. Clinicians and pharmacists must work together to prevent clinically significant drug interactions that could affect patients' health.

References

1. Azzam, A. A. H., McDonald, J., & Lambert, D. G. (2019). Hot topics in opioid pharmacology: mixed and biased opioids. *British Journal of Anesthesia, 122*(6), e136–e145.
2. Bolton, A. E., Peng, B., Hubert, M., Krebs-Brown, A., Capdeville, R., Keller, U., & Seiberling, M. (2004). Effect of rifampicin on the pharmacokinetics of imatinib mesylate (Gleevec, STI571) in healthy subjects. *Cancer Chemotherapy and Pharmacology, 53*(2), 102–106.
3. Bortolussi, S., Catucci, G., Gilardi, G., & Sadeghi, S. J. (2021). N- and S-oxygenation activity of truncated human flavin-containing monooxygenase 3 and its common polymorphic variants. *Archives of Biochemistry and Biophysics, 697*, 108663.
4. Boyland, E., & Chasseaud, L. F. (1969). The role of glutathione and glutathione S-transferases in mercapturic acid biosynthesis. *Advances in Enzymology and Related Areas of Molecular Biology, 32*, 173–219.

5. Colizzi, M., Weltens, N., McGuire, P., Van Oudenhove, L., & Bhattacharyya, S. (2019). Descriptive psychopathology of the acute effects of intravenous delta-9-tetrahydrocannabinol administration in humans. *Brain Sciences, 9*(4), 95. https://doi.org/10.3390/brainsci9040095.

6. Commandeur, J. N., Stijntjes, G. J., & Vermeulen, N. P. (1995). Enzymes and transport systems involved in the formation and disposition of glutathione S-conjugates. Role in bioactivation and detoxication mechanisms of xenobiotics. *Pharmacological Reviews, 47*(2), 271–330.

7. El-Haj, B. M. (2021). Metabolic N-dealkylation and N-oxidation as elucidators of the role of alkylamino moieties in drugs acting at various receptors. *Molecules, 26*(7), 1917. https://doi.org/10.3390/molecules26071917.

8. Guengerich, F. P. (2001). Common and uncommon cytochrome P450 reactions related to metabolism and chemical toxicity. *Chemical Research in Toxicology, 14*(6), 611–650.

9. Lakshmanan, M. (2019). Drug metabolism. In *Introduction to Basics of Pharmacology and Toxicology* (Vol. 1, pp. 99–116). Singapore: Springer.

10. Marchitti, S. A., Brocker, C., Stagos, D., & Vasiliou, V. (2008). Non-P450 aldehyde oxidizing enzymes: The aldehyde dehydrogenase superfamily. *Expert Opinion on Drug Metabolism & Toxicology, 4*(6), 697–720.

11. Meyer, U. A., & Zanger, U. M. (1997). Molecular mechanisms of genetic polymorphisms of drug metabolism. *Annual Review of Pharmacology and Toxicology, 37*, 269–296.

12. Nebert, D. W., & Dalton, T. P. (2006). The role of cytochrome P450 enzymes in endogenous signaling pathways and environmental carcinogenesis. *Nature Reviews Cancer, 6*(12), 947–960.

13. Patilea-Vrana, G. I., Anoshchenko, O., & Unadkat, J. D. (2019). Hepatic enzymes relevant to the disposition of (-)-Δ9-Tetrahydrocannabinol (THC) and its psychoactive metabolite, 11-OH-THC. *Drug Metabolism and Disposition, 47*(3), 249–256.

Chapter

NATURAL PRODUCTS AND HERBAL MEDICINES

8

Contents

Introduction

Since ancient times, natural products and herbal medicines have been essential components of human healthcare systems, providing cures and treatments for a wide range of illnesses. These natural products, which are derived from plants, minerals, and other sources, have been widely used in traditional medicine across various cultures globally. Due to their perceived safety, efficacy, and potential benefits, natural products and herbal medicines are becoming more and more popular in today's world of pharmaceutical advancements. The organic origin of natural products is one of their main selling points; they are frequently thought to be safer and less likely to have side effects than synthetic drugs. Particularly herbal medicines make use of the many bioactive compounds found in plants, which have therapeutic qualities of their own. These substances have intricate interactions with the body, providing a comprehensive approach to well-being and recovery. Furthermore, the holistic approach of herbal medicine frequently targets the root causes of illnesses in addition to their symptoms, with the goal of promoting long-term wellness as opposed to merely providing temporary relief. Natural products and herbal medicines are praised not only for their apparent safety but also for their historical and cultural significance. Herbal remedies have long been used in many traditional medical systems, including Traditional Chinese Medicine (TCM), Ayurveda, and Indigenous healing practices. The foundation of modern herbal medicine practices is the knowledge that has been transmitted through these traditions. Additionally, the rich biodiversity of plant species found in various regions, each of which offers a unique set of therapeutic benefits, is reflected in the cultural diversity of herbal medicines.

Growing worries about the effects of conventional pharmaceuticals on the environment are another factor contributing to the renewed interest in natural products and herbal remedies. Synthetic drug extraction and production frequently require the use of harsh chemicals and produce large amounts of waste, which contaminate the environment. On the other hand, because they come from renewable resources and are frequently made using environmentally friendly practices, natural products are thought to be more environmentally sustainable.

Furthermore, pharmacological mechanisms and potential applications of natural products and herbal medicines have been clarified by the growing body of scientific research on these subjects. Numerous bioactive compounds with a wide range of therapeutic effects, including antioxidant and anti-inflammatory qualities as well as antimicrobial and anticancer effects, have been found through studies. The increasing amount of data not only supports the conventional applications of herbal remedies, but it also creates new avenues for their incorporation into conventional medical practice.

But even with their growing appeal and possible advantages, natural goods and herbal remedies are not without problems. It is still a concern to standardize herbal preparations to guarantee their efficacy, safety, and quality. Different regions have very different regulatory frameworks, which causes variations in the quality and labeling of products. To avoid negative reactions, it is also important to thoroughly research the interactions that occur between herbal remedies and conventional medications. Natural products and herbal remedies, which combine custom, cultural legacy, and scientific innovation, constitute an important part of healthcare. Their resurgence in popularity is a result of people's desire for sustainable alternatives to traditional pharmaceuticals as well as their growing appreciation for holistic approaches to health. To fully realize the potential of natural products in enhancing global health and well-being, more research, standardization, and regulatory initiatives will be necessary in the future.

Orientation and Directional Terms

Term	Definition	Illustration
Pharmacognosy	Pharmacognosy is the study of medicines or crude drugs produced from natural sources such as plants, microbes, and animals.	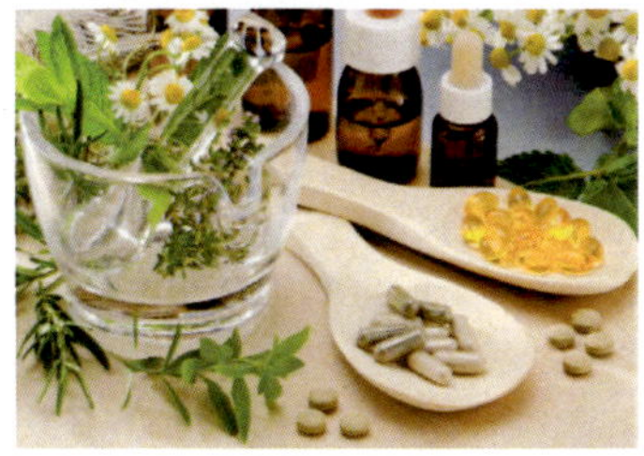
Paraherbalism	It is the pseudoscientific use of extracts of plant or animal origin as supposed medicines or health-promoting agents.	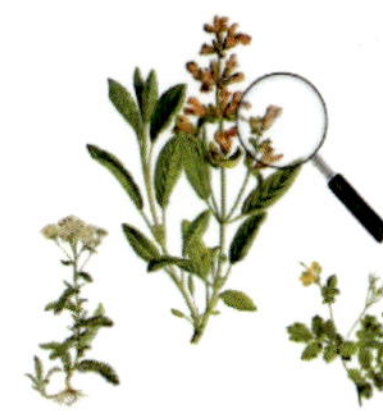
Arterolane	Arterolane is a substance that was tested for antimalarial activity by Ranbaxy Laboratories.	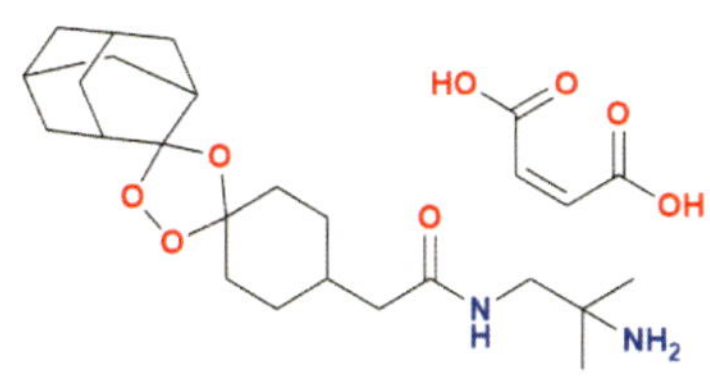
Drug discovery	Drug discovery is the process by which new candidate medications are discovered.	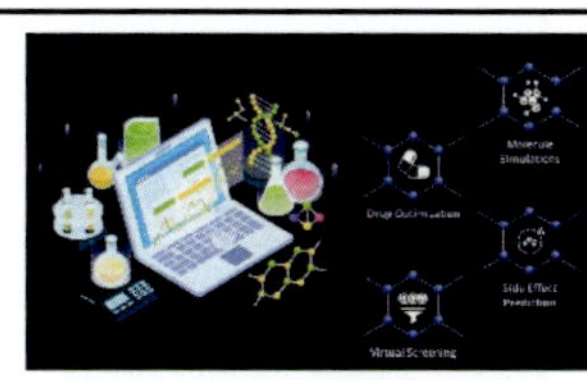
Epigallocatechin gallate	Epigallocatechin gallate, also known as epigallocatechin-3-gallate, is the ester of epigallocatechin and gallic acid, and is a type of catechin.	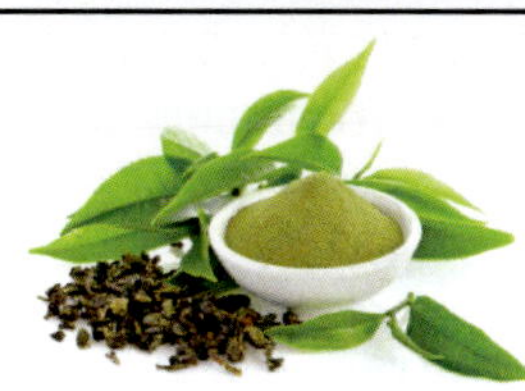

8.1. Overview of Natural Products and Herbal Medicines

Natural goods and conventional medical treatments are very significant. For a long time, natural products and their derivatives have been acknowledged as a source of structural diversity and therapeutic agents. Natural products possess a vast array of diverse multidimensional chemical structures. Simultaneously, they have garnered significant attention for their potential use as biological function modifiers. Drug discovery, which is nothing more than the process flow from a screening of natural product to a new isolate that requires expertise and experience, is turning into a challenging scientific task to find robust and viable lead candidates. But in addition to their diversity in chemical structures and biodiversity, the emergence of new technologies has completely changed how natural products are screened to find new therapeutics. Using these technologies presents a special chance to revive natural products as a leading drug discovery source. To find new and effective drug compounds, the process known as "natural product in drug discovery" focuses on the success of pharmacological activity. The chapter tries to describe the process of isolating, characterizing, and using bioactive compounds derived from natural products as drug candidates, or lead.

The study of pharmacognosy and the application of medicinal plants, which form the foundation of traditional medicine, is known as herbal medicine. Some herbal medicines have been transformed into contemporary treatments thanks to extensive pharmacological research conducted worldwide. One such example is the anti-malarial class of medications known as artemisinin, which was isolated from the herb Artemisia annua, which was used in Chinese medicine to treat fever. The safety and effectiveness of many plants used in 21st-century herbalism, which typically lacks standards for purity or dosage, are supported by scant scientific data. Herbal medicine can also use minerals, shells, certain animal parts, and products from fungi and bees. Using raw plant or animal extracts as unproven medications or health-promoting agents is known as pseudoscientific and alternative herbalism. The foundation of paraherbalism is the unsupported assumption that preserving different substances from a particular source with minimal processing is safer or more efficient than manufactured goods.

8.1.1. Natural Products in Drug Discovery

Historically, natural products and their structural analogs have played a significant role in pharmacotherapy, particularly in the treatment of infectious diseases and cancer. Natural products do, however, also pose difficulties for drug discovery, including technological obstacles to screening, isolation, characterization, and optimization. As a result, the pharmaceutical industry began to pursue natural products less actively in the 1990s. Improved analytical tools, genome mining and engineering techniques, and advancements in microbial culturing are just a few of the scientific and technological advancements that have recently addressed these issues and created new opportunities. As a result, there is renewed interest in using natural products as drug leads, especially to combat antibiotic resistance.

8.1.1.1. Sources of Drugs

The combination of synthetically prepared chemicals determines the therapeutic agents' level of complexity. Depending on their source, therapeutic agents can be classified as natural, synthetic, or semi-synthetic. Novel therapeutic agent compounds continue to have a significant source in the natural environment. Natural therapeutic agents are made from substances that are found in nature and contain extracts of active ingredients derived from a variety of sources, such as microorganisms, minerals, plants, and animals. Because of the diversity of their components' chemical and structural makeup, plants are the most common source of natural medicine. Aspirin (found in the bark of willow trees), digoxin (found in the flower *Digitalis lanata*), and morphine (found in opium) are a few examples of medications made from plants. In fact, it is estimated that > 60% of medications in industrialized countries are either natural products or their secondary metabolites. Notwithstanding obstacles posed by various, cutting-edge drug discovery techniques, natural products keep yielding more clinical candidates and therapeutic compounds. These substances continue to serve as a crucial basis for innovative pharmaceuticals, especially those aimed at treating infections with drugs like azitromycin, amphotericin B, acyclovir, and romidepsin. Many of them have since moved on to clinical trials or the marketplace. Because of the diversity and complexity of natural products' structures and chemicals, as well as their high throughput, automated separation techniques, and combinatorial chemistry, the screening of natural products has changed dramatically as a result of the development of novel technologies in drug discovery.

8.1.2. Importance of Natural Product Drugs

The introduction of novel, chemical, diverse entities with their application as patterns for semi-synthetic and total synthetic modification; the number of diseases treated by these diverse compounds; and their rate of use in the treatment of diseases are some ways to assess the significance of natural products used in the prevention and treatment of human diseases. Pharmaceutical research still focuses on natural products because alternative approaches to drug discovery have not been successful in producing many lead compounds for important therapeutic areas like metabolic and anti-infective diseases. Natural product research keeps coming up with new ways for the pharmaceutical industry to find lead compounds for drugs. It is now undeniable that natural products have been and will continue to be important sources of novel pharmaceutical therapeutic agents. The metabolites of synthetic drugs have fewer negative side effects and less therapeutic effect. Small chemical building blocks, known as synthetic therapeutic agents, are created through computer-based research techniques like computational chemistry and by utilizing a variety of chemical sources, including the anti-malaria medication arterolane. These building blocks are not found in nature. Natural sources of therapeutic agents, on the other hand, may not have adverse effects because they have pharmacological and physiological effects on living cells. Furthermore, the distribution of molecular properties in natural products is wider and includes lower molecular mass, partition coefficient, and structural diversity. Additionally, natural products interact with other biological molecules, proteins, and enzymes more frequently. Furthermore, when compared to synthetic compounds and combinatorial libraries, natural products have higher molecular rigidity and fewer heavy metals.

8.1.3. The Successful of Natural Products in Drug Discovery

The secret to successful natural product drug discovery and development will undoubtedly lie in an integrative strategy that combines the many discovery tools with the recently established field of integrative biology. It is foreseeable that natural products will continue to play a crucial role in the hunt for novel, affordable, and safe medications. In this situation, the pharmaceutical industry needs to wake up, shift its perspective, and reallocate its resources to natural product-based drug discovery initiatives. Not only do natural products enhance synthetic molecules, but they also possess drug-relevant characteristics that no synthetic compound can match. The great structural and chemical diversity of natural products is one of their main characteristics. Actually, modern medicinal chemistry lacks about 40% of the chemical scaffolds present in natural products, making synthetically produced molecules complementary to those found in them. Given that 45% of the top-selling medications on the market today are derived from natural products or their derivatives, it is highly likely that this is one of the factors contributing to their past success in drug discovery.

The biological past of natural products is another significant benefit. Natural products are made by repeatedly interacting with enzymes that modulate their biosynthesis. Additionally, many natural products have biological functions that involve binding to other proteins. Therefore, one could argue that natural products' capacity to interact with other molecules—a necessary precondition for creating a medicine that works—has been biologically validated. When compared to synthetics, many natural products show superior binding properties, which is a predictable but frequently ignored fact. The sterically more complex structures found in natural products most likely play a part in this.

In addition, natural products are more complex sterically, containing more bridgehead tetrahedral carbon atoms, rings, and chiral centers; they also have higher molecular weights and contain less nitrogen, halogen, or sulfur atoms but more oxygen atoms.

The effectiveness of natural products is directly linked to the various fields of natural products chemistry, molecular and cellular biology, synthetic and analytical chemistry, biochemistry, and pharmacology. These disciplines collectively work to harness the wide range of chemical structures and biological functions found in natural products. Furthermore, analyzing extensive databases filled with diverse chemotypes and information on target genes and proteins can aid in the development of novel chemical compounds through computational molecular modeling for pharmacological testing.

Currently, about half of all prescribed medications in developed countries come from natural products, the only sources of which are plants, animals, marine life, and microorganisms. It is believed that terrestrial plants provide a special and renewable resource for the discovery of possible new medications and biological entities because of the structural and biological diversity of their constituents.

There is no proof that naturally occurring products, which have a greater degree of structural diversity than synthetic compounds, have served as the main source of biologically active agents or will continue to play a major role in the development of novel medications. The usefulness of natural products in the treatment and prevention of human diseases can actually be measured in three ways: 1) by counting the number of diseases these substances treat or prevent; 2) by counting the number of new chemical entities of a wide structural diversity that are introduced on a regular basis; and 3) by counting the frequency with which these substances are used in the treatment of diseases.

Natural products are good lead compounds that can be further modified during the drug development process, and they are also important sources for new drugs. The varied structures and complex carbon skeletons of natural products have led to the significant use of natural products in drug discovery. Natural secondary metabolites are thought to exhibit greater "drug-likeness and biological friendliness than totally synthetic molecules" because they have developed within living systems, which makes them attractive candidates for additional drug development. Beyond the success of natural products as pharmaceuticals, one possible explanation could be the categorization of natural compounds as "privileged structures.". This idea is based on the observation that chemical agents produced by living things—especially secondary metabolites—have evolved over millennia under the pressure of evolution and are thus more likely than "randomly" assembled, synthetic chemicals made by humans to have a particular biological activity. Only a small portion of the world's living species have ever been examined for bioactivity, despite the immense potential. For example, only about 10% of all plant species that exist today have been tested; the percentage is even lower for microbes.

Drug discovery is the process of finding and/or creating new drugs in the fields of pharmacology, biotechnology, and medicine. Most medications have historically been found by chance discovery or by figuring out the active component from conventional treatments. Targeting particular entities based on an understanding of how disease and infection are regulated at the molecular and physiological levels is a novel strategy.

The lengthy process of finding new drugs involves identifying potential candidates, synthesizing, characterizing, testing, and assaying them for therapeutic efficacy. Before going through clinical trials, a compound will start the drug development process once these tests have demonstrated its value.

8.2. Sources and Classification of Natural Products

Natural products are a wide range of substances that come from living things, such as fungi, animals, plants, and microbes. They can be classified based on their source, chemical structure, or biological activity. An overview of the classification and sources of natural products:

1. ***Plant-Derived Natural Products***

   i. **Alkaloids**: Nitrogen-containing compounds found in plants, known for their diverse pharmacological activities. Examples include morphine from opium poppy and caffeine from coffee beans.

   ii. **Terpenoids**: Derived from the isoprene unit, terpenoids are abundant in essential oils and have various medicinal properties. Examples include menthol from mint and artemisinin from Artemisia annua.

   iii. **Phenolic Compounds**: These compounds are characterized by their phenol rings and include flavonoids, tannins, and lignans. They exhibit antioxidant and anti-inflammatory properties. Examples include quercetin from onions and resveratrol from grapes.

   iv. **Glycosides**: Compounds containing a sugar molecule attached to another moiety. Many plant-derived glycosides have medicinal properties, such as cardiac glycosides like digoxin from foxglove.

   v. **Polyphenols**: These compounds include flavonoids, phenolic acids, and stilbenes, known for their antioxidant and anti-inflammatory effects. Examples include curcumin from turmeric and epigallocatechin gallate (EGCG) from green tea.

vi. ***Animal-Derived Natural Products***

vii. **Peptides and Proteins**: Some peptides and proteins found in animals have therapeutic potential. Examples include insulin from pigs and venom peptides from snakes and spiders.

viii. **Marine Natural Products**: Compounds sourced from marine organisms, including sponges, algae, and corals, have diverse biological activities. Examples include cytarabine from sea squirts and halichondrin from sponges.

2. ***Microbial-Derived Natural Products***

   i. **Antibiotics**: Microorganisms produce various antibiotics to compete with other organisms. Examples include penicillin from Penicillium fungi and streptomycin from Streptomyces bacteria.

   ii. **Secondary Metabolites**: Microorganisms produce secondary metabolites with diverse biological activities. Examples include statins produced by fungi and cyclosporine from *Tolypocladium inflatum*.

3. ***Mineral-Derived Natural Products***

   i. **Clay Minerals**: Certain clay minerals have been used in traditional medicine for their detoxifying properties.

   ii. **Sulfur Compounds**: Sulfur-containing minerals like sulfur springs have been historically used for therapeutic purposes.

Scientific journals, books on pharmacognosy and natural product chemistry, databases like PubMed and SciFinder, respectable educational institutions, and research groups with a focus on natural product research are some of the sources used to classify and provide information on natural products.

8.2.1. Medicinal Properties of Plant-Derived Compounds

Compounds derived from plants have many therapeutic uses, which makes them an important source of therapeutic agents for both conventional and modern medicine. Here are some of the key medicinal properties of plant-derived compounds:

1. **Anti-inflammatory**: Many plant-derived compounds exhibit anti-inflammatory properties, reducing inflammation and associated pain. Examples include curcumin from turmeric, resveratrol from grapes, and gingerol from ginger.
2. **Antioxidant**: Plant compounds such as flavonoids, polyphenols, and carotenoids act as antioxidants, scavenging free radicals and reducing oxidative stress. Examples include quercetin from onions, catechins from green tea, and lycopene from tomatoes.
3. **Antimicrobial**: Numerous plant-derived compounds possess antimicrobial properties, inhibiting the growth of bacteria, fungi, and viruses. Examples include allicin from garlic, berberine from goldenseal, and tea tree oil from Melaleuca alternifolia.

4. **Anticancer**: Certain plant compounds have been shown to exhibit anticancer properties, inhibiting the growth and proliferation of cancer cells. Examples include paclitaxel from the Pacific yew tree, vincristine from periwinkle, and sulforaphane from broccoli.
5. **Analgesic**: Plant-derived compounds can act as analgesics, reducing pain perception. Examples include capsaicin from chili peppers, salicin from willow bark (which is converted to salicylic acid in the body, similar to aspirin), and menthol from mint.
6. **Antidiabetic**: Some plant compounds have demonstrated antidiabetic properties, helping to regulate blood sugar levels. Examples include berberine from various plants, cinnamon polyphenols, and gymnemic acids from *Gymnema sylvestre*.
7. **Cardioprotective**: Certain plant-derived compounds have cardioprotective effects, supporting heart health and reducing the risk of cardiovascular diseases. Examples include resveratrol from grapes, omega-3 fatty acids from fish oil, and flavonoids from cocoa.
8. **Neuroprotective**: Plant compounds like flavonoids and polyphenols exhibit neuroprotective properties, supporting brain health and potentially reducing the risk of neurodegenerative diseases. Examples include epigallocatechin gallate (EGCG) from green tea and curcumin from turmeric.
9. **Hepatoprotective**: Some plant-derived compounds have hepatoprotective effects, supporting liver health and protecting against liver damage. Examples include silymarin from milk thistle, curcumin from turmeric, and quercetin from onions.

The various phytochemicals found in plants, such as glycosides, phenolic compounds, terpenoids, and alkaloids, are frequently credited with these therapeutic benefits. The mechanisms of action and therapeutic potential of compounds derived from plants are still being discovered by research, which encourages more investigation and application in the medical field.

8.2.2. Standardization and Quality Control of Herbal Medicines

To guarantee the efficacy, safety, and consistency of herbal medicines, standardization and quality control are essential procedures. Herbal remedies, which come from organic sources like plants, are complex mixtures with widely differing amounts of potency, active ingredients, and bioavailability. To preserve the quality and medicinal effectiveness of herbal products, standardization entails creating consistent requirements. Quality control measures aim to reduce variability and guarantee adherence to regulatory standards by encompassing multiple aspects of production, ranging from raw material selection to the finished product.

The variability of plant material, which is influenced by various factors including geographical location, climate, cultivation practices, and post-harvest processing, presents a significant challenge in the standardization of herbal medicines. To overcome this difficulty, standardization processes frequently entail the detection and measurement of marker compounds, which function as authenticity and quality markers. To examine the chemical makeup of herbal extracts and ascertain the existence and concentration of particular bioactive compounds, analytical techniques such as gas chromatography (GC), mass spectrometry (MS), and high-performance liquid chromatography (HPLC) are frequently employed.

The identification of plants using techniques like chemical fingerprinting, DNA barcoding, and macroscopic and microscopic inspection is another facet of standardization. These techniques assist in confirming the veracity of plant material and identifying any contamination or adulteration. To guarantee that products contain the right species of plants and prevent substitution with potentially hazardous or ineffective substitutes, authenticity of herbal ingredients is crucial.

Standardization includes not only the identification of botanical materials but also the quantification of phytochemical content and concentration of active ingredients. This entails measuring the concentrations of bioactive substances that give herbal medications their therapeutic effects. Standardized herbal extracts are frequently made with particular extraction techniques and standardized to have a fixed concentration of active ingredients. However, choosing the right markers for standardization can be difficult because some bioactive compounds might only be found in specific plant species or might vary in concentration depending on the surrounding conditions.

Beyond chemical analysis, quality control of herbal medicines also involves testing for heavy metals and microbes, as well as physical attributes like appearance, taste, and odor. From the procurement of raw materials to packaging and labeling, good manufacturing practices (GMP) are crucial to guaranteeing the quality and safety of herbal products throughout the production process. GMP guidelines set forth protocols for maintaining equipment, maintaining cleanliness, ensuring product consistency, and documenting processes to reduce the risk of contamination.

Furthermore, before herbal medicines can be marketed, regulatory bodies in many nations demand that they go through a rigorous testing and evaluation process. Preclinical research is used to evaluate safety and toxicity, and clinical trials are used to determine the best dosage regimens and assess efficacy. Labeling requirements, such as the ingredients list, dosage guidelines, and any possible side effects or contraindications, are also governed by regulatory standards.

There are still issues in the global trade and distribution of herbal products, despite efforts to standardize and regulate the quality of herbal medicines. Differences in the requirements and implementation of regulations in various areas can result in disparities in the safety and quality of products. In addition, the extensive accessibility of herbal products via unofficial and online marketplaces poses further difficulties for maintaining public health and consumer protection.

To guarantee the safety, effectiveness, and consistency of herbal medicines, standardization and quality control procedures are crucial. Standardization procedures support the preservation of product quality and authenticity by setting uniform specifications, confirming botanical identity, and quantifying active ingredients. To address the complexities and difficulties involved in the standardization and quality control of herbal medicines, however, continued efforts are required, especially in light of international trade and regulatory harmonization.

8.2.3. Safety and Efficacy Considerations of Herbal Remedies

It's important to be aware of both the possible advantages and disadvantages of herbal remedies when evaluating their safety and effectiveness. Since ancient times, people have used herbal remedies—which are made from natural sources like plants—to treat a wide range of illnesses and advance health. Like any medication, they do have certain drawbacks, though, such as the possibility of side effects, potential conflicts with prescription medications, and variations in potency and quality.

Risk of side effects is one of the main safety concerns with herbal remedies. While many herbs are safe when used as directed, some people may experience allergic reactions or adverse effects from certain herbs. As an illustration, herbs like St. Ephedra, kava, and John's wort have all been linked to negative side effects, including liver damage and cardiovascular issues. In addition, the absence of standards and regulations in the production of herbal products can result in inconsistent product quality and contamination with heavy metals, pesticides, or other dangerous materials.

Potential herb-drug interactions are another cause for concern regarding safety. Pharmacologically active substances found in many herbs have the ability to interact with medications, either amplifying or decreasing their effects. Herbs such as ginkgo biloba, garlic, and ginger, for instance, have the potential to interact with anticoagulant medications and raise the risk of bleeding. In the same way, herbs like St. Antidepressants, immunosuppressants, and other drugs may interact with John's wort and lessen their effectiveness or cause negative side effects. Healthcare providers, especially those who treat patients with multiple medications or chronic medical conditions, should be informed about potential interactions between herbs and drugs and advise patients accordingly. To guarantee the therapeutic benefits of herbal remedies, assessing their efficacy is crucial, in addition to safety concerns. Although many herbs have been traditionally used to treat particular medical conditions, there is a wide range of scientific evidence regarding their effectiveness. While some herbs lack conclusive evidence or have conflicting study results, others have undergone rigorous clinical trials that demonstrate their effectiveness for specific indications. Herbs such as echinacea, elderberry, and zinc, for instance, have been investigated for their possible ability to lessen the duration and intensity of colds and influenza, with varying degrees of success.

Furthermore, variations in plant species, growing environments, harvesting practices, and preparation methods can all have an impact on the potency and therapeutic effects of herbal products. It is imperative to standardize herbal extracts and implement quality control measures to guarantee consistency and reproducibility of outcomes. Due to the complexity and diversity of plant constituents, uniform standards for herbal products continue to present difficulties.

Despite these obstacles, there is still a growing demand for herbal remedies due to things like a desire for more individualized healthcare, a preference for natural therapies, and dissatisfaction with conventional treatments. In many healthcare settings, integrative medicine approaches—which blend conventional treatments with evidence-based complementary therapies like herbal medicine—are becoming more popular. But both patients and medical professionals must use caution when using herbal remedies, taking into account both their possible advantages and disadvantages.

The assessment of herbal remedies as a component of a healthcare regimen must take into account both safety and efficacy concerns.

Although many herbs have been used for centuries as traditional medicines, there is conflicting scientific evidence regarding the safety and effectiveness of these remedies. To make well-informed decisions regarding the use of herbal products, healthcare professionals should possess knowledge regarding herb-drug interactions, potential adverse effects, and the quality of herbal products. In the rapidly changing field of healthcare, more investigation, standardization initiatives, and regulatory monitoring are required to guarantee the security, effectiveness, and caliber of herbal remedies.

8.2.4. Screening and Design

Not only has the number of molecular targets increased, but shorter drug discovery timelines have also been required due to advances in the fields of molecular mechanisms, cellular biology, and genomics. Pharmaceutical companies are turning to synthetic chemical libraries as a result of the development of more advanced combinatorial synthesis and computational techniques, as well as the inability of natural products to keep up with the rapidly expanding market for novel drug classes. Even though the pharmaceutical industry respects the science found in natural products and acknowledges nature's role as their chief architect, they are afraid to conduct research in this field. However, the failure of combinatorial chemistry and high throughput screening (HTS) to produce effective chemical entities is about to make a rethinking of new approaches more and more prominent.

The numbers needed to meet the HTS requirements could not be produced by the outdated, time-consuming extraction and isolation procedures. For natural product-based drug discovery (NPDD) programs, almost all organizations use fungi and actinomycetes as screening sources. Next are plants, bacteria, and therapeutic herbs. Some people use microalgae and invertebrates for screening. Seldom are insects taken advantage of. However, some people look for microbes in strange places. Many nations will be prevented from participating in the drug discovery process due to unrealistic expectations of financial investment, as initial natural products are rarely introduced as drugs unaltered.

The ability to recognize, choose, and prepare natural products intended for medical application is made possible by pharmacognosy. Such a structure can function as a lead compound (not to be confused with compounds containing the element lead). Typically, the natural product compound has some kind of biological activity, and that compound is known as the active principle. A large number of medications used today come straight from natural sources.

HTS is typically used in the process of discovering a new medication against a selected target for a specific disease. Here, a sizable chemical library is examined to determine whether or not it can alter the target. The ability of HTS to demonstrate a compound's selectivity for the selected target is another crucial feature. Finding a molecule that will only interfere with the selected target and not other, related targets is ideal. To achieve this goal, additional screening runs—a process known as cross-screening—will be conducted to determine whether the "hits" against the selected target will conflict with other related targets. Cross-screening is crucial because a compound is more likely to cause off-target toxicity in a clinic setting if it hits multiple unrelated targets.

A perfect drug candidate is not likely to come out of these early screening runs. It is more common to find that multiple compounds exhibit some level of activity. If these compounds have similar chemical properties, one or more pharmacophores may be created. Medicinal chemists will now try to enhance specific aspects of the lead compound through the application of structure-activity relationships. It is anticipated that the properties of the new molecular entities will improve throughout the several iterative screening runs required for this process, enabling the preferred compounds to move on to in vitro and in vivo testing for activity in the preferred disease model.

Although HTS is a popular approach for finding new drugs, it is not the only one. Starting with a molecule that already possesses some of the desired qualities is frequently an option. Such a molecule could be taken out of a natural product or even an existing medication that has room for improvement. Other techniques are also frequently employed, such as virtual high throughput screening, which uses computer-generated models to screen data and tries to "dock" virtual libraries to a target. Drug design is a crucial technique for finding new drugs. It involves analyzing the target's physical and biological characteristics to predict what kinds of compounds would bind to an active site. These exercises can lead to the rapid emergence of novel pharmacophores.

One or two compounds will be suggested for drug development after a lead compound series with adequate target potency, selectivity, and desirable drug-like qualities has been established. The superior of these is typically referred to as the "lead compound," and the other as the "backup". Combinatorial chemistry may have only expanded the haystack's volume, concealing the needle. In their native environments, natural substances undoubtedly exhibit biological activity. However, studying natural products requires extensive experience, especially in taxonomy, which is not something that can be acquired quickly. This knowledge cannot be retrieved in the future if it is abandoned. Outsourcing the work will be one of the solutions because NPDD will be heavily influenced by many technologically sophisticated biotech businesses.

Recent developments in combinatorial biosynthesis, microbial genomics, and screening procedures are revolutionizing the field of natural product research. Furthermore, by using dereplication processes—combinations of techniques to avoid the compounds that have already been reported—access to hyphenated techniques like Liquid Chromatography-Mass Spectrometry and Liquid Chromatography-Nuclear Magnetic Resonance has raised the prospect of significantly reducing the time and cost involved in natural product research.

To enhance the biological activity or drug-like qualities of natural compounds, combinatorial libraries can be designed with their distinct molecular diversity in mind. This can be done by partially synthesizing the parent molecule or by completely synthesizing it after computer-assisted drug design techniques have defined and refined the essential structural components needed for biological activity from libraries. Compared to earlier times, more focused objectives and effective in vitro and in vivo models are now accessible and usable. Natural product research currently employs a broad strategy that combines biological, molecular, botanical, and phytochemical methods.

The multi-constituent mainstay of bioactive extracts can be highlighted for antagonistic and synergistic investigations at the cellular and molecular levels, representing a paradigm shift from the discovery of single bioactive molecules. Of the 250,000 species of higher terrestrial plants known to exist, only 5 to 15 % are thought to have undergone systematic chemical and pharmacological research. The perceived threat of biodiversity extinction today is also very high, owing to environmental factors such as global warming. Determining the native natural resources and thoroughly researching them for use in drug discovery is therefore imperative. Moreover, both the practice of traditional medicine and the development of natural product drugs depend on a sustainable supply of medicinal plants.

The pharmaceutical industry must take advantage of the knowledge pertaining to traditional medicines. These later ones require scientific validation but may offer a cure for various diseases and disorders. Since the distinction between modern and traditional therapies is still ill-defined, evaluating the therapeutic value of herbal medicines objectively must come first to concentrate research on traditional medicines to further national interests.

Making a distinction between rational and empirical medication and accounting for the notable psychodynamic effects connected to both the active ingredients and their typical indications can facilitate the evaluation of quality. It is encouraging to see that businesses are beginning to apply traditional knowledge to both drug discovery initiatives and formulation development. Good Manufacturing Practices and Best Quality Practices are used in the formulations that these companies will be producing to guarantee standardized, safe, and effective herbs as well as completed phytomedicines that can be commercialized globally, much like Chinese medicines. For the development of natural products, the therapeutic areas of obesity, metabolic disorders, and inflammation might get more focus. At the molecular level, inflammation is thought to be the primary cause of nearly all diseases, including cancer. Obesity and metabolic disorders are examples of lifestyle diseases that are silent killers that have not received enough attention. Traditional medicine already has a wealth of knowledge regarding their treatments. Numerous plants and their secondary metabolites have already been studied in these fields, and it is time for the pharmaceutical industry to make use of this important knowledge.

8.2.5. Chemical Diversity of Natural Products

Complex molecular structures, including cyclic semi-rigid scaffolds, multiple chiral centers, more than five H-bond donors, more than ten H-bond acceptors, more than five rotatable C-C bonds, a large polar surface area, and a molecular weight above 500, are frequently found in natural products. This might result in moderate levels of bioavailability and matching dosage schedules to attain the necessary efficacy, but as has been previously proposed, there might be a latent advantage in such complex structures. There have been sporadic suggestions that this complexity may be a limitation on the amount of time and resources available to complete the chemical synthesis of libraries based on natural products.

Since biological and geographic diversity form the foundation of chemical diversity in nature, scientists travel the globe to collect samples for bioassays and drug discovery screens. Bioprospecting is the term for this search for natural products. Conversely, some medications are created using a lead compound that was first found in nature. This indicates that the lead compound can be synthesized entirely, serve as a precursor or starting point for a semi-synthetic compound, or serve as a template for a total synthetic compound with a distinct structure.

This is because secondary metabolites with extremely intricate structures make up the majority of biologically active natural product compounds. This has the benefit that they are incredibly unique compounds, but the complexity also makes it challenging to synthesize many lead compounds, and the compound must typically be extracted from its natural source, which is a time-consuming, costly, and ineffective process. Therefore, there is typically a benefit to creating simpler analogs. In the past, natural products have been the source of the majority of drugs; however, with the growing popularity of molecular approaches to drug discovery, their use has decreased. However, they are a valuable source of novel lead compounds against recently identified therapeutic targets due to their structural diversity. Utilizing natural products is now simpler than it was thanks to technological advancements in analytical methods.

It has long been known that the high chemical diversity, biochemical specificity, and other molecular properties of natural products set them apart from libraries of synthetic and combinatorial compounds and make them attractive as lead structures for drug discovery. Furthermore, compared to synthetic drugs or combinatorial libraries, natural products usually have a higher steric complexity and a larger number of chiral centers.

8.2.6. Isolation and Purification

It is necessary to separate and purify the lead compound, also known as the active principle if it is found in a mixture of other compounds derived from a natural source. The compound's structure, stability, and amount all have a significant impact on how simple it is to isolate and purify the active principle. The effective isolation and purification of penicillin and other natural products was previously impossible until new experimental techniques like freeze drying and chromatography were developed.

8.2.7. Identification of Biologically Active Material

Finding novel bioactive chemical entities from natural sources can be accomplished in two ways: either by selecting materials at random and screening them, or by applying ethnopharmacological knowledge to the process. The former method is based on the observation that only a very small portion of the biodiversity of the world has ever been investigated for biological activity; on the other hand, organisms that live in environments rich in species have a greater need for defense and competition mechanisms to survive. Therefore, the isolation of novel biological activities may result from the collection of plant, animal, and microbiological samples from rich ecosystems. The National Cancer Institute in the United States began doing antitumor agent screening in the 1960s, and this is one instance of a successful application of this strategy. During this campaign, cytostate paclitaxel (taxoid) from the Pacific yew tree *Taxus brevifolia* was identified. With its previously unidentified mechanism of action (microtubule stabilization), paclitaxel demonstrated antitumor activity and is currently licensed for clinical use in the treatment of ovarian, breast, and lung cancers as well as Kaposi sarcoma.

In addition to random selection, gathering information about the application of plants and other natural products as herbal medicines can help identify possible biological activities. It's important to keep in mind that a sizable portion of humanity still gets their only medication from plants. This means that ethnobotany—the study of how plants are used in society—and ethnopharmacology—a subfield of ethnobotany that focuses on the use of plants for medicinal purposes—may offer a wealth of information. One such example is artemisinin, an antimalarial compound derived from the sweet worm tree, *Artemisia annua* that has been used in Chinese medicine since 200 BC and is currently being used to treat the multi-resistant malarial protozoa *Plasmodium falciparum*.

8.2.8. Structure-Activity and Structure-Property Relationships of Natural Products

Natural products are characterized by their frequent occurrence as complexes or suites of structurally related analogs. It is unclear what this expressed molecular diversity means biologically, especially since some of the members of the suite (often major) don't seem to have any biological activity or function. Essentially, the question is: Why would an organism use its resources to synthesize multiple analogs of a molecule that it needs for only one purpose? The "screening hypothesis" provides a potential answer, based on the idea that biological activity is a rare quality that all molecules must have and that an organism may have a selective advantage if it can produce and maintain chemical diversity at a low cost. The necessity for an organism to produce its own chemical diversity to maximize the activity of its secondary metabolites—basically, to perform its own structure–activity relationship (SAR) optimization—may thus account for the existence of congeners within a natural product series.

8.2.9. Development of New Technologies in Pharmaceutical Discovery Research: Modern Methods of Drug Discovery

The popularity of natural products gave screening for new, physiologically active metabolites from these products a new impetus. In the field of pharmaceutical discovery research, new technologies like combinatorial chemistry, high-throughput screening, proteomics, genomics, and bioinformatics have emerged since the 1990s and are being widely integrated. The chemical diversity of natural products can be greatly exploited by these technologies. Other methods have only recently been developed and are still developing quickly. These include physicochemical ideas, computer-aided drug toxicity and metabolism prediction, protein 3D structures, NMR-based screening, molecular diversity, compound library design, and 3D QSAR in contemporary drug design.

Drug discovery technologies underwent significant advancements and diversification during that time. Activities related to NPDD are in direct competition with genomics, combinatorial chemistry, and HTS. It is anticipated that advances in lead structure discovery and drug target elucidation will lead to new methods for enhancing and expediting the combined drug discovery and development processes. Drug discovery is being revolutionized by powerful new technologies.

Effective technologies to support the acquisition and inventory of the natural product sources must be included in discovery programs when using natural products to support HTS. In this process, handling information is essential. Every step of this process will require more information handling, and computer technology can keep up with the demand.

Up to 100,000 test substances can now be evaluated weekly against multiple targets thanks to advancements in screening technologies. Only a few micrograms of the test material are needed for each assay. Natural products acquisition programs are currently designed to gather a large variety of tissue samples in small wet weight increments, in accordance with these trends. With this format, collectors can supply a large number of samples for screening, and for subsequent studies, they rely on recollection. This implies that a larger number of samples need to be tracked by discovery programs that are actively testing natural products. In an attempt to keep the costs of follow-up studies within reasonable bounds, information on the chemistry of known natural products must also be taken into account.

Recollection and dereplication are basic requirements for an information handling system. There's a commonality among these requirements. Using satellite navigation technologies, it is simple to determine the latitude and longitude location of a source organism collection and plot it on a map. Similar mappings of previous collections' locations are possible, though these data's accuracy will differ. These locations can be mapped in a geographic information system (GIS), which connects conventional text/field database records to computer-based mapped data. It would be simple for investigators to see the spatial relationships between collection points in a GIS by utilizing an extensive dataset of natural products chemical discoveries. Additionally, based on available data, expeditions for new acquisition efforts could be efficiently scheduled to target particular regions and prevent repeating previously collected data.

Using spatial data and GIS technology is one of the most potent components of a comprehensive information management system that supports programs for the acquisition of natural products. The system can go beyond what is required for a normalized data model in a relational database design thanks to GIS technology. Data with a spatial component can be added as an overlay using GIS. The addition of these diverse data does not alter the logical design or data model, which is crucial. Additionally, spatial data can be added selectively based on the need to know basis.

HTS is a sector that relies heavily on information. A growing dataset is a result of the variety of information currently in existence that must be taken into account during the discovery process, the rise in sample submissions for testing, and the development of discovery screen models. Technologies currently in use are capable of meeting the information handling needs for programs aimed at acquiring natural products. But before these technologies can be used, they must be realized well. GIS technology, for instance, is a potent instrument that is usually supplied with expanded capabilities that go beyond the general requirements for this application as stated. Again, these technologies need to be realized for the application to develop an efficient solution. The GIS capability must be delivered in a customized format that offers only those features required by the natural products investigator.

On the other hand, these information management requirements can be leveraged as a resource to direct the data collection process and raise the likelihood of success. It's not always necessary to use a random method when screening extracts from natural products. For a range of biological tests, examples of structure/activity relationships are starting to appear. Publicly available data on the chemistry of natural products and associated biological activity can direct a collection effort to focus on, but avoid duplicating, collections from known-property organism groups. Modern drug discovery programs need sophisticated information handling capabilities.

In addition to new approaches like HPLC and capillary electrophoresis for separation, proteomic diagnostics, target discovery, and validation, a brief discussion is given to the application of mass spectrometry (MS) and genomics-derived sequence databases for protein characterization.

As a "theoretical, computer-based science dedicated to the extrapolation of biological knowledge from biological information," bioinformatics is covered next. Today, the primary focus of bioinformatics is the screening and evaluation of potential drug targets, particularly those originating from genomic applications. Numerous sequences are produced by genomics, but to find the regions of identity and/or similarity that may be of therapeutic interest, those genetic sequences must be analyzed. A renewed interest in natural products in drug discovery has resulted from unmet expectations from current lead-generation strategies combined with recent technological advancements that help to address these issues. The latter ought to be employed as one of the drug discovery strategies based on genomics.

Nevertheless, natural products continue to be an important source of starting materials for drug discovery, even in the face of combinatorial chemistry's ascent to prominence in the lead discovery process. Engaging in natural product-based drug discovery (NPDD) puts high-throughput screening (HTS), combinatorial chemistry, and genomics in direct competition. Biological resource centers and newly emerging biotech ventures based on NPDD are anticipated to play a major role in this field, while genomics and CBD have recently had a significant impact on NPDD.

The chemical diversity of natural products can be greatly exploited by these technologies. It is stated right away that none of these techniques are a panacea that will end the drug discovery cycle in a matter of years; rather, they are complementary instruments with various advantages and disadvantages that need to be used sparingly and in concert.

8.2.9.1. Combinatorial Chemistry

While natural products have a much higher hit-rate in high throughput screening with high chemical diversity, combinatorial chemistry produces larger libraries, but the compounds within are relatively simple planar molecules. Furthermore, the pharmaceutical industry's interest has been revived due to advancements in isolation, purification, and characterization protocols that have accelerated the output of natural product research.

From its beginnings as a haphazard approach to creating molecular diversity, combinatorial chemistry has developed into a potent design tool for creating and refining therapeutic candidates. There is an urgent need for technologies that can shorten the time it takes for new products to reach market due to the pressure to find, optimize, develop, and commercialize novel drugs more quickly and affordably. The molecular diversity of materials, both natural and artificial, offers a useful source of compounds for finding and refining novel therapeutic candidates. Producing libraries of small molecules to screen for novel bioactivities is now feasible thanks to the rapidly developing field of combinatorial chemistry. Pharmaceutical companies can now find new drug candidates more quickly, save a significant amount of money on preclinical development costs, and ultimately change their basic approach to drug discovery thanks to this potent new technology.

Combinatorial chemistry and molecular diversity in drug discovery, which brings together the work of the foremost experts in the fields of molecular diversity and combinatorial chemistry, emphasizes the key ideas and problems associated with using combinatorial chemistry to build chemical libraries.

As was already indicated, combinatorial chemistry played a significant role in making it possible to efficiently generate large screening libraries to meet the demands of high-throughput screening. After twenty years of combinatorial chemistry, it has been noted that no progress has been made in terms of lead or drug candidates, despite the increased efficiency in chemical synthesis. This has prompted comparisons between the chemical properties of combinatorial chemistry products and those of currently available medications and/or natural products. The distinction between combinatorial chemistry libraries and natural products is frequently explained by the chemo-informatics notion of chemical diversity, which is defined as the distribution of compounds in the chemical space according to their physicochemical properties. In contrast to existing drugs and especially natural products, which show much greater chemical diversity and distribute more evenly throughout the chemical space, synthetic compounds from combinatorial libraries appear to cover only a small and relatively uniform chemical space. The number of chiral centers (much higher in natural compounds), structure rigidity (higher in natural compounds), and number of aromatic moieties (higher in combinatorial chemistry libraries) are the most notable distinctions between natural products and compounds in combinatorial chemistry libraries. The nature of heteroatoms (O and N enriched in natural products, and S and halogen atoms more frequently present in synthetic compounds) and degree of non-aromatic unsaturation (higher in natural products) are two other chemical distinctions between these two groups. Given that chirality and structural rigidity are two well-established aspects of medicinal chemistry that are known to improve the specificity and therapeutic efficacy of a compound, it has been proposed that natural products make good lead molecules when compared to today's combinatorial chemical libraries.

8.2.9.2. High-Throughput Screening

A common technique for finding hits in scientific experiments, High-Throughput Screening (HTS) is particularly useful in drug discovery and has applications in biology and chemistry. HTS enables a researcher to quickly perform millions of biochemical, genetic, or pharmacological tests using robotics, data processing and control software, liquid handling equipment, and sensitive detectors. By using this method, active substances, antibodies, or genes that alter a specific biomolecular pathway can be quickly identified. The outcomes of these studies serve as a basis for developing new drugs and for comprehending the function or interplay of specific biochemical processes in biology.

To facilitate High Throughput Screening (HTS) with natural products, discovery programs need to incorporate efficient technologies that facilitate the procurement and cataloging of the sources of natural products. In this process, handling information is essential. Every step of this process will require more information handling, and computer technology can keep up with the demand.

Fundamentally, HTS employs a brute-force strategy to gather a significant volume of experimental data—typically observations regarding the responses of a biological entity to exposure to diverse chemical compounds—in a comparatively short amount of time. This larger experiment, called a screen, has a single objective, which is typically testing a scientific hypothesis.

All of this data can then be applied to this screen. A screening facility usually contains a library of stock plates, each of which may have been produced in-house by the lab or acquired from a commercial source. The contents of the library are meticulously cataloged. Separate assay plates are made as needed and are used in experiments instead of these stock plates directly. By pipetting a small amount of liquid—typically measured in nanoliters—from the wells of a stock plate into the corresponding wells of a completely empty plate, an assay plate is essentially a duplicate of a stock plate.

Automation plays a significant role in the utility of HTS. During the course of a single assay plate, a specialized robot is frequently in charge of most of the procedure, from creation to final analysis. An HTS robot can typically prepare and analyze multiple plates at once, which expedites the process of gathering data even more. There are currently HTS robots that can test up to 100,000 compounds in a single day.

HTS is a relatively new invention that has recently been made possible by advancements in high-speed computer technology and robotics. However, maintaining an HTS operation still requires a highly specialized and costly screening lab, so rather than setting up an HTS facility from scratch, small-to-medium sized research institutions frequently use the services of an existing one.

The people interested in a natural product simply want to know what it is, where it came from, whether it is novel, and how to obtain more when it registers as a confirmed "hit" in a discovery screen. Thus, there are two types of general information handling system requirements: dereplication and recollection.

Any program for acquiring natural products must be based on recollection; additional information about the source organism must be obtainable for subsequent research. For discovery screens, dereplication against the expanding list of recognized chemical compounds is becoming more and more crucial. To compare and dereplicate against known chemical compounds, a chemical substructure-based database search can be carried out based on the initial chemical characterization of an active fraction or fractions. When a laboratory chemist can produce a list of potential chemical structures to compare with an extract containing unidentified compounds, they have a significant advantage. Then, a chemist can assess the extract's potential for containing recognized compounds with ease and decide whether or not to pursue it further as a source of novel bioactive compounds. This quick procedure can boost a program's effectiveness and reduce the cost of subsequent isolation and structural elucidation studies.

8.2.9.3. Bioinformatics, Proteomics and Genomics

Proteomics encompasses methods for identifying particular proteins and characterizing their entire structure and functional role, as well as technologies for protein mapping, which involves separating, distinguishing, and quantifying the proteins present in individual samples. Two-dimensional polyacrylamide gel electrophoresis (2D-PAGE), the predominant protein mapping technology currently in use, can resolve up to 2000 proteins on a single gel, which is a significant improvement over previous separation techniques but still short of the 6000 proteins expressed by typical tissues.

Recent advances in information technology, instrumentation, and molecular biology have made it possible to screen compounds at throughputs that were unthinkable just a few years ago. The utilization of robotics for sample handling and assay execution, coupled with the availability of molecular targets and the capacity to engineer them into basic reporter systems like yeasts, render random screening of chemical diversity an appealing method for uncovering novel activity. The ability to gain a molecular understanding of physiological processes is made possible by molecular cloning techniques. At present, more than 250 gene products associated with major neurotransmitters are identified, and hundreds of distinct ion channel subtypes have also undergone genetic characterization. The understanding of intracellular signaling pathways has also increased, potentially leading to the discovery of numerous new drug targets.

Lead discovery is a bigger bottleneck for these companies, which continue to be "target rich" but "lead poor" due to the increasingly complex and capital-intensive drug discovery process. Under such circumstances, the process of finding new drugs is becoming more industrialized. While there is much hope for high throughput screening (HTS) and combinatorial chemical synthesis, most companies' investments in these technologies have not yielded the expected results in terms of new lead discovery.

Drug discovery is being revolutionized by powerful new technologies such as combinatorial chemistry and HTS. However, natural products continue to offer unparalleled structural variety, particularly as novel environmental niches are investigated. By manipulating the proteins that generate them, natural products can also be used to investigate biological pathways.

The pharmaceutical industry has benefited greatly from the human genome by having a wealth of new drug discovery avenues to choose from. Nevertheless, the anticipated deluge of novel chemical entities has not materialized. However, the sequencing of many pathogen genomes as well as the human genome has created a previously unheard-of chance to identify novel targets for pharmaceuticals. Chemogenomics is a new technology that uses active compounds as probes to characterize proteome functions, allowing for the initial discovery of targets. The best probes for this kind of research are natural products. A potent chemogenomic descriptor for describing small molecules and pharmacologically significant proteins is the binding affinity fingerprint.

8.3. Natural Drugs Available in Market: Anti-Inflammatory

More and more diseases are posing a threat to the general public worldwide in the modern era. As a result, while the percentage of diseases varies globally, diseases themselves are not new; rather, the detection of new diseases is a result of global warming. By 2000 AD, the WHO had vowed to provide "Health for all," believing that prevention is always preferable to treatment.

8.3.1. Himalaya Boswellia

Boswellia is the source of the pure herb extract used to create Himalaya Herbals. Boswellic acid was the bioactive molecule found in Shallaki's gum resin, also known as *Boswellia serrata*. The lead molecule pyrazoline is found in boswellic acid. It functions by supplying healthy joints and muscles, reducing inflammation, and bolstering the body's natural immune response. Because it takes gentle care of the joints, Boswellia is a safe and natural herb for joint health. Boswellia offers numerous health advantages, including immune-modulating properties and the promotion of healthy cholesterol and triglyceride levels. In Ayurveda, Boswellia is widely used to treat arthritis and promote general well-being.

8.3.2. Ginger

Ginger has been praised by herbal medicine for its immune-boosting properties for many years. Ginger is thought to be used on a daily basis because of its significant warming effect on the body. Due to its breakdown in the body, it can aid in clearing the body of toxins that have accumulated. Our body's sewage system, the lymphatic system, is also known to be cleaned by it. Ginger keeps toxins from building up and greatly protects against bacterial, fungal, and viral infections. Ginger, a medicinal plant, has numerous health advantages as well. It is specifically utilized as a natural pain reliever and nausea reducer due to its anti-inflammatory qualities and ability to prevent diabetes.

8.3.3. Licorice Root

Research on the use of licorice in the treatment and prevention of illnesses like hepatitis C, HIV, and influenza is growing in visibility. According to a study, the triterpenoid content of licorice root supports its antiviral properties. It mentions the immune-stimulating, free radical-scavenging, and antioxidant properties of licorice. Pain relief is one of the benefits of licorice root.

- **Olive Leaf:** The olive leaf has antiviral properties, giving it the ability to treat the common cold and dangerous viruses.
- **Oregano:** The advantages of oregano

oil are becoming more widely recognized. It can be used in daily life, has no negative health effects, and is superior to certain antibiotics. The bioactive compounds that have been identified, investigated, and shown to have potent qualities and applications are thymol and carvacrol. They affect viral infections, allergies, tumors, parasites, and inflammation brought on by disease (Figure 8.1).

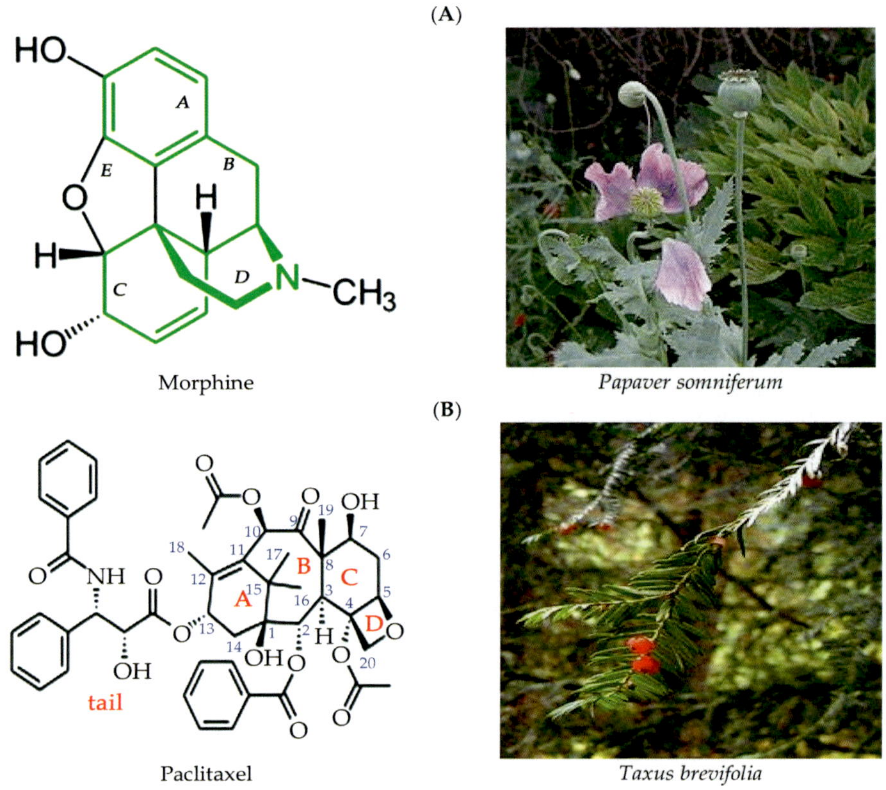

Figure 8.1. *Two examples of successful stories of plant natural products that are being used in hospitals and clinics for disease treatment. (A) Morphine is isolated from Papaver somniferum also called opium poppy (B) Paclitaxel is isolated from Taxus brevifolia also called pacific yew.*

Source: *Thomford NE, Senthebane DA, Rowe A, Munro D, Seele P, Maroyi A, Dzobo K. Natural products for drug discovery in the 21st century: Innovations for novel drug discovery. International Journal of Molecular Sciences. 2018; 19(6):1578. https://doi.org/10.3390/ijms19061578.*

8.3.4. Novel Drug Targets and Natural Product Inhibitors

In their pursuit of new drugs, Novartis has not wavered in their commitment to the development of natural products. This dedication has produced valuable clinical compounds as well as new targets and pathways in the disease process. A novel compound, NVP-LBM-415, a derivative of the natural product actinonin, was found by screening samples of natural products against this target. Its Ki was 0.3 nM. The substance has good tissue distribution, strong antibacterial activity, and oral bioavailability. Phase I research is currently underway.

In inflammatory environments, vascular cell adhesion molecule-1 (VCAM-1) is essential for controlling leukocyte migration and cell-to-cell interactions. Proteins with a signal peptide sequence, such as VCAM-1, are synthesized on the ribosome. The signal recognition particle (SRP) identifies this signal peptide sequence for translocation. Novartis has discovered a fungal metabolite called HUN-7293 that specifically inhibits the translocation of VCAM-1 to the luminal side of the endoplasmic reticulum. This is achieved by blocking the connection between the VCAM-1 signal peptide and the highly conserved protein-conducting Sec61β complex. It is possible to block translocation dependently on signal peptides without affecting the translocation of other proteins, which opens up new therapeutic options.

Despite the fact that certain natural products cannot be turned into pharmaceuticals, they are important tools for validating pathways and are the main candidates for compounds that can disrupt protein-protein interactions. For instance, the WNT pathway is crucial for cell survival, proliferation, and differentiation; mutations in the pathway's protein, B-catenin, are linked to colon cancer. T cell factor (Tcf) transcription factors interact with B-catenin. The natural product toxoflavin was discovered at Novartis during a screen for inhibitors of this protein-protein interaction. Treating *Xenopus* sp. with B-catenin mRNA resulted in an aberrant body type. Toxoflavin reversed this transformation.

Radiation therapy and conventional chemotherapy are ineffective against hypoxic tumor cells. Elevated patient mortality is positively correlated with hypoxia inducible factor-1 (HIF-1) levels. Chetomin, a natural product inhibitor, was discovered through screening for inhibitors of the protein–protein interaction of HIF-1 with the CH1 domain of p300 at Harvard Medical School and Dana-Farber Cancer Institute. This cancer target was validated by systemic administration of chetomin, which inhibited hypoxia-inducible transcription within tumors and inhibited tumor growth.

Because they modify the structure of the chromatin, histones are essential for the expression of genes. Acetylation controls the conformation of histones. Many cancers are linked to histone deacetylase dysregulation. Histone deacetylase inhibition causes hyperacetylation and increased transcription of growth-inhibiting genes. A number of newly discovered natural products and their derivatives are undergoing preclinical and clinical development.

Many times, the biological characteristics of natural product compounds lead to the discovery of novel biological processes. A metabolite of the ascomycete *Isaria sinclairii*, myriocin has strong anti-proliferative and immunosuppressive properties. The serious GI side effects of myriocin limited its usefulness. An analog known as FTY720 was created, which eliminated the GI toxicity while retaining the immunosuppressive and serine-palmitoyl-transferase activity. The mode of action was novel in that it involved the sequestration of lymphocytes from the bloodstream into the lymphatics. Novartis is developing FTY720, which has shown promise in Phase II clinical trials as the first oral treatment for multiple sclerosis.

Natural products have been very important in the drug-discovery process. Compounds derived from natural products have been the source of numerous medications for the treatment of human disease over the past 75 years. the most recent advancements in natural product compounds and enabling technologies in the treatment of cancer, antivirals, antibiotics, and immunosuppressive drugs. These natural remedies are being developed to treat resistant viruses and bacteria, enhance cancer therapy, and extend immunosuppressive therapy to illnesses like multiple sclerosis.

In addition to being directly used as medications or drug templates, natural product compounds frequently result in the discovery of novel biology that improves our understanding of the targets and pathways involved in the pathophysiology of disease. These anticancer targets and pathways have been validated by compounds that interact with novel targets, such as protein–protein complexes, B-catenin in the WNT pathway, and HIF-1/p300. These compounds open up new avenues for the identification and exploitation of drug targets in these pathways.

To ensure the success of natural product drug discovery going forward, novel and creative methods are needed. Using genomics advancements, looking for natural product compounds in areas that haven't been mined effectively before, and utilizing new screening technologies are a few of these novel approaches (Table 8.1).

Table 8.1. Marketed Drugs of Marine Origin Along With Their Trade Name, Source of Origin, Mechanism of Action, and Disease Treatment Indications

Name (Drug Bank ID)	Brand Name (Company)	Source Organism	Type (MW)	Mechanism of Action	Treatment Indications, Approving Agency (Year)
Spongonucleosides					
Cytarabine, ara-C (DB00987)	CYTOSAR-U® (Pfizer, New York City, NY, USA) and DEPOCYT® (Pacira Pharma, San Diego, CA, USA; Bedford Lab, Seattle, WA, USA, Enzon Pharmaceuticals, Piscataway, NJ, USA)	*Cryptotethia crypta* (sponge)	Small molecule (243.22 Da)	Synthetic spongonucleoside analog, arrests cells in S phase by inhibiting DNA synthesis	Remission induction in acute nonlymphocytic leukemia, FDA (1969) Lymphomatous meningitis, FDA (1999)
Vidarabine, ara-A (DB00194)	VIRA-A® (King Pharmaceuticals, Bristol, FL, USA)	*Cryptotethia crypta* (sponge)	Small molecule (267.24 Da)	Synthetic spongonucleoside analog, stops the replication of herpes viral DNA	Acute keratoconjunctivitis and recurrent superficial keratitis caused by HSV-1 and HSV-2, FDA (1976)
Fludarabine, F-ara-A (DB01073)	FLUDARA® (Sandoz, Basel, Switzerland) and OFORTA® (Sanofi-Aventis, Paris, France)	*Cryptotethia crypta* (sponge)	Small molecule (285.23 Da)	Synthetic spongonucleoside analog, inhibits DNA synthesis by inhibiting DNA polymerase alpha, ribonucleotide reductase, and DNA primase	B-cell CLL, FDA (1991)

Nelarabine (DB01280)	ARRANON® (GSK, Brentford, UK) ATRIANCE® (Novartis, Basel, Switzerland)	*Cryptotethia crypta* (sponge)	Small molecule (297.27 Da)	Synthetic spongonucleoside analog, is metabolized into ara-GTP, competes with dGTP, and is incorporated into the DNA, inhibiting DNA elongation	T-cell acute lymphoblastic leukemia and T cell lymphoblastic lymphoma, FDA (2005)
Histochrome	Pacific-Ocean Institute of Bioorganic Chemistry, Vladivostok, Russia	*Scaphechinus mirabilis* (sea urchin)	Small molecule (220 Da)	The drug prevents DNA damage and regulates apoptosis under oxidative stress condition	Used to treat degenerative diseases of the retina and cornea, macular degeneration, etc., myocardial ischemia/reperfusion injury etc., Russia (1999)
Microtubule Inhibitors					
Eribulin mesylate (DB08871)	HALAVEN® (Eisai, Bunkyo, Japan)	*Halichondria okadai* (sponge)	Small molecule, orphan (826.00 Da)	Polyether macrolide, arrests cells in G2/M phase by inhibiting microtubule growth after direct interaction	Metastatic breast cancer, FDA (2010), unresectable or metastatic liposarcoma, FDA (2016)
DNA Alkylating Agent					
Trabectedin, ET-743 (DB05109)	YONDELIS® (PharmaMar SA, Madrid, Spain)	*Ecteinascidia turbinata* (tunicate)	Small molecule, orphan (761.80 Da)	DNA alkylating agent, forms adducts with DNA guanine residue in the minor groove, bends the DNA helix toward the major groove, and disrupts the association of DNA binding proteins	Soft-tissue sarcoma and relapsed platinum-sensitive ovarian cancer, EMA (2007), unresectable or metastatic liposarcoma or leiomyosarcoma, FDA (2015)
Lurbinectedin (DB12674)	ZEPZELCA™ (PharmaMar SA, Madrid, Spain)	*Ecteinascidia turbinata* (tunicate)	Small molecule, orphan (784.90 Da)	DNA alkylating agent, forms adducts with DNA guanine residue in the minor groove, bends the DNA helix toward the major groove, and disrupts the association of DNA binding proteins	Metastatic SCLC, FDA (2020)

Antibody-Drug Conjugates					
Brentuximab vedotin (DB08870)	ADCERTIS® (Seattle Genetics, Bothell, Wahington, WA, USA)	*Dolabella auricularia* (mollusk)	Biotech (~153 kDa)	The antibody component (IgG1) targets CD30 and MMAE disrupts the microtubules after internalization	Hodgkin lymphoma and systemic anaplastic large-cell lymphoma, FDA (2011)
Polatuzumab vedotin (DB12240)	POLIVY™ (Genentech, San Francisco, CA, USA)	*Dolabella auricularia* (mollusk)	Biotech (~150 kDa)	The antibody component targets CD79b and MMAE disrupts the microtubules after internalization	Relapsed or refractory diffuse large B-cell lymphoma, FDA (2019)
Enfortumab vedotin (DB13007)	Padcev® (Astellas Pharma US Inc., Northbrook, IL, USA)	*Dolabella auricularia* (mollusk)	Biotech (~153 kDa)	The antibody component (IgG1) targets nectin-4 and MMAE disrupts the microtubules after internalization	Treatment of patients with advanced, treatment-resistant urothelial cancer, FDA (2019)
Belantamab mafodotin (DB15719)	Blenrep® (GlaxoSmithKline, Brentford, UK)	*Dolabella auricularia* (mollusk)	Biotech (~153 kDa)	The antibody component (IgG1) targets BCMA (B-cell maturation antigen) and MMAF disrupts the microtubules after internalization	Treatment of adult patients with relapsed or refractory multiple myeloma who have received at least 4 prior therapies, including and anti-CD38 monoclonal antibody, a proteasome inhibitor, and an immunomodulatory agent, FDA (2020)
Peptides or Proteins Used as Drugs or in Drug Preparations					
Plitidepsin (DB04977)	APLIDIN® (PharmaMar SA, Madrid, Spain)	*Aplidium albicans* (sea squirt)	Small molecule, orphan ⍰ (1110.30 Da)	Binds to the gene product of eEF1A2, thus inhibiting cancer cell viability	Tumors in pancreatic, stomach, bladder, and prostate cancers, TGA (2018)
Ziconotide (DB06283)	PRIALT® (Azur Pharma, Dublin, Ireland)	*Conus magus* (marine snail)	Small molecule (2639.20 Da)	Blocks excitatory neurotransmitter release by inhibiting the N-type calcium channels of primary nociceptive afferent nerves and relieves pain	Severe chronic pain, FDA (2004) and EMA (2005)

Protamine sulfate (DB09141)	PROSULF® (CP Pharm, Hong Kong, China; Wockhardt Mumbai, India; etc.) PROTAM® (Eipico, Ramadan City, Egypt)	Salmon sperm heads	Biotech (~4.3 kDa)	Reversal of the anticoagulant effect of heparin by forming an inactive complex with heparin	Heparin overdose, FDA (1939) [**22**,**23**]
Keyhole limpet hemocyanin (DB05299)	IMMUCOTHEL® VACMUNE® (Biosyn Corporation, Carlsbad, CA, USA)	Keyhole limpet (marine mollusk)	Biotech (350 to 390 kDa)	An immunomodulator	IMMUCOTHEL® for bladder cancer, , VACMUNE® as protein carrier for vaccine development , the Netherlands (1997), Austria and South Korea (2001), Argentina (2004/2005)
Fish Oil and its Components Used as Drugs					
Omega-3-acid ethyl esters (DB09539)	LOVAZA® (GSK, Brentford, UK), OMACOR® (GSK, Brentford, UK), and OMTRYG® (Trygg Pharma, Oslo, Norway)	Fish	Small molecule (330.51 to 356.55 Da)	Reduces triglyceride synthesis by inhibiting 1,2-diacylglycerol acyltransferase	Reduce triglyceride (TG) levels, FDA (2004) [**27**,**28**,**29**]
Icosapent ethyl (DB00159)	VASCEPA® (Amarin Pharma, Dublin, Ireland)	Fish	Small molecule (330.51 Da)	Reduces triglyceride synthesis by inhibiting 1,2-diacylglycerol acyltransferase	Reduces the risk of myocardial infarction, stroke, coronary revascularization, and unstable angina, FDA (2012)
Omega-3-carboxylic acids (DB09568)	EPANOVA® (AstraZeneca Pharmaceuticals, Landon, UK)	Fish	Small molecule (302.45 to 328.49 Da)	Reduces triglyceride synthesis by inhibiting 1,2-diacylglycerol acyltransferase	Reduce triglyceride (TG) levels, FDA (2014)
Fish oil triglycerides (DB13961)	OMEGAVEN® (Fresenius Kabi, Bad Homburg, Germany)	Fish	Small molecule (mixture of fatty acids, 700 to 1000 Da each)	Source of calories and essential fatty acids	PNAC, FDA (2018)

Source: *Haque N, Parveen S, Tang T, Wei J, Huang Z. Marine natural products in clinical use. Marine Drugs. 2022; 20(8):528. https://doi.org/10.3390/md20080528.*

8.4. Future Directions for Natural Product Drug Discovery

In the 21st century, biological diversity and contemporary genomics will likely be the two main subjects driving bioscience, and biodiversity is thought to be becoming more and more significant in this domain. Natural products do indeed contain a wealth of biodiversity, the study of which necessitates a great deal of in-depth experience, especially in taxonomy, which takes time to acquire. To treat clinical conditions that are not treatable with conventional therapies, pharmaceutical and biotechnology companies need to quickly adjust to the urgent need for new medications and implement innovative approaches. Therefore, investigating the structure-activity relationships of active ingredients that occur naturally may provide a way around such medical obstacles. On the other hand, industries need to develop methods, like computational chemistry, to make more sustainable use of their natural resources if they hope to benefit from and contribute to the drug discovery process. It is imperative for industries to acknowledge that while natural products serve crucial biological purposes and are valuable components of ecosystems, their economic worth may be diminished until their primary purpose is identified and validated. Pharmaceutical companies need to be ready to actively and financially support drug discovery torecognize the significant advantages and usefulness of this process. For the production of different precious lead components, ranging from simple chemical structures to extremely complex structures, natural products are thought to be especially valuable. When comparing secondary metabolites to their natural counterparts, natural metabolites consistently exhibit greater biochemical and pharmacological activities. The isolation, purification, screening, and discovery of novel drug candidates are the main goals of the current natural resource-based drug discovery processes. Potential lead compounds must be produced on a large-scale using biotechnology or extraction techniques to advance and become clinically viable.

Natural products can mimic unique metabolites of biological functionality, such as hormones and naturally occurring ligands, and also possess great structural diversity, which is essential for the drug discovery process in the highly competitive and revolutionized field of modern pharmaceutical research. To remain competitive with other cutting-edge drug discovery methods and to pique the interest of the pharmaceutical industry, natural product research needs to continuously improve the effectiveness of screening (computational or not), isolation, robotic separation, and purification. To identify compounds of interest and advance them into clinically applicable therapies, additional research is needed in the areas of drug stability and formulation, efficacy, pharmacokinetics, and metabolic engineering. Their survival is also being threatened by the rising demand for medicinal plants in herbal and traditional medicine. It is essential to grow medicinal plants under controlled, scientific conditions to produce the desired, high-quality medicinal plants and to enhance biodiversity worldwide.

Furthermore, the biological ecosystem is significantly impacted by the production process' toxic waste, which is especially detrimental to plants and aquatic life in streams. Toxic waste that contains both unpleasant, odor-producing chemicals and toxic elements needs to be treated and separated separately to protect the environment. By preserving the natural flora, we can contribute to the sustainability of ecosystems and safeguard any natural resource that might be utilized in the search for novel biological and medicinal metabolites.

8.4.1. Automating Natural Product Drug Discovery

Automation is typically linked to negative emotions; many people associate it with job loss and erroneous outcomes, such as robots taking over the world. Automation has, however, been effectively applied to expedite the drug discovery process. Indeed, high-throughput assays are already widely employed in the drug discovery process by pharmaceutical companies. Computers and a variety of software programs help with both the synthesis and the design of the majority of synthetic compounds. Software used in target and hit finding during drug design includes ADAM and EVE. In addition to lowering material consumption during compound design, synthesis, and biological testing, new software and hardware are being developed. For instance, laboratories and pharmaceutical companies are designing integrated microfluidics systems that can handle liquids and heat, which is required for purification and analyzes during synthesis. These systems are intended for compound synthesis and screening. This has made it possible to test multiple theories in a matter of days. With the help of artificial intelligence (AI) and "organ-on-chip" technologies, even more sophisticated technologies are now fully integrated into the drug discovery process, supporting scientists in the design of new drugs and process optimization. With the help of these technologies, drug design and optimization mistakes and biases have been reduced, the quantity of candidate compounds required for testing has decreased, testing times for candidate compounds have been shortened to a few days, and disease biology has been recapitulated more accurately than with in vitro assays. Innovation and technical advancements have frequently given rise to unmet expectations and false hopes. Drug discovery automation and innovation need to be quick, but they also need to be long-lasting. A number of things are taken into account when designing a compound or molecule. These consist of the products' ultimate biological activity as well as the properties of ADMET (absorption, distribution, metabolism, excretion, and toxicity). As a result, there are several aspects to the drug discovery process optimization. To obtain the best compound activity and properties, a balance must ultimately be struck. Automation will make it possible for scientists to choose the best compound design with the desired ADMET properties and pertinent biological activity. Over the past few years, a number of concepts have been developed to help with compound design and increasing compound collections with new chemical structures and constituents. Examples of these concepts are the biology-oriented synthesis (BIOS) and the diversity-oriented synthesis (DOS). An even more sophisticated idea is function-oriented synthesis, which aims to replicate a promising compound's function to produce basic scaffolds and simplify and ease their synthesis.

Numerous deep learning-based automated compound generators have been developed, enabling automated analysis of the compounds produced to produce even better designs of compounds with desired properties and biological activity. Deep learning models are helpful in predicting the ADMET characteristics of new candidate drugs, even though their primary applications are in drug-target interaction prediction and the synthesis of new molecules. During the drug discovery process, a number of deep learning models have also been utilized to forecast the binding affinity for candidate compounds. Using automated computer-assisted de novo design, a number of compounds based on the imidazopyridine scaffold have been synthesized, leading to the discovery of numerous ligands for antagonists of G protein-coupled receptors. To design a compound library and choose building blocks, a virtual library enumeration in parallel to target panel prediction is also an option. Scientists were able to identify ligands with distinct binding profiles by combining microfluidics-assisted synthesis with computational activity prediction. Therefore, bioactivity-focused compound libraries can be produced quickly and effectively using computer-aided target prediction and microfluidics synthesis.

The availability and utilization of building blocks as well as chemical reactions that can produce a variety of byproducts are crucial components of compound synthesis automation. In the end, the development of novel machines to synthesis complex structures that recapitulate the biosynthesis of most natural compounds was facilitated by the use of small volumes of the starting compounds and compact synthesis combined with in-line purification and analyzes. Crucially, the construction of various microfluidic devices with multiple complex and specialized algorithms to track product synthesis is made possible by 3D printing. Since the majority of microfluidics systems are specially designed for a particular purpose, 3D printing is crucial for microfluidics platforms. Using remote control, some of the most recent automated robotic synthesis techniques increase efficiency. Certain automated methods for compound synthesis are highly adaptable, requiring a minimal number of building blocks to produce an extensive array of secondary products. Compounds can be synthesized continuously rather than in batches thanks to microfluidics-based synthesis. It is now possible to simulate the oxidation of drugs by cytochrome P450, which means that in the future, on-chip chemotransformations of compounds may take the place of in vitro metabolite identification. Automation of drug discovery is being revolutionized by the synthesis of compounds using microfluidics in conjunction with in-process analysis and purification. Microfluidics not only permits the use of minimal quantities of compounds and reagents, but also, obviously, prevents human exposure to hazardous solutions and chemicals. Because the majority of animal models do a very poor job of predicting how humans will react to medications and biological tests, microfluidic systems that incorporate organoid-based techniques can help recapitulate human and species-specific functions. As a result, physiologically relevant environments can be created inside of the microfluidic devices, and these environments have the potential to stabilize over time. A number of systems that replicate human tumors and their microenvironments have been developed, utilizing either 3D cancer models or cancer cells. For continuous flow systems like compound synthesis through microfluidics, there are a number of limitations. Because certain reagents and solutions used in compound synthesis are incompatible with the microfluidic systems, there is a risk of fluidic surface instability during the synthesis and eventual deposition of reactive reagents and by-products. Another significant issue with the microfluidic system is channel clogging.

A number of integrated platforms for microfluidics-assisted synthesis and testing are currently accessible. These platforms combine the selection of reagents and compounds and can adjust according to the materials that are available for the compounds' subsequent steps in synthesis and testing. Finding the best and most creative path to compound synthesis is made easier by a number of computational tools and networks that have been developed for automated compound synthesis and contain millions of reactions and pathways. To have a sustainable drug discovery process, artificial intelligence must be used in drug design. When machines generate hypotheses, it can lead to the simultaneous design of compounds based on multiple criteria. These standards may include synthesizability, side effects, and biological activity. Additionally, machine-guided hypothesis generation or compound structure generation is far faster and capable of producing multiple designs simultaneously. Thus, artificial intelligence is an enabling technology that helps scientists recognize patterns and can be enhanced to do so.

8.4.2. Computer-Aided Drug Design from Natural Products

Although many of the world's health problems can be resolved by synthetic compounds with structures modeled after natural products, many of the novel synthetic compounds would have been rejected as unsuitable for use in drug development. The "rule of three" and "rule of five" criteria, which are frequently applied when making decisions about drug leads, are overly rigid, and some of the new designs would not have succeeded. In actuality, a large number of the guidelines utilized in the process of designing drugs exhibit human bias, which limits their applicability and efficacy, particularly with regard to natural products. Using computer-aided designs, numerous therapeutic synthetic compounds, including several anticancer agents, have been developed. For example, complex natural products were made simpler using the Scaffold Hunter software to create virtual fragments of small, chemically appealing molecules. Such computational software must preserve the biological activity of the mother compound in the simple molecules it visualizes. In fact, the pyruvate kinase activators and inhibitors have previously been found using this technique. Simple molecules derived from natural products might, nevertheless, also show less activity than the parent compound. With notable success, the biological activities of simple structures or chemical structures derived from the mother compound have been predicted using the PASS software. A number of marine alkaloids' anti-tumor properties have been predicted by the PASS software.

In fact, it was also correctly predicted that a number of St. John's wort constituents would have cytochrome P450 modulating properties. Numerous databases, web servers, and computational software programs have been created with the ability to forecast compound-target associations. The majority of these softwares, if not all of them, infer target and typical ligand-receptor docking based on how a novel compound resembles well-known medications. If the new compound does not resemble any known drug, the SPIDER software can predict the new compound's target by comparing computed features between natural products and the new compound. Identifying G-protein coupled receptor ligands was one of the SPIDER software's achievements. Drug development will continue to be impacted by the application of computational target prediction and drug design in the near future. Predictions can only be made for targets or proteins that have already been studied. In the process of discovering new natural products, computer-based quantitative structure activity approaches can be used to forecast potential derivatives that may enhance activity as well as to elucidate the molecular basis of the products' therapeutic values. The benefit of computer-aided drug design is that it directs lead compound optimization, helping to determine whether to improve affinity or pharmacodynamic and pharmacokinetic characteristics.

Early in the drug discovery process, new systems are being developed to identify the toxicity of lead compounds or candidates. Throughout the drug discovery process, strategies utilizing in silico methods can be employed to identify drug toxicity early on. When paired with in vitro and in vivo biological testing, these methods can significantly reduce the time and expense associated with drug discovery while also enhancing safety assessment. The goal of quantitative structure–activity relationship models is to comprehend the connection between a compound's toxicity and structure. Properties of the drug's metabolism, including adsorption, distribution, metabolism, and excretion, must be assessed to comprehend the possibility of drug accumulation. Environmental toxicity must be taken into account, which exacerbates the problem of candidate compound toxicity. Thus, the possibility of a drug's presence in the environment needs to be considered during the drug discovery process. Other animals may be poisoned by these lead compounds or candidate compounds.

With the development of sophisticated technologies, researchers have been able to determine the extent of tumor heterogeneity and the variations in patient responses to therapy. Nevertheless, the "one drug-one target" approach is the foundation of drug discovery. Combination therapy is undoubtedly the gold standard in today's medical field. As a result, combinatorial drug design is required, in which two or more medications work together to either target the same pathway or produce a cure. Kinase inhibitors and other targeted therapies can be used in conjunction with conventional chemotherapeutic agents. Currently being developed are a few methods for computer-based screening for combinatorial drug design and therapy.

8.4.3. Natural Products and Precision Medicine

Over the last few years, genomics has been used to inform drug discovery; however, most of the resulting drugs have not been very effective in the clinic. This is mostly because diseases are complex entities. The quick identification and interpretation of genetic variations causing patient-specific disease features is now possible thanks to developments in genomics technology and analytical tools (Figure 8.7). The goal of precision medicine would then be to treat these particular characteristics. The need to comprehend how genetics affects disease and vice versa is at the core of the Human Genome Project. The potential of genetics to revolutionize drug discovery has excited oncologists and scientists studying cancer. The analysis of the genomes of both patients and healthy individuals is now possible thanks to the quick development of numerous new techniques (Figure 8.7). It is noteworthy that a patient's clinical presentation and genome can be connected. Many of the medications used today are the result of studies into whether particular proteins are drug targets. However, as there were fewer distinct new drug targets, productivity in terms of drugs produced decreased over time. The "gene to screen" strategy was founded on the understanding that the majority of a cell's overall phenotypic is determined by the genes expressed within that cell. A neutral and affordable method of genotyping and comparing genomic variations between healthy individuals and disease patients is through genome-wide association studies (GWAS). The genetic determinants of disease and the underlying mechanisms guiding the development of disease have been identified thanks to GWAS (Figure 8.2).

Innovative drug development strategies necessitate a paradigm shift due to the low success rate of drug discovery. The first step in developing novel drugs is to take inspiration from natural products that can be used to treat diseases. It is impossible to overstate the importance of using natural products to develop novel medications for both communicable and non-communicable diseases. Thanks to technological advancements, it is now possible to comprehend the profiles of these intricate natural products, which may lead to the discovery of novel therapeutic agents. Natural product lead compounds have been used to isolate or synthesize an astounding number of blockbuster medications. This presents the discovery of new therapeutic drugs through natural products as a highly effective approach. Innovative drug discovery from natural products has the potential to raise the success rate of new therapeutic moieties in this era of rapidly developing scientific technology. Drug discovery from natural products is a key factor in addressing global health issues and accomplishing sustainable development objectives related to health.

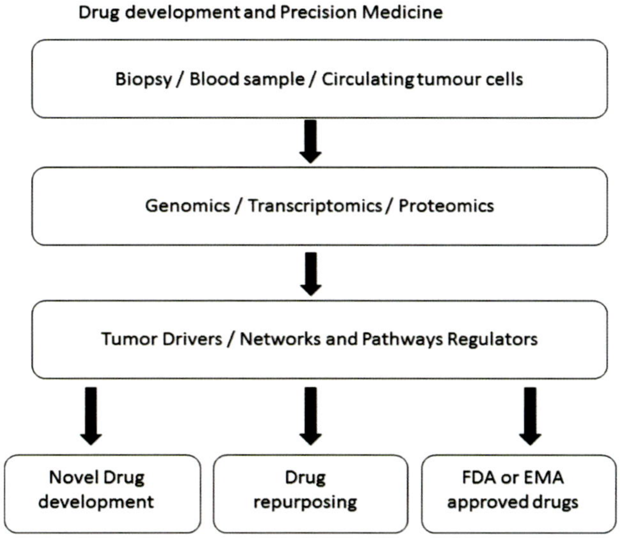

Figure 8.2. *Precision therapies in oncology can be designed to only affect cancer cells. Biomarkers can be identified through next-generation sequencing, gene expression profiling and proteomics. Drivers and regulators of important pathways involved in cancer cell proliferation, survival and chemoresistance can be identified. Only with this knowledge can the development of novel drugs be achieved.*

Source: Thomford, N. E., Senthebane, D. A., Rowe, A., Munro, D., Seele, P., Maroyi, A., & Dzobo, K. Natural Products for drug discovery in the 21st century: Innovations for novel drug discovery. International Journal of Molecular Sciences. 2018; 19(6), 1578. https://doi.org/10.3390/ijms19061578.

A Closer Look

Herbal Medicines

Herbal medicine has a long history that spans thousands of years and is practiced in many different cultures and traditions all over the world. Herbal medicines have been used for their therapeutic qualities, frequently as treatments for a variety of illnesses. They are made from plants or plant extracts. This method of healing is based on the profound conviction that a variety of substances found in nature can both prevent and cure disease.

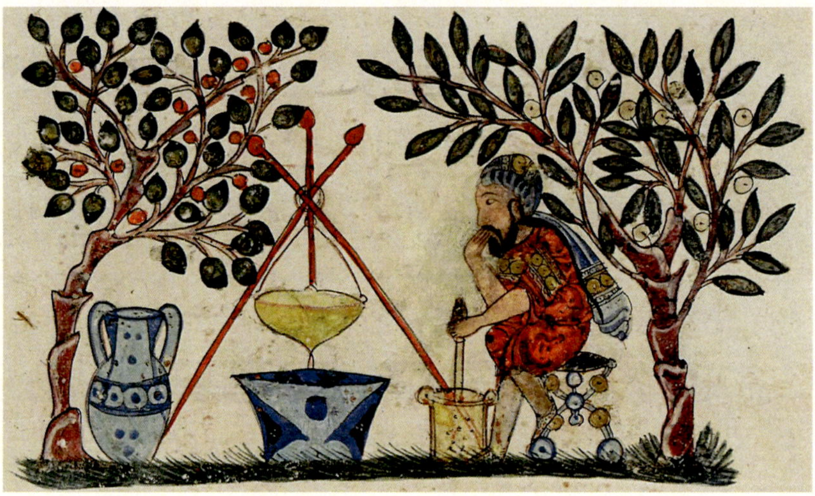

Source: By Marie-Lan Nguyen (2011), Public Domain, https://commons.wikimedia.org/w/index.php?curid=63136870.

The wide variety of active ingredients found in herbal remedies—among them phenolic compounds, alkaloids, flavonoids, and terpenes—is one of their main selling points. These bioactive ingredients have complex interactions with the body that affect physiological functions and have anti-inflammatory effects. For instance, certain herbs may function as antioxidants or antimicrobials, while others may have anti-inflammatory qualities. Furthermore, herbal remedies can be used in a variety of ways because they are frequently prepared and administered as teas, tinctures, pills, and topical ointments, among other forms. In addition to empirical data obtained via observation and experimentation, traditional herbalists frequently rely on centuries-old knowledge that has been passed down through the generations.

Herbal medicines have a long history and are widely used, but there is still ongoing discussion and research regarding their safety and efficacy. Certain herbal remedies have been scientifically proven effective for specific ailments, but there is insufficient clinical evidence to back up the claims made for other remedies. Furthermore, there may be variations in the strength and purity of herbal products, which raises questions regarding their consistent quality and possible negative effects.

Integrative medicine approaches have emerged as a result of growing interest in combining herbal medicines with traditional healthcare practices in recent years. This trend is a reflection of an understanding of the possible advantages of fusing the best aspects of modern medicine with the restorative powers of nature. It also emphasizes how crucial it is to carry out additional research to clarify the mechanisms of action and maximize the application of herbal remedies in clinical settings.

Summary

- Natural products and traditional medicines are of great importance. Natural products and their derivatives have been recognized for many years as a source of therapeutic agents and structural diversity.
- The introduction of novel, chemical, diverse entities with their application as patterns for semi-synthetic and total synthetic modification; the quantity of diseases treated by these diverse compounds; and their rate of use in the treatment of diseases.
- Standardization and quality control of herbal medicines are crucial processes to ensure their safety, efficacy, and consistency. Herbal medicines, derived from natural sources such as plants, have a complex composition, varying significantly in their active ingredients, potency, and bioavailability.
- Quality control of herbal medicines extends beyond chemical analysis to include physical characteristics, such as appearance, taste, and odor, as well as microbiological and heavy metal testing.
- When considering the safety and efficacy of herbal remedies, it's essential to recognize both their potential benefits and risks. Herbal remedies, derived from natural sources such as plants, have been used for centuries to treat various ailments and promote health.
- Chemical diversity in nature is based on biological and geographical diversity, so researchers travel around the world obtaining samples to analyze and evaluate in drug discovery screens or bioassays. This effort to search for natural products is known as bioprospecting.
- General information handling system requirements are recollection and dereplication. These requirements share a common feature. The latitude-longitude location of a source organism collection can be easily obtained using satellite navigation technologies and placed on a map.

References

1. Bhanu, P. S., & Sagar, Z. R. (2003). Herbal drugs. *The Indian Pharmacist, 2*(12), 13–16.
2. Gupta, A. K., & Chitme, H. R. (2000). Herbal medicine for health. *The Eastern Pharmacist, 23*(512), 41–44.
3. Hemalatha, S., Manda, V., & Mohan, Y. (2007). Microwave assisted extraction – An innovative and promising extraction tool for medicinal plant research. *Pharmacognosy Reviews, 1*(1), 7–17.
4. Kar, A. (2006). *Pharmacognosy and Pharma Biotechnology* (pp. 5–11). New Delhi: New Age International Ltd.
5. Littleton, J. (2007). The future of plant drug discovery. *Expert Opinion on Drug Discovery, 2*(5), 673–683.
6. Mukherjee, P. K. (2002). Quality Control of Herbal Drugs: An Approach to Evaluation of Botanicals. India: Business Horizons.
7. Panda, H. (2004). Handbook on Medicinal Herbs With Uses. India: Asia Pacific Business Press.
8. Samanta, M. K., Mukherjee, P. K., Prasad, M. K., & Suresh, B. (2000). *The Eastern Pharmacist. 2000;23(512):23-27.*

9. Spreeman, R., & Gaedcke, F. (2000). Herbal drugs. *The Eastern Pharmacist, 23*(512), 29–37.

10. Tyagi, K., Bhanu, P. S., & Sagar, Z. R. (2003). Failures and successes of herbal medicines. *The Indian Pharmacist, 2*(12), 17–23.

11. Vogel, G. H. (2008). *Drug Discovery and Evaluation, Pharmacological Assays*, Springer-Verlag Berlin Heidelberg 2008, https://doi.org/10.1007/978-3-540-70995-4.

Chapter 9

ANALYTICAL TECHNIQUES IN PHARMACEUTICAL CHEMISTRY

Contents

Introduction

The pharmaceutical industry heavily relies on analytical chemistry, particularly in the drug development process where it ensures the safety, effectiveness, and quality of new medications. The pharmaceutical industry uses a variety of analytical techniques, but chromatography techniques like HPLC, LC-MS, GC, and GC-MS are frequently employed. These methods are the industry norm for examining polymorphism in novel medications. However, because of its accuracy and speed of measurement, spectroscopic instrumentation is also utilized in the industry. An inventive drug molecule that has therapeutic potential to treat or prevent disease is the first step in the drug development process.

It is crucial to successfully synthesize and characterize these drug molecules—also referred to as active pharmaceutical ingredients, or APIs—to find treatment candidates that can be made available to the general public for the treatment or prevention of disease. Therefore, it is essential to have efficient analytical techniques to streamline the drug manufacturing process and characterize drug candidates at every stage.

Orientation and Directional Terms

Term	Definition	Illustration
Chromatography	Chromatography is a laboratory technique for the separation of a mixture into its components.	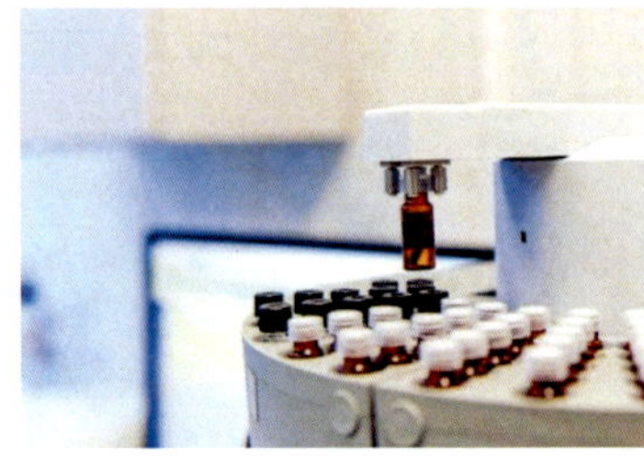
Spectroscopy	Spectroscopy is the field of study that measures and interprets electromagnetic spectra.	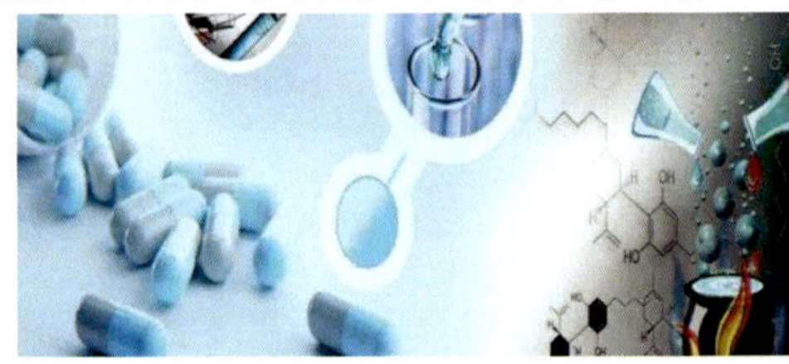
Sparfloxacin	Sparfloxacin belongs to the class of medicines known as antibiotics. It is used to treat bronchitis and pneumonia caused by bacterial infections.	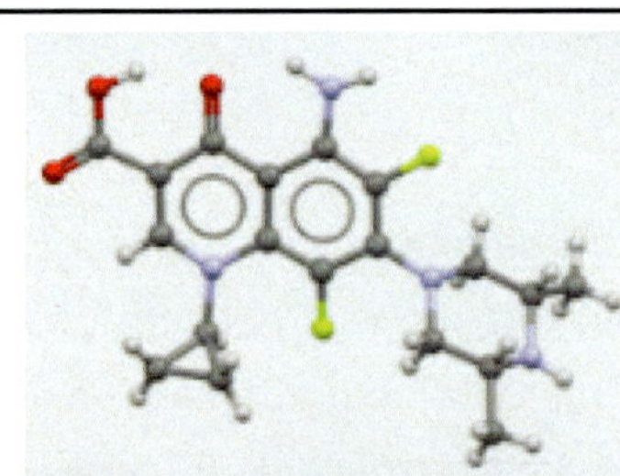
Pharmacological spectrum	Pharmacological spectrum refers to the range of pharmacological activities of a drug or substance.	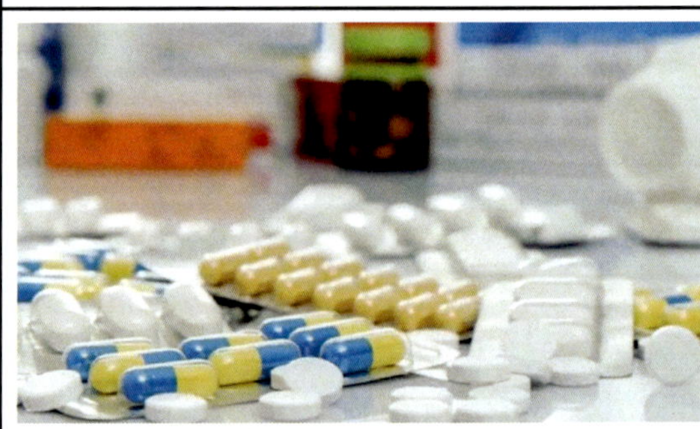
Nutraceuticals	Nutraceuticals are substances that have physiological benefits and are used as medicine in addition to nutrition.	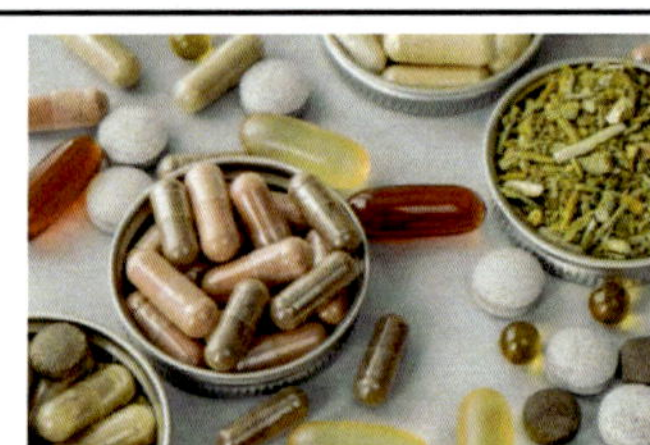

9.1. Analytical Chemistry

Analytical chemistry employs tools and techniques for matter separation, detection, and quantification. Each of the three approaches can be applied alone or in conjunction with another approach. Some molecules are isolated through separation. Analytes are identified and detected using qualification methods, and their concentration is ascertained using quantitative methods.

Additionally, analytical chemistry makes use of instrumental and classical wet chemistry techniques. Traditional qualitative techniques for separation include distillation, extraction, and precipitation. Differentiations based on color, melting or boiling points, solubility, or radioactivity are some other techniques for identification. Furthermore, the amount is quantified by mass or volume changes in common quantitative analytical techniques.

The primary instrumental techniques for separation are usually field-flow fractionation, electrophoresis, or chromatography. Concentration can be ascertained using both qualitative and quantitative techniques after the target analyte has been isolated. This is frequently accomplished by employing different spectroscopic techniques for additional characterization and analysis, or by utilizing the same instrument following separation. The same instrument is frequently used in classical instrumental methods for sample separation, detection, and quantification (Figure 9.1).

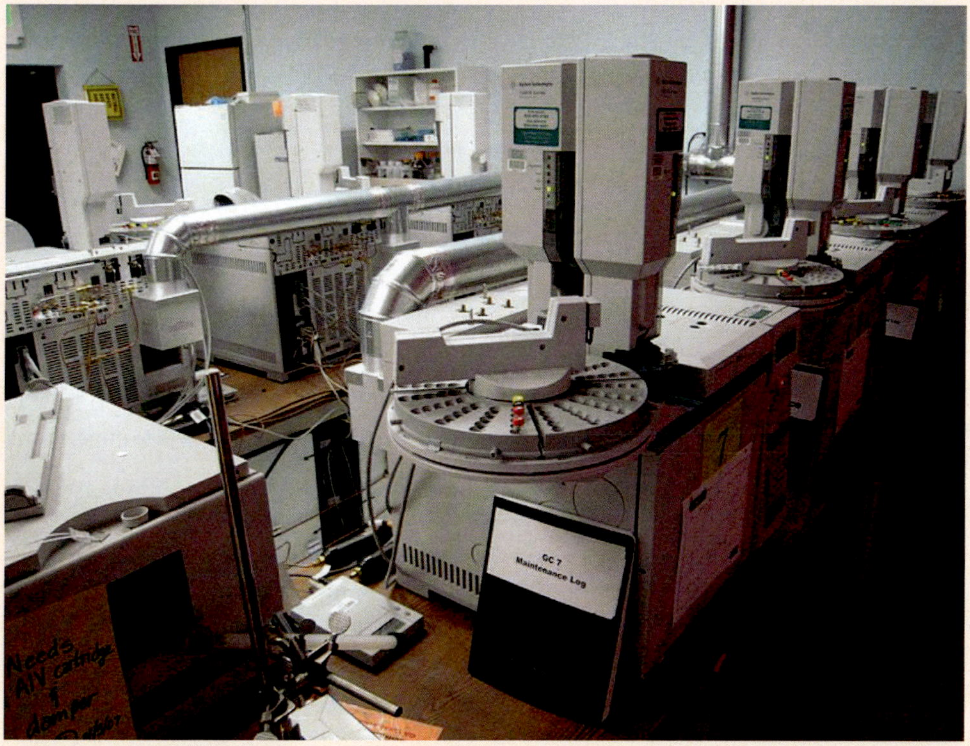

Figure 9.1. *Analytical techniques.*

Source: By Hey Paul from Sacramento, CA, USA – IMG_0068, CC BY 2.0, https://commons.wikimedia.org/w/index.php?curid=18244416.

However, because it can distinguish between molecules with different molecular characteristics but the same elution time using chromatography, spectroscopic instrumentation is frequently used as a complementary technique. In addition, these methods are combined with chemometrics and multivariate statistics to uncover additional structural details and identify principal components at low concentrations. This holds particular significance in the pharmaceutical sector.

9.1.1. Analytical Techniques in Pharmaceutical Industry

Three general analytical methods are used in the pharmaceutical industry to quantify target molecules, separate analytes, and determine structure. These include spectroscopy, chromatography, and traditional analytical chemical techniques. The titrimetric method, a rapid qualitative technique for detecting the presence of a specific analyte or pharmaceutical ingredient, is a popular classical analytical approach.

Reaction rates can now be determined by analyzing kinetic measurements through the optimization of function group procedures. Using these techniques, the pharmaceutical industry has been able to determine the presence of specific pharmaceutical ingredients in commercial dosage forms, including captopril, gabapentin, and sparfloxacin.

Because chromatography methods are accurate in both separation and detection, they are widely used in the pharmaceutical industry. Using thin-layer chromatography (TLC), one can filter out unidentified substances from large batches of medication. Due to the separation of all likely drug constituents, it offers a qualitative approach. High-performance TLC is an advanced version of the method that can analyze complex mixtures, multiple samples, or drugs faster due to its faster run time. Moreover, complex mixtures can be separated using high-performance liquid chromatography (HPLC), which has excellent specificity, accuracy, and precision. While there are a number of detectors used in HPLC, the UV detector is one of the most widely used ones because it can monitor multiple wavelengths simultaneously.

HPLC is a technique that has dominated the pharmaceutical industry and is capable of analyzing multiple drugs during the formulation process. Furthermore, it has become the industry's new gold standard for quality assurance and control when combined with mass spectrometry (LC-MS). Gas chromatography is another common chromatography separation method in the industry for identifying volatile organic compounds. It is employed in the pharmaceutical sector for the analysis of leftover solvents and contaminants.

On the other hand, because spectroscopic techniques are quick, inexpensive, and extremely accurate, they are widely used in the pharmaceutical industry. Typical analytical methods include infrared and Raman spectroscopy.

The pharmaceutical industry is the one that uses near-infrared spectroscopy (NIRS) the most because it is a quick, non-destructive method that can analyze nearly any matrix. It is primarily employed in process monitoring, quality control, and raw material testing. Because it is simple to prepare samples for and allows for the detection of physicochemical properties from a single spectrum, it is widely accepted in the pharmaceutical industry.

To maintain high-quality assurance and quality control, analytical chemistry's primary function in the pharmaceutical industry is the efficient and effective detection and characterization of pharmaceutical ingredients.

9.2. Chromatographic Techniques in Pharmaceutical Analysis

Bioactive compounds, whether natural or synthetic, can be used to categorize all pharmaceuticals. It is important to note that the scientific literature does not agree on a definition of a bioactive substance. Their role in the development of novel medications and more potent pharmaceutical formulations that can be used to treat a variety of diseases is also significant due to the broad pharmacological spectrum of natural and synthetic bioactive compounds, some of which have anti-cancer properties. Bioactive compounds, both natural and synthetic, are utilized in the manufacturing of pharmaceuticals, nutraceuticals, dietary supplements, and cosmetics. Testing the purity and amount of a biologically active ingredient, whether synthetic or natural, in pharmaceutical preparations is a crucial component of chemical analysis. Chromatographic techniques are a great tool for analyzing bioactive substances that are taken out of plants and included in pharmaceutical preparations. Planar methods, high-performance liquid and gas chromatography, and both enable the systematic analysis of the qualitative and quantitative composition as well as the comparison of distinct plant substances according to compositional differences and similarities. Chromatography is a method used to separate mixtures of multiple components into individual components based on how quickly each component migrates along the stationary phase's bed. It enables compound separation without requiring detailed knowledge about the kind of substances to be separated, in contrast to other traditional separation methods (like crystallization, extraction, or distilation), i.e., both the quantity and proportion of each in the mixture. Chromatography is an excellent analytical technique that is widely used for scientific, industrial, and medical purposes due to its versatility and resolving power. It is a vital component of many scientific studies' methodology as well as a tool for keeping an eye on the environment's condition and the chemical and pharmaceutical industries' production of pure compounds. Chromatography is most commonly used in the analysis of pharmaceuticals (30%), biochemical and clinical chemistry (25%) food and cosmetics (10%), environmental protection (15%), and inorganic substances (5%); the remaining 15% of applications are in other fields. Chromatography, on the other hand, is typically employed in 75% of all analyzes that are created for different pharmacopeias.

9.2.1. Thin Layer Chromatography

The TLC method was used to examine the bioactive substances, both synthetic and natural. Pharmaceutical preparations primarily consist of artificially manufactured medicinal substances. A variety of medications were examined, including antidiabetic medications (metformin, saxagliptin, dapaglifloxin, linagliptin), antibiotics (gatifloxacin, ofloxacin, cefoperazone, chloramphenicol), steroid compounds (dexamethasone, prednisone, clobetasol, estradiol, norethisterone, estrone, estriol, testosterone), vitamins (D and K), alkaloids, non-steroidal anti-inflammatory medications belonging to different groups (ibuprofen, meloxicam, celecoxib, etoricoxib, firocoxib, robenacoxib, and cimicoxib), and antihypertensive medications (reserpine, lupeol, scopoletine, bacoside A, piperine in Cardimap tablet). Raw materials and plant preparations are used in herbal medicine, also known as phytotherapy. Thus, natural bioactive compounds, mostly found in plants, were the focus of the research. These included phenolic compounds (gallic acid), steroidal (diosgenin, stigmasterol, ecdysteroids, β-sitosterol), and phenolic compounds (diosgenin, arctigenin), tannins, saponins, coumarins, alkaloids (trigonelline, berberine, barbamine, palmitine, magnoflorine, jatrorrhizine, ephedrine), flavonoids (i.e., triterpenes (betulinic acid), hydroquinone, p-tyrosol, rosavin, diosmin, and essential oils; and antidepressants (salidroside, rosavin, and hydroquinone).

Parys and team employed the TLC-densitometric method to identify non-steroidal anti-inflammatory medicines and meloxicam. Numerous chromatographic plate types were used, including silica gel 60 and 60F254, neutral aluminum oxide 60F254 and 150F254, a combination of silica gel 60 and Kieselguhr 60F254, and silica gel RP-18F254 and RP-8F254. The NP-TLC analysis was performed using the mixtures of ethyl acetate-ethanol-toluene-25 % NH4OH (6:3:1:0.06, v/v/v/v) and ethyl acetate-toluene-n-butylamine (2:2:1, v/v/v). An 8:2 v/v methanol-water mixture was used for the RP-TLC analysis. Several visualization agents, including rhodamine B, Janus blue, methyl green, brilliant green, crystalline violet, alkaline blue, gentian violet, methylene violet, fuchsine, and brilliant cresyl blue, were used to carry out the processes of spot visualization of meloxicam. The mixture of ethyl acetate-toluene-n-butylamine (2:2:1, v/v/v) in NP-TLC, as well as silica gel 60F254 and neutral aluminum oxide plates, turned out to be the most effective chromatographic conditions among all those examined. Meloxicam was detected in RP-TLC at the lowest concentration level thanks to the use of RP-8F254 and RP-18F254 plates and a methanol-water (8:2, v/v) mixture. Furthermore, of all the visualization agents examined, crystalline violet and gentian violet were discovered to be new visualization agents on silica gel 60F254 and neutral aluminum oxide 150F254, respectively, due to meloxicam's smallest limit of detection.

Applications of thin-layer chromatography include bioactivity, identification, and separation. e. antioxidant activity and toxicity of specific steroids, as well as novel renewable bioactive compounds derived from plant material—such as Indonesian-cultivated algae—and bioactive compounds. The red algae *Chlorella* sp. and Eugleuma cottonii were used to extract steroids. originating from Indonesia have been divided onto a silica gel plate F254, activated by heating it in an oven with the eluent n-hexane-ethyl acetate in the appropriate volume composition. They have then been identified under UV light at 254 and 366 nm, in addition to using Liebermann-Burchard reagent.

9.2.2. Column Liquid Chromatography

The most common method for analyzing different bioactive compounds in phytochemical and pharmaceutical research is high-performance liquid chromatography (HPLC). Pharmaceutically active compounds (APIs) in various samples (matrices), such as synthetic drug products and plant materials, can be qualitatively and quantitatively analyzed with high sensitivity and accuracy using high-performance liquid chromatography (HPLC) as opposed to other analytical techniques.

In a single HPLC run, RP-HPLC could detect multiple NSAIDs in combination pharmaceutical formulations simultaneously. For example, an RP-HPLC method has been applied as a stability-indicating assay for the newly synthesized codrug (indomethacin-paracetamol) and the active ingredients indomethacin, famotidine, and paracetamol. In a different study, Al-Khateeb and colleagues describe a straightforward, quick, effective, and environmentally friendly way to use high-temperature liquid chromatography (HTLC) for the simultaneous separation and measurement of a few NSAIDs (ibuprofen, ketoprofen, naproxen, and sodium dichlorophenol) in pharmaceuticals as well as NSAID traces in water samples. expanding body of study on the simultaneous analysis of NSAID combinations, i.e., the following two publications by Hassan and Nam are also confirmed by the isocratic RP-HPLC method employing short column for aspirin, paracetamol, and naproxen. It is said that using HPLC methods to identify NSAIDs in a mixture is an affordable option.

In pharmaceutical formulations of some drugs that affect the autonomic nervous system, such as ephedrine in the presence of naphazoline and neostigmine methylsulfate, an RP-HPLC technique was also applicable as a stability-indicating method for the analysis of active ingredients and their impurities. Neostigmine methylsulfate in bulk medication and injection formulation can be simultaneously subjected to quality control, forced degradation, and stability studies thanks to the RP-HPLC analysis that Parab and colleagues have developed.

Profiling of possible antioxidants using HPLC-MS/MS by Al-Jaber and colleagues have presented some phenolic acids and flavonoids in extracts of Salvia species from Jordan. The presence of seven additional flavonoids, including luteolin-7-O-glucoside, apigenin, apigenin-7-O-glucoside, rutin, nariginin, hesperidin, and quercetin, as well as four bioactive phenolic acids, including gallic acid, caffeic acid, rosmarinic acid, and salvianolic acid B, was found to be responsible for the good antioxidant activity, according to the obtained results.

When HPLC analysis is coupled with SEC-MALS, a combination comprising SEC column and phosphate buffered saline (PBS) as the mobile phase, i.e., either polymer- or silica-based are frequently employed. As an example, Fu et al. employed this method in a high-quality investigation into recombinant anti-interleukin-23 monoclonal antibodies as possible targets for anticancer medications. Size-exclusion chromatography's usefulness in maintaining the purity of upcoming antibody-drug conjugates (ADCs) as anticancer agents is demonstrated by another study. Using trastuzumab as a model, a novel method was presented in this work to derive homogeneous ADCs with a drug-to-antibody ratio of 2 from any human immunoglobulin 1 (IgG1). Farras and colleagues presented a related study about the search for functional monoclonal antibodies (mAbs) based on the structure of trastuzumab. Another study demonstrates that using HPLC in conjunction with SEC-MALS was a quick way to determine the capsid content of AAV-containing samples and, consequently, to aid in the creation of therapeutic AAV-based medications.

9.2.3. RP-TLC/RP-HPLC and Lipophilicity

Młodawska Morak et al. used the RP-TLC method to examine the lipophilic characteristics of 1,2,3-triazole-dipyridothiazine with antitumor activity. The logP that was computed was compared with the lipophilicity parameters that were obtained using the TLC technique. They discovered that the lipophilicity parameters measured experimentally using the RP-TLC technique were not well approximated by the computation methods. In a different study, the chromatographic parameters RF and RM are used to calculate the lipophilicity descriptor for twenty-one newly synthesized chalcones using the Soczewiński–Wachtmeister methodology. Three binary phases—acetonitrile–water, ethanol–water, and acetone–water—and reversed phase silica gel 60 RP-18F254 plates (RP-TLC) were used for the thin-layer chromatography analysis. The acetonitrile-water mobile phase was the most effective of all the phases that were utilized. With the use of this mixture, it was possible to predict the lipophilicity chromatographic parameter (C_0) that correlated with calculated logP the best.

Furthermore, the quantitative structure-retention relationship (QSRR) analysis conducted between C_0 and specific molecular descriptors was useful in identifying the descriptors that had the greatest impact on C_0 and, consequently, on the lipophilicty parameter of the compounds under investigation. Utilizing thin layer chromatography and the Soczewiński–Wachtmeister method, spirohydantoins used to treat diabetes and epilepsy were also evaluated for lipophilicity. There were reported strong relationships between lipophilicity and the blood–brain barrier and between lipohilicity and plasma protein binding. Dołowy and associates. examined the lipophilicity of antidiabetic medications, specifically metformin and phenformin, using NPTLC and RPTLC techniques. The lipophilicity results were compared with the partition coefficient theoretical values of the drugs under study. They had trouble getting accurate lipophilicity values. They suggested that new procedures for determining the lipophilicity of metformin and phenformin could be based on theoretical techniques based on the Gutman and Randic topological indexes.

9.2.4. Gas Chromatography

Gas chromatography (GC) coupled to single or tandem mass spectrometric approaches (GC-MS, GC-MS/MS) or with different detection systems (GC-FID) proved to be an efficient tool for identifying a variety of bioactive compounds in phytochemical and pharmaceutical analyzes.

Because of their diverse biological effects, essential oils are a promising class of natural products derived from aromatic plants. GC is a useful technique for testing any volatile substances, including these. i.e., the antitumor, antibacterial, antimicrobial, and antioxidant properties of these substances.

The suitability of GC analysis in identifying contaminants in pharmaceuticals. For instance, the delgocitinib methyl, ethyl, and isopropyl methanesulfonate impurities (MMS, EMS, and IPMS) were successfully determined using GC-FID. Helium was used as the carrier gas at a flow rate of 5 points0 mL/min for the analysis on the DB-624 UI column (30 m × 0.25 mm × 1.4 μm). From 1 to 5 ppm, the developed method demonstrated good linearity, accuracy, and precision. For MMS, the LOD and LOQ were 0.1 and 0.3 ppm, and for EMS and IPMS, they were 0.05 and 0.1 ppm, respectively. Ahirrao and team employed the GC-MS/MS technique to estimate genotoxic contaminants, i.e., the active ingredients of alalevonadifloxacin mesylate (ALA), a new antibiotic licensed in India to treat infections brought on by Gram-positive bacteria, are methyl methane sulfonate (MMS), ethyl methane sulfonate (EMS), and isopropyl methane sulfonate (IMS). Helium was used as the carrier gas in the study, and the Rtx-624 column (30 m × 0.32 mm × 1.8 μm) was used. The flow rate of helium was 1.5 mL/min. With LOQs of 5, 10, and 20 ng/g of ALA for MMS, EMS, and IMS, respectively, the suggested method was extremely sensitive.

The phytocomponents found in *Clerodendrum serratum* Linn roots, which are used in Indian Ayurvedic and Siddha medicine to treat a variety of ailments including cough, asthma, rheumatism fever, and cephalalgia ophthalmia, were identified using GC-MS analysis. Squalene was then determined to be one of the constituents using the GC-FID method. Helium was used as the carrier gas for the GC-MS measurements, which were carried out on an Elite-5MS column (30 m × 0.25 mm × 1 μm). On the other hand, nitrogen was used as the carrier gas and the flow rate was 12 points7 mL/min for the GC-FID measurements, which were carried out on the Zebron DB column (30 m × 0.25 mm × 0.50 μm). The obtained data indicated that the main components were stigmasterol, methyl palmitate, hexadecenoic acid, and squalene. The squalene purity within and between days was found to be 1.154 · 1.819 percent and 1.510 ÷ 1.861 percent, in that order.

The squalene under analysis had a LOD of 0.79 μg/mL and a LOQ of 1.89 μg/mL.

9.2.5. Combined Techniques

Current developments in the identification of bioactive substances found in diverse complex matrices center on what are known as coupled techniques, or combined techniques. These methods combine different detection techniques with separation techniques. Chromatography techniques (e.g., GC) are primarily employed as techniques for separation, and spectroscopic approaches (MS, NMR) are employed as techniques for detection. Combinations of multiple chromatographic techniques can also be considered combined techniques. The combined method should allow for the best possible identification of the substances to be determined, be sensitive over a broad range of concentrations, and be selective for the analytes to be determined. The selection of the most suitable combined technique should be based on the type of analyte, how simple it is to combine different methods, how sensitive the required determinations must be, and whether the necessary equipment is available.

High-performance liquid and thin-layer chromatography were employed to analyze the flavonoids and phenolic acids present in *Flos Lamii albi*. Si 60F254 plates were subjected to HPTLC analyzes utilizing a multiple gradient development program. The following materials were used for the analysis of flavonoids at a 3 cm distance: 6 mL of solution A (toluene: hexane: formic acid, 7: 3: 0.1), 3 mL of ethyl acetate, and 1 mL of methanol. Next, at a distance of 9 cm, 5 mL of solution A (toluene: hexane: formic acid, 7: 3: 0.1), 2 mL of ethyl acetate, and 2 mL of methanol were used. The following materials were used in development steps 1 and 2 of the phenolic acid analysis: 3 mL solution B (heptane: dichloromethane, 7: 3), 2 mL diisopropyl ether, 0 point 1 mL 85 % formic acid, and 1 mL distiled water. However, 4 mL of solution B (heptane: dichloromethane, 7:3), 1 mL of diisopropyl ether, and 0.1 mL of 85 % formic acid were utilized for development from step 3 to step 7. *Flos Lamii albi* was found to contain protocatechuic, vanillic, and cafeic acids. The extract that underwent basic hydrolysis had the highest concentration of caffeic acid. Using an RP-18 column and a water-methanol-formic acid (75: 25: 0.5, v/v/v) mobile phase, HPLC was utilized to separate the phenolic acids, with UV detection at 254 nm. Nine acids—protocatechuic, vanillic, caffeic, syringic, gallic, gentisic, p-coumaric, and chlorogenic acids—as well as trace amounts of ferulic acid were found in esterified forms.

In addition to phenolics, flavonoids, and glycoside derivatives, the ethyl acetate fraction of the methanolic extract from the leaves of *Casearia arborea* contained flavonoid-3-O-glycosides, which were identified using UHPLC-DAD-ESI-HRMS/MS in conjunction with molecular networking-based dereplication and NMR. This plant is a major source of cytotoxic highly oxidized clerodane diterpenes. Through the use of NMR spectroscopy for metabolite isolation and characterization or co-injection of standards in HPLC-DAD, the researchers discovered compounds that are not annotated in the Global Natural Products Social Molecular Networking (GNPS) platform. On the RP Zorbax Eclipse Plus column, HPLC-DAD analysis was carried out using gradient elution of acetonitrile and water (0.01 percent acetic acid). A measurement was made at λ = 352 nm. Six flavonoid-3-O-glycosides were annotated as a molecular family in the molecular networking formed by the GNPS platform. A quercetin-3-O-pentoside cluster, rutin, isoquercitrin, quercitrin, and avicularin were among them. With the exception of identifying quercetin-3-O-robinobioside and kaempferol, the annotations with standard compounds by HPLC-DAD co-injection three flavonoid-3-O-pentosides and characterization via 1D and 2D NMR were confirmed. Moreover, 1D and 2D NMR spectroscopy was used to isolate and characterize three flavonoid-3-O-pentosides. These were recognized as avicularin, guaijaverin, and reynoutrin.

Scientists investigated the usefulness of high-speed countercurrent chromatography (HSCCC) and offline 2,2-diphenyl-1-picrylhydrazyl (DPPH)-gas chromatography (GC)-mass spectrometry (MS) for the screening and identification of antioxidant separation in *Curcuma wenyujin* essential oil. H. Chen and Co. Ling. The HP-5 5 percent phenyl methyl siloxane capillary column and GC chromatograph with a flame ionization detector (FID) were used to analyze the essential oil. Using DPPH-GC, the five compounds were identified as antioxidants, and GC-MS was then used to confirm this identification. The following solvents were used in the HSCCC method to successfully isolate eucalyptol, camphor, δ-elemene, β-elemene, and curzerene: n-hexane-acetonitrile-ethanol (5:3:2, v/v) and n-hexane-acetonitrile-acetone (4:3:1, v/v). Finally, the DPPH scavenging assay has verified the antioxidant property of *Curcuma wenyujin*.

The furanosesquiterpenoids from bark exudates of *Communiphora swynnertonni* or the Burrt tree, which is used by ethnic groups in Tanzania and Kenya to treat a variety of human diseases and eradicate ectoparasites infesting livestock, were analyzed using the HPLC-SPE-NMR technique. A silica-based Apollo C18 column was used for the separation, and the mobile phase consisted of water, acetonitrile, and 0.1 percent formic acid in a gradient elution method. A measurement was made at λ = 246 nm. The exudate was found to contain four furanosesquiterpenoids that are known to exist: 6-oxodendrolasin, (E)-6-oxoisodendrolasin, (Z)-6-oxoisodendrolasin, crassifolone, and one new one called 7,8-dihydroisodendrolasin (Table 9.1).

Table 9.1. Application, Advantages, and Disadvantages of Chromatographic Methods in Clinical Trials and Participation Rate

Method	Separation Basis	Advantages	Disadvantages	Separatable Compounds
PC	Different rates of separation across paper	Cheap, simple, and user-friendly method	Separate low number of samples, no quantitative analysis	Complex and volatile compounds
CC	Size, polarity, or hydrophobicity	Compatible with most complex mixtures, user friendly method	Expensive, time consuming, no quantitative analysis	Nanovesicles
GPC	Sieving molecules based on their size	Simple and reliable method	Limitation in volume of sample, low capacity for separation	Proteins, polysaccharides, enzymes, and polymers

TLC	Capillary force	Simple, cheap, and user friendly	Limitation for volatile samples and low accuracy and pression	Non-volatile pharmaceutical compounds
AC	Reversible interaction between analyte and specific ligand	High reliability, great sensitivity and specificity	Complicated maintenance, costly	Purification of enzymes, protein and analyzing vaccines
DLC	Reversible interaction between analyte and specific DYE ligand	Inexpensive and user-friendly	Limitation in selectivity of dye legends	Proteins, enzymes, coenzymes, cofactors, antibodies, and amino acids
HIC	Interacts with the hydrophobic ligand	High efficiency and sensitivity	Costly buffer (salt)	Separate proteins
GC	Vaporise samples and sperate through column	Fast and very high efficiency	Only compatible for volatile and thermally stable analytes	Volatile and thermally stable analytes
IEC	Charge of chemical and biological groups	Efficient and cheap in column price	Costly buffer	Proteins, enzymes, peptides, amino acids, and antibodies
RP-HPLC	Pressurising the mixture of mobile phase and sample through the column	Fast, reproducible, and efficient method with high accuracy and precision	Costly and complicated maintenance	Most pharmaceutical compounds

Source: Tavana, B., & Chen, A. Determination of drugs in clinical trials: current status and outlook. Sensors. 2022; 22(4), 1592. https://doi.org/10.3390/s22041592.

9.3. Spectroscopic Techniques

The study of how matter absorbs and emits electromagnetic waves is known as spectroscopy. The definition encompasses the investigation of particle interactions, including those involving protons, ions, and electrons. The development of pharmaceuticals has relied heavily on spectroscopic analysis to investigate a wide range of topics, including antibiotic patents, drug identity and purity, crystalline structures of drugs, interactions between active ingredients and excipients, and much more.

Pharmaceutical spectroscopy equipment is available in a multitude of configurations, catering to a wide spectrum of researchers with varying financial constraints.

9.3.1. UV-VIS Spectrophotometry

Spectrophotometric techniques, which rely on chemical reactions and natural UV absorption, are another significant category of methods that are frequently included in pharmacopeias. The quantitative measurement of a material's transmission or reflection characteristics as a function of wavelength is known as spectrophotometry. These techniques have the benefit of requiring little time and labor. Additionally, these techniques have outstanding precision. Over the past few years, there has been a significant increase in the use of UV-Vis spectrophotometry, particularly in the analysis of pharmaceutical dosage forms. The colorimetric methods are usually based on the following aspects:

- Complex-formation reaction.
- Oxidation-reduction process.
- A catalytic effect.

It is noteworthy to mention that bulk material assay frequently employs colorimetric methods. One method for determining corticosteroid drug formulations is the blue tetrazolium assay. The European Pharmacopoeia presents the colorimetric method, which is also utilized for the determination of cardiac glycosides. There have been several reported methods for determining the active pharmaceutical ingredients in bulk drugs and formulations using spectrophotometry.

9.3.2. Near Infrared Spectroscopy

NIR spectroscopy is a method that makes use of the near-infrared region of the electromagnetic spectrum (from about 700 to 2500 nanometers). By measuring light scattered off of and through a sample, NIR reflectance spectra can be used to quickly determine a material's properties without altering the sample.

NIR converts measured data into actionable information to help optimize processes or improve research. Capable of examining irregular surfaces with the same ease as a carefully prepared sample, NIR is non-destructive, and requires little or no sample preparation. It can also be used to analyze multiple constituents in a single scan.

9.3.3. Nuclear Magnetic Resonance Spectroscopy

The field of NMR-based screening has advanced quickly since the first report detailing the use of NMR spectroscopy to screen for drug molecules appeared in 1996. Numerous cutting-edge methods have been introduced in recent years and have been widely used in academic and pharmaceutical research. Recently, NMR has been used in quantitative analysis to quantify drugs in pharmaceutical formulations and biological fluids, characterize the composition of drug products, and ascertain the impurity of the drug.

9.3.4. Ion Mobility-Mass Spectrometry

Because it is coupled to a high mass accuracy time-of flight mass analyzer and has the unique ability to separate ions based on size, shape, or charge, ion mobility-mass spectrometry (IM-MS) has drawn the interest of many researchers. For glycopeptide analysis, a variety of ion mobility techniques have been applied. The most widely used commercially available IM-MS instrument, traveling wave ion mobility-mass spectrometry (TWIMSMS), has been used to identify the glycopeptides of each glycoform and to thoroughly characterize the glycozylation heterogeneity profile of an IgG1 mAb. Li and team discovered that ion mobility reduced chemical noise to enable the detection of lower abundant ions. They also observed that TWIMS could separate peptides from glycopeptides into distinct trend lines that could be used to predict the glycozylation status of other peptides. Additionally, Muc 2-derived epimeric glycopeptides have been distinguished using TWIMS-MS. Using TWIMS-MS, two isomeric glycopeptides with identical peptide backbones that differ only in α-GlcNAc or α-GalNAc attachment were partially separated; remarkably, multiple overlapping conformers were found for each glycopeptide. The authors used CID-IMS-MS to confirm the identity of each glycopeptide; TWIMS-MS was used to separate the diagnostic oxonium ions, emphasizing the usefulness and significance of characterizing product ions. It has also been possible to quickly separate coeluting isomeric O-linked glycopeptides that differ only in the glycozylation site using high-field asymmetric wave ion mobility spectrometry (FAIMS). By adjusting the correction voltage used, the coeluting peptides were separated. Electron transfer dissociation (ETD) was used to confirm the glycozylation sites; the two glycozylation sites can be easily distinguished by their diagnostic product ions. The utilization of FAIMS for isobaric peptide separation and ETD for glycozylati site confirmation has demonstrated significant utility in the analysis of intricate glycopeptide mixtures.

9.3.5. Mass Spectrometry

Among many other fields, environmental and forensic scientists, biologists, chemists, and medical researchers utilize mass spectrometry (MS), a potent analytical technique. Using mass spectrometry (MS), we can examine a molecule's mass or the masses of various molecule fragments.

9.3.5.1. The Basics of a Mass Spectrometry Experiment

MS instruments come in a wide variety of forms, but they all share three fundamental elements. An ionization source is the first component, where a proton or an electron is added to give the molecule a positive electrical charge. The ionized molecule might or might not fragment into a population of smaller pieces, depending on the ionization technique employed. Certain sample molecules in the Figure 9.2 break up into smaller pieces, while others stay whole. The cationic fragments are separated based on their mass in the mass analyzer that comes next in line.

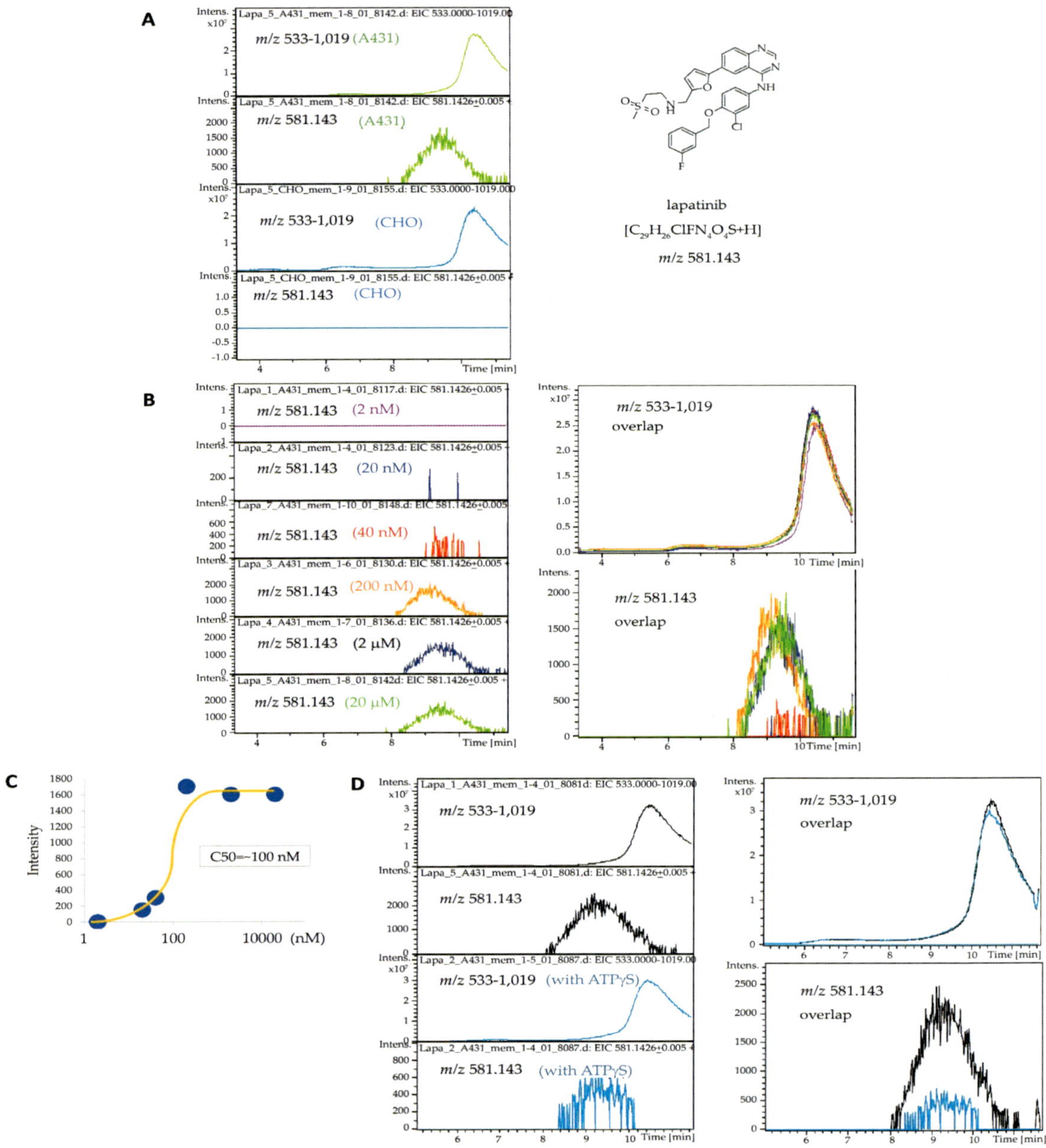

Figure 9.2. *Mass spectrometry: detection of interaction between the A431 cell membrane protein fraction and EGFR inhibitor, lapatinib.*

Source: Ogiso, H., Suno, R., Kobayashi, T., Kawami, M., Takano, M., & Ogasawara, M. A liquid chromatography-mass spectrometry method to study the interaction between membrane proteins and low-molecular-weight compound mixtures. Molecules. 2022; 27(15), 4889. https://doi.org/10.3390/molecules27154889.

The detector that finds and measures the separated ions comes last. Electron ionization is one of the more popular MS techniques used in the organic laboratory. A high-energy electron beam is used in the ionization source to bombard the sample molecule, which causes the molecule to lose one of its valence electrons and become a radical cation. As a result of the intense energy transfer caused by this bombardment process, the radical cation soon starts to disintegrate into smaller pieces, some of which are neutral and some of which are positively charged. Either a vacuum source removes the neutral fragments or they are adsorbed onto the chamber walls. An electric field accelerates the positively charged fragments and any unfragmented molecular ions down a tube in the mass analyzer component (Figure 9.3).

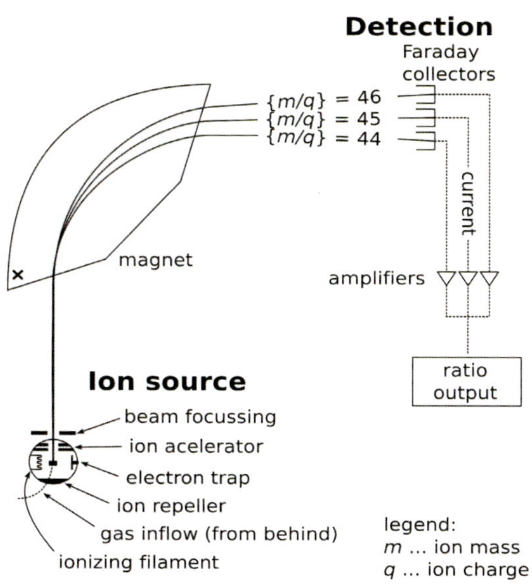

Figure 9.3. *Mass spectrometry.*

Source: By Devon Fyson – https://commons.wikimedia.org/w/index.php?curid=5082916.

The ions in this curved tube are deflected by a powerful magnetic field. Since almost all ions have charges of z = +1, sorting by the mass to charge ratio is the same as sorting by mass. Ions with different mass to charge (m/z) ratios are deflected to a different extent, resulting in a "sorting" of ions by mass. The sorted ions are quantified and recorded by a detector at the end of the curved flight tube.

Gas chromatography (GC) is a separation method that is used in conjunction with mass spectrometry. When working with a sample that is a mixture of two or more distinct compounds, the combined GC-MS procedure is very helpful because the different compounds are separated before being submitted to individual MS analysis. We won't go into the specifics of gas chromatography here, but if you are enrolled in an organic laboratory course, you may have the opportunity to experiment with GC and will most likely learn about the theoretically similar processes of thin layer and column chromatography. To put it succinctly, helium gas is used in GC to push a very tiny amount of vaporized liquid sample through a long, coiled metal column.

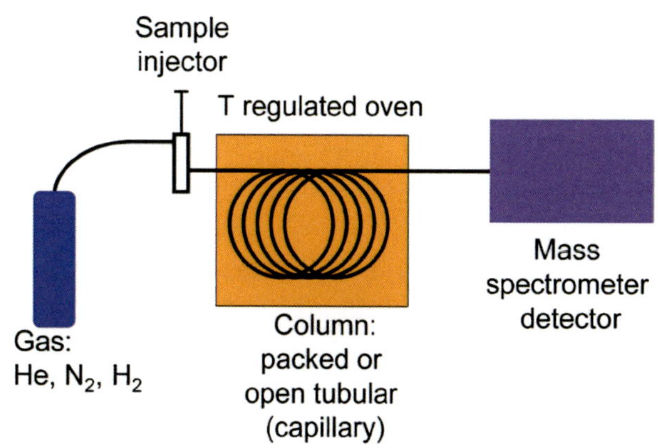

Figure 9.4. *Mass spectrometry (GC-MS).*

Source: By K. Murray (Kkmurray) – Own work, CC BY-SA 3.0, https://commons.wikimedia.org/w/index.php?curid=1935816.

Different compounds in the sample adhere to the column walls to varying degrees along the way. As a result, they move through the column at varying speeds and emerge from the end of the column independently. Every purified compound in GC-MS is fed straight into the MS instrument from the end of the GC column, resulting in a unique mass spectrum for every compound in the initial mixed sample.

We can tell the device to search an MS database and identify every compound in the sample because an MS spectrum is a very dependable and repeatable "fingerprint" of a compound (Figure 9.4).

Modern GC-MS equipment has a sensitivity so great that it can identify and detect minuscule trace amounts of organic compounds. Environmental chemists are using GC-MS more frequently to find harmful organic contaminants in food and water samples. High-speed GC-MS instruments are another tool used by airport security screeners to search checked luggage for bomb-making chemical residue.

9.3.5.2. Mass Spectrometry of Proteins – Applications in Proteomics

Biomolecules are typically difficult to analyze using electron ionization mass spectrometry (EIMS) due to their high polarity, which makes it challenging to get them into the vapor phase. Over the past few decades, a revolution in mass spectrometry of biomolecules has occurred due to the development of numerous new techniques for ionization and separation. The general approach to biomolecule analysis is soft ionization, which imparts significantly less energy to the molecule under study during the ionization process (in comparison to methods like EIMS). Adding protons is typically used in soft ionization instead of taking electrons out, resulting in much less energetic cations than radical cations created by taking an electron out. Since there is little to no fragmentation as a result of soft ionization, the mass being measured is that of an intact molecule. Large biomolecules are usually broken down into smaller pieces by enzymatic or chemical means, and their masses are then ascertained by'soft' mass spectrometry.

Proteins that are present in biological samples in extremely small amounts can now be more easily found and identified thanks to recent advancements in soft ionization mass spectrometry technology. When a protein sample is sprayed into a tube for electrospray ionization (ESI), an electric field causes the molecules to absorb additional protons from the solvent. "Matrix-assisted laser desorption ionization" (MALDI) is another popular "soft ionization" technique. Here, a laser is used to achieve protonation after the protein sample has been adsorbed onto a solid matrix (Figure 9.1).

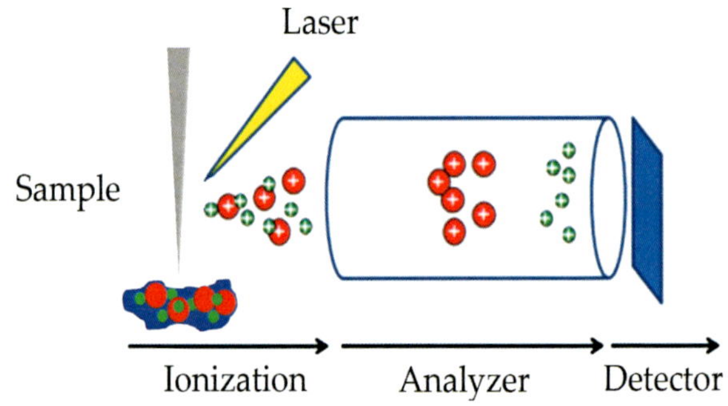

Figure 9.5. *Both electrospray ionization and MALDI are used in conjunction with a time-of-flight (TOF) mass analyzer component.*

Source: By Carson Szot, Antony Croxatto, Guy Prod'hom & Gilbert Greub – https://commons.wikimedia.org/wiki/File%3AMALDI-TOF_MS.png, CC BY-SA 4.0, https://commons.wikimedia.org/w/index.php?curid=64032426.

Lighter ions move more quickly than heavier ions with the same overall charge, which allows for the separation of the proteins when they are accelerated by an electrode through a column. Thus, a complex biological sample (blood plasma, urine, etc.) containing numerous proteins can be processed. can be distinguished from one another and their respective masses precisely calculated. Thanks to the extreme sensitivity of modern protein MS, researchers were recently able to identify Tyrannosaurus rex protein in a fossilized skeleton! In the field of proteomics, soft ionization mass spectrometry has grown in importance in recent years. Protein biochemists have historically focused on the composition and properties of individual proteins. On the other hand, proteomics researchers are more interested in understanding the interactions and reactions of a vast number of proteins within a living system to changes in the organism's state. The search for protein "biomarkers" for human disease, or proteins that are more abundant in the tissues of diseased individuals than in healthy ones, is a significant area of proteomics. When a known biomarker for a disease, like diabetes or cancer, is found in a healthy individual, doctors may be able to take preventive action to delay or prevent the disease's onset, as it may indicate that the patient may be particularly vulnerable to the illness.

In a 2005 study, fluid samples from lung transplant recipients who experienced tissue rejection were compared to samples from recipients who did not experience rejection using MALDI-TOF mass spectrometry. It was discovered that, particularly in the tissue rejection samples, three peptides (short proteins) were present at elevated levels. These peptides are thought to have potential as biomarkers to identify patients who are more likely to reject their lung transplants.

9.4. Applications of Analytical Techniques in Pharmaceutical Analysis

Worldwide, High-performance liquid chromatography (HPLC) has established itself as a key analytical method for both qualitative and quantitative drug analysis. The foundational element for the development of this method, which is directly in charge of the chromatographic separations, is the column packing material. The Van Deemter equation, an empirical formula that characterizes the relationship between linear velocity (flow rate) and plate height (HETP, column efficiency), provides the fundamentals of compound separation. The efficiency of chromatographic separation, speed, and resolution all increase with decreasing column material particle size, according to the HPLC separation principle. The HPLC is the most widely used, straightforward, affordable, and dependable method for pharmaceutical analysis.

Nevertheless, HPLC technology is not able to meet all analytical needs. When determining complex samples using HPLC, such as formulation excipients, biological samples, drug metabolites, degradation products, impurities, and drug isomers, a number of issues with low-level analyte determination (0 point 1 percent), analysis speed, and resolution per unit time come up. The researchers are working on creating sub-2μm particles to meet the need for high-resolution separation. The sub-2μm polymeric particles, non-porous silica, and porous silica that were created each have unique separation properties. Compared to non-porous packings, porous packing materials have a much higher sample capacity and can withstand higher pressure.

UHPLC is currently developing into a cutting-edge, contemporary method that offers liquid chromatography a new path. Ultra-high-performance liquid chromatography, or UHPLC, is primarily improved in three areas: sensitivity, resolution, and speed. When compared to HPLC, UHPLC offers superior resolution, speed, and sensitivity for particles with a diameter of less than 2 μm. Pharmaceutical companies are looking for innovative ways to boost economy and speed up drug development in the twenty-first century. Under extremely high pressure (up to 100M Pa), separation and quantification are carried out in UHPLC. In contrast to HPLC, it has been observed that high pressure has no detrimental effects on the analytical column. Additionally, UHPLC uses less time and solvent overall. Waters created the hybrid particle technology (HPT) HPLC column for the first time in 1999. Combining organic polymeric packings with inorganic silica results in the HPT, which has a peak shape, high mechanical strength, efficiency, and pH stability for basic compounds. The second generation hybrid material particle, which offers enhanced strength, pH range, and efficiency, is made up of a bridged ethylsiloxane/silica hybrid (BEH) structure. In addition, high strength silica (HSS) particle technology has been applied, which improves the mechanical stability of silica and, in comparison to hybrid particles, increases compound selectivity and retention time. The most recent development in hybrid materials is called Charge Surface Hybrid (CSH) Technology, which incorporates surface charge into the packing materials to improve peak shape and selectivity across the whole range of ionic mobile phases. Following the aforementioned advancements in particle size and column packing material, Waters Company was renamed UHPLC, formerly known as UPLC. This review paper aims to give an overview of UHPLC, its pharmaceutical applications, and some examples of the most cutting-edge work in pharmaceutical analysis. UHPLC improves the selectivity, sensitivity, and range of LC analysis; requires less sample quantity; shortens the total run time for separation; increases resolution performance; uses less solvent; allows for quick resolution and quantification of related and unrelated compounds; and is inexpensive to analyze. The disadvantages of UHPLC include: Lack of variety in commercial columns at sub-2 μm particle size; higher pressure requires more maintenance; higher pressure shortens the life of the columns; complex design and development of sub-2 μm stationary phase; non-regenerable and limited use of stationary phase; and difficulties in providing higher pressure for solvents. With an HPLC column (3 point 0 to 4 point 6 mm), frictional heating of the mobile phase occurs at high operating pressure. This causes non-uniform flow, which reduces separation efficiency. Smaller diameter columns (1 to 2 point 1 mm) used in UHPLC have reduced frictional heating. Initially, the HPLC was transformed into a UHPLC, which could analyze proteins at pressures of up to 17,500 psi and 1 μm particles. UV/TOF detection was initially used in the UHPLC to separate different pharmaceutical compounds. Numerous studies on UHPLC have been published, detailing all of its benefits over HPLC as well as its features and applications.

9.4.1. Method Development and Validation

Establishing documented evidence that offers a high degree of assurance that a particular process will consistently produce a product meeting its predetermined specifications and quality attributes is the FDA's definition of validation. To obtain a strong, dependable separation for each activity, laboratories must assess combinations of mobile phase, pH, temperature, column chemistries, and gradient profiles. This is a laborious and complex process that takes time to develop and validate. With UPLC, methods can be optimized in as little as one or two hours, and analysis times can be as short as one minute. This greatly reduces the amount of time needed for method development and validation.

9.4.2. Manufacturing and QA/QC

When manufacturing a drug product, identity, purity, quality, safety, and efficacy are crucial considerations to make. Purity requirements for both raw materials and completed pharmaceutical products must be met for the successful production of high-quality pharmaceutical products. As part of quality assurance and control, material stability must also be continuously monitored. In QA/QC laboratories, highly regulated quantitative analyzes are carried out using UPLC. A registered analytical method relies heavily on the reliable and high-quality products that are consistently supplied.

9.4.3. Determination of FDC Products

A formulation of two or more medications combined in a single dosage form that is offered in specific fixed doses is known as a fixed dose combination (FDC) product. If the solubility differs significantly, developing a method for two or more drugs becomes extremely complicated. As a result, more advanced methods of analysis like UPLC-PDA and UPLC-QTOF/MS are required. Because of the short analysis times, a large number of samples can be analyzed daily.

9.4.4. Stability testing/Stress Testing

ICHQ1A (R2) states that forced degradation studies, or forced degradation studies of the drug substance, are conducted to identify degradation products, ascertain the molecule's intrinsic stability, and enhance the analytical methods' capacity to indicate stability. The primary disadvantage of HPLC-UV and/or HPLC-MS analytical techniques, which are typically employed for forced degradation studies, is their time-consuming nature and their inability to yield sufficient information about the resolution of all contaminants and degradation products. Changeable collision energy values provided by the UHPLC/Q-TOF-MS system enable the generation of mass information with acceptable accuracy and precision, which is ultimately beneficial in elucidating the structure, identifying drug fragmentation patterns, identifying degradation products, and establishing degradation mechanisms. The UPLC method has been effectively utilized by the authors to determine the contents of tablets containing aceclofenac, paracetamol, and their breakdown products.

9.4.5. Detection and Identification of Impurities

A drug product's efficacy, safety, and quality are all directly correlated with impurity profiling, which is required by many regulatory bodies. The related substances that arise in drugs during formulation or storage are known as impurities. When it comes to finding contaminants, mass spectrometry is among the best methods. The presence of impurities can be identified by the fragmentation pattern, additional peaks, and the highest mass peak value compared to the compound itself. Molecular fragments are produced by a fast change in collision energy, facilitating the quick identification of compounds and their associated impurities. One can easily propose the structure of the compound based on different fragments of the compound.

9.4.6. Dissolution Testing

Dissolution testing is a crucial step in the formulation, development, and production processes for quality control and drug release. The dissolution profile serves as evidence of the active ingredient's dependability and consistency from batch to batch. Dissolution testing is a crucial step in the formulation, development, and production processes for quality control and drug release. Testing more potent medications is crucial for sustained-release dosage formulations because dissolution may be the rate-limiting step in the delivery of the medication. The dissolution profile serves as evidence of the active ingredient's dependability and consistency from batch to batch. Additionally, enhanced analytical sensitivity is needed for more recent and powerful formulations. Accurate and dependable automated online sample acquisition is offered by UPLC. Dissolve testing is fully automated, starting with the drop of the pill and continuing through data collection, aliquot analysis, test result distribution, and publication management.

9.4.7. Pharmacokinetic and Bioequivalence Studies

A crucial component of development programs is the quantification of a drug in biological samples for pharmacokinetic, toxicity, and bioequivalency studies. Statistical pharmacokinetics (PK) analysis is one of the many uses for accurate and dependable data produced by UPLC-PDA's sensitivity and selectivity at low detection levels. Preclinical and clinical studies are used to test the drugs, which are typically low molecular weight.

9.4.8. Identification of Metabolites

Any chemical compound must have its metabolites identified once it has reached the development stage. To fully understand the compound's therapeutic efficacy, it is imperative to identify all associated metabolites. It has been effectively applied to metabolite studies by quantifying molecular ions and product ions in sample matrices through specific MS/MS transitions. Using TOF-MS, sub-2 μm particle UPLC columns and HPLC monolithic columns, the human metabolites of paracetamol were identified. In comparison to the HPLC system, the UHPLC system produced three times more sensitivity and detected metabolites. Metabolite profiling in a range of biological samples has been studied using MetaboLynx™ software in conjunction with UHPLC/Q-TOF. Drug discovery requires the biotransformation of new chemical entities (NCE). The process of metabolite identification becomes regulated when a compound enters the development stage.

9.4.9. Metabonomic Studies

Metabonomics is the study of how a drug product's biochemistry changes when it comes into contact with the human body. Drug metabolites can be discovered with the aid of metabolic studies. Its therapeutic and toxic aspects can be ascertained through metabolite identification. It has been used in the development of pharmaceuticals, especially in the quick in-vitro and in-vivo testing of medicinal products. Labs conduct metabolic studies to expedite the creation of novel medications. This method was used to determine the chemical structures of various components of red and white ginseng used in Chinese formulations. Metabonomics enhances comprehension of possible toxicity and permits efficacy monitoring by offering a quick and reliable way to identify these alterations. The biotechnology and chemical industry businesses benefit from similar discovery, development, and manufacturing processes when metabonomic and metabolomic information is properly applied. Amino acid analysis using UPLC is precise, dependable, and repeatable in the fields of protein characterization, cell culture observation, and food nutritional analysis.

9.4.10. Peptide Mapping

Peptide mapping is the process of determining the chemical structure of the linked peptide within a protein. When used to analyze complex molecules like proteins, this technique yields accurate results. The use of time-of-flight mass detection can facilitate the structural identification of proteins.

9.4.11. Analysis of Natural Products and Herbal Medicine

Complex samples derived from herbal traditional medicines and natural products have been identified. Using this technique, for instance, Asian ginseng and adulterated American ginseng preparations were separated through qualitative and quantitative analysis. The technique is useful for identifying and elucidating the structure of different isomeric compounds, including pseudoginsenoside and ginsenoside. Using fingerprinting, the chemical components of a well-known Chinese herbal remedy for stomach and intestinal injuries were investigated. To identify active compounds in extremely complex samples derived from natural products and traditional herbal medicines, UPLC offers high-quality separations and detection capabilities.

9.4.12. Screening of Antibiotics in Surface and Wastewater

Antibiotics have been found in surface water, influent, and effluent wastewaters using this technique. During the manufacturing process, these compounds are carried by the washing of machinery and transferred into the wastewater. Numerous antibiotics, including ciprofloxacin and ofloxacin, among others, have been identified and their residues in pharmaceutical industry wastewater have been confirmed. Using the multi-residue method, numerous pharmaceutical compounds from different therapeutic classes—such as beta-blockers, cholesterol-lowering agents, psychiatric medications, anti-ulcer agents, analgesics, and anti-inflammatory drugs—were identified and quantified. For every compound, the separation time was 10 minutes. By choosing different collision energy values for the compounds to fragment, the collision induced dissociation (CID) method was used to measure the masses of the compounds.

9.4.13. Therapeutic Drug Monitoring

The tracking of patients' plasma β-lactam antibiotic concentrations based on their individual pharmacokinetic profiles. In human plasma, the UPLC-MS/MS method was utilized to simultaneously estimate two β-lactamase inhibitors and seven β-lactam antibiotics. The technique's primary advantage is its ability to analyze data more quickly than other methods for this kind of multiple analytes. These days, a lot of biological specimen toxicological analyzes use this technique. These toxicants can be produced by the biotransformation of medications, excipients from drug products, by-products, intermediates, isomers, impurities, and degradation products. These substances can be found in blood, plasma, and urine at very low concentrations, all of which were simple to identify and measure.

9.4.14. Screening of Synthetic Compounds

The method is now a vital tool for high-throughput quality control screening of artificial pharmaceuticals. These high throughput analytical demands cannot be met by using more traditional techniques like NMR because of their relatively low sensitivity, high sample purity requirements, need for operator expertise, and usage of expensive solvents. It is shown that automation, when combined with the use of software for precise mass measurement, can streamline analytical procedures.

9.4.15. Identification of Unknown Pesticides

The technique is employed to detect pesticides in fruits and vegetables. Pesticides that contain both organic and inorganic compounds with complex chemical structures. The public's health depends on the identification of these hazardous substances in vegetables, which can be done using this delicate technique. Methods were employed to analyze the extremely low concentration of pesticide residue that was extracted from fruit packaging materials.

9.4.16. Analysis of Doping Agents

The approach has been used to analyze and control doping agents from different classes, including stimulants, narcotics, diuretics, and β-blockers. On the other hand, the developed methods were first applied for quantification and then used for doping agent screening. The World Anti-Doping Agency (WADA) determined that the method was reliable for identifying these restricted drugs. The World Anti-Doping

Code's guidelines were followed in the validation of the applied method.

9.4.17. Screening of Organic Pollutants in Water

It is used to identify organic pollutants in waste and natural water. The solid-phase extraction process produced the samples. The analysis was performed using the common addition method. This method was used to analyze organic pollutants that were mixed with water samples in a range of concentration levels, sourced from different sources. The created technique was used to identify and detect a number of organic pollutants as well as antibiotics, analgesics, and anti-inflammatory medications.

9.4.18. High-throughput Screening (HTS)

High-throughput screening (HTS) is a methodical approach to screening and assaying organic, synthetic, and pharmaceutical compounds. The HTS method has been extensively employed in drug discovery and design for the purpose of identifying, characterizing, and quantifying chemical compounds. The therapeutic, metabolic, pharmacokinetic, toxicological, analytical, and degradation data of novel drugs can be obtained by using the HTS methods. During the drug development process, it lowers costs, time, material consumption, and solvent consumption. Complete knowledge of a drug's therapeutically useful metabolites and derivatives is essential for both drug design and discovery. The compound's ability to treat depends on all of its metabolites being formed during the biotransformation process, and it is crucial to identify each of these metabolites. Metabonomics is the study of how drugs are metabolized and how metabolites and their derivatives are formed. The UHPLC/Q-TOF-MS technique is a relatively new method in the era of developed and modified chromatographic techniques, and it is used in drug discovery and development worldwide.

9.4.19. Iodinated Byproducts in Drinking Water (IBP)

The structures of a number of iodinated byproducts in water (IDBPs) treated with chlorine and chlorine-ammonia have been proposed and quantitatively analyzed with the aid of UPLC coupled to electrospray ionization-triple quadrupole mass spectrometer (ESI-tqMS).

9.4.20. Toxicity Studies

Toxicological problems during the drug development process lead to a drop in drug candidates, which costs the company money. Assessing potential medications for toxicity, drug-drug interactions, and potential inhibition or initiation of metabolizing enzymes in the body is a challenging task. Because of its high resolution, UPLC enables accurate detection. Furthermore, peaks at low concentrations can be detected thanks to its sensitivity. These elements reduce sample analysis failure rates and analysis times.

A Closer Look

Nonsteroidal Anti-inflammatory Drugs (NSAIDs)

NSAIDs, known as non-steroidal anti-inflammatory drugs, are widely used medications that help decrease pain, inflammation, and fever. They achieve this by blocking the action of enzymes called cyclooxygenase (COX), with a focus on COX-1 and COX-2. These enzymes play a role in producing prostaglandins, which are lipid compounds responsible for causing inflammation, pain, and fever.

NSAIDs are commonly used to treat a wide range of ailments, such as headaches, menstrual cramps, acute injuries, and musculoskeletal pain (such as arthritis and back pain). They are available in different forms such as tablets, capsules, creams, gels, and patches, and can be obtained over-the-counter or with a prescription.

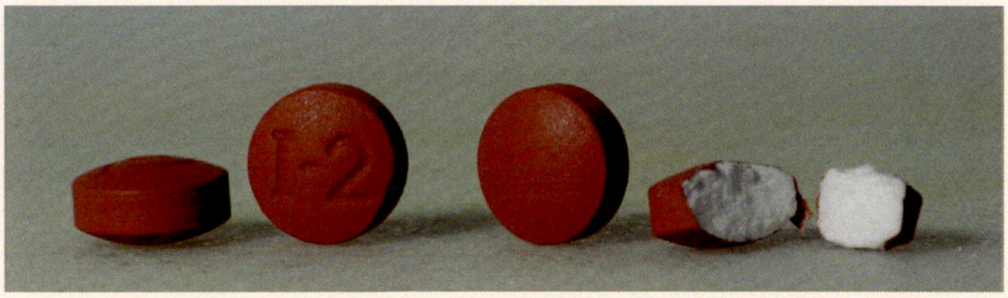

NSAIDs: By Ragesoss – Own work, CC BY-SA 3.0, https://commons.wikimedia.org/w/index.php?curid=3530009.

Inhibiting COX enzymes reduces the synthesis of prostaglandins, which is the main mechanism of action of NSAIDs. Prostaglandins stimulate pain receptors, increase vascular permeability, and promote vasodilation, all of which contribute to inflammation. NSAIDs help to relieve pain, lower fever, and reduce inflammation by decreasing prostaglandin synthesis.

The way NSAIDs are categorized depends on how well they select for COX enzymes. Conventional nonsteroidal anti-inflammatory drugs (NSAIDs) like aspirin, ibuprofen, and naproxen inhibit the enzymes COX-1 and COX-2, which results in a wide range of anti-inflammatory, analgesic, and antipyretic effects. However, because they inhibit the cytoprotective effects of COX1 on the gastric mucosa, they are linked to gastrointestinal (GI) side effects like ulcers and bleeding.

Celecoxib is one example of a selective COX-2 inhibitor that targets COX-2 enzymes specifically while maintaining the gastroprotective properties of COX-1. They have a lower risk of gastrointestinal adverse effects, but they may raise the risk of cardiovascular events, like heart attacks and stroke, especially in people who already have cardiovascular risk factors or who use them for an extended period of time.

NSAIDs are effective at treating pain and inflammation, but they do have some drawbacks. Renal failure, cardiovascular issues, and gastrointestinal discomfort are typical side effects. Hypertension, gastrointestinal bleeding, and kidney damage are additional risks linked to long-term NSAID use.

Summary

- Analytical chemistry has a significant presence in the pharmaceutical industry, especially in the drug development process providing quality assurance, safety, and efficacy of new medicines.
- Within the pharmaceutical industry, there are three broad analytical techniques adopted for determining structure, separating analytes, and quantifying target molecules.
- Chromatography methods have a strong presence in the pharmaceutical industry due to their accuracy of separation and detection.
- The natural and synthetic bioactive compounds are analyzed by the TLC technique.
- High-performance liquid chromatography (HPLC) is the dominant technique in pharmaceutical and phytochemical analysis of various bioactive compounds.
- GC is a useful technique for testing any volatile substances, such as essential oils, which are a promising group of natural products of the aromatic plants, as a result of their various biological effects, i.e., their antioxidant, antibacterial, antimicrobial, and antitumor activities.
- Pharmaceutical spectroscopy equipment comes in many forms, and its variety makes it accessible to a broad range of research professionals working within diverse budgets.
- Near-infrared spectroscopy (NIRS) is a rapid and nondestructive procedure that provides multi-component analysis of almost any matrix.
- Mass spectrometry (MS) is a powerful analytical technique widely used by chemists, biologists, medical researchers, and environmental and forensic scientists, among others.
- Identity, purity, quality, safety and efficacy are the important factors to be considered while manufacturing a drug product.

References

1. Ahirrao, V. K., Jadhav, R. A., Rane, V. P., Bhamare, H. R., & Yeole, R. D. (2020). Time-dependent selected reaction monitoring-based GC-MS/MS method for estimation of genotoxic impurities in new antibacterial agent: Alalevonadifloxacin mesylate. *Journal of Analytical Science & Technology, 11*, 22.
2. Al-Jaber, H. I., Shakya, A. K., & Elagbar, Z. A. (2020). HPLC profiling of selected phenolic acids and flavonoids in *Salvia eigii*, *Salvia hierosolymitana* and *Salvia viridis* growing wild in Jordan and their in vitro antioxidant activity. *PeerJ*, 8, e9769.
3. Al-Khateeb, A. L., & Dahas, F. H. (2021). Green method development approach of superheated water liquid chromatography for separation and trace determination of non-steroidal anti-inflammatory compounds in pharmaceutical and water samples and their extraction. *Arabian Journal of Chemistry, 14*, 103226.
4. Almeida, R. S., Freitas, P. R., Araújo, A. C. J., Alencar Menezes, I. R., Santos, E. L., & Ferreira, V. A. (2020). GC-MS profile and enhancement of antibiotic activity by the essential oil of *Ocotea odorífera* and safrole: Inhibition of *Staphylococcus aureus* efflux pumps. *Antibiotics, 9*, 247.
5. Aranaz, P., Navarro-Herrera, D., Zabala, M., Romo-Hualde, A., López-Yoldi, M., Vizmanos, J. L.,

Milagro, F. I., & González-Navarro, C. J. (2020). Phenolic compounds reduce the fat content in Caenorhabditis elegans by affecting lipogenesis, lipolysis, and different stress responses. *Pharmaceuticals, 13*, 355.

6. Assali, M., Abualhasan, M., Zohud, N., & Ghazal, N. (2020). RP-HPLC method development and validation of synthesized codrug in combination with indomethacin, paracetamol, and famotidine. *International Journal of Analytical Chemistry*, *2020*, 1894907.
7. Bobakulov, K., Ozek, G., Ozek, T., Asilbekova, D. T., Abdullaev, N. D., Sagdullaev, S. S., & Başer, K. H. C. (2020). Essential oils and lipids from the flowers of two varieties of *Ocimum basilicum* L. cultivated in Uzbekistan. *Journal of Essential Oil Research, 32*, 323–330.
8. Boukhatem, M. N., Sudha, T., Darwish, N. H. E., Chader, H., Belkadi, A., & Mousa, S. A. (2020). A new eucalyptol-rich lavender (*Lavandula stoechas* L.) essential oil: Emerging potential for therapy against inflammation and cancer. *Molecules, 25*, 3671.
9. Cherfia, R., Zaiter, A., Akkal, S., Chaimbault, P., Abdelwahab, A. B., & Chaouche, N. K. (2020). New approach in the characterization of bioactive compounds isolated from *Calycotome spinose* (*L.*) Link leaves by the use of negative electrospray ionization LITMSn, LC-ESI-MS/MS, as well as NMR analysis. *Bioorganic Chemistry, 96*, 103535.
10. Dobričić, V., Turković, N., Ivković, B., Csuvik, O., & Vujić, Z. (2020). Evaluation of the lipophilicity of chalcones by RP-TLC and computational methods. *Journal of Planar Chromatography, 33*, 245–253.
11. Dołowy, M., Jampilek, J., & Bober-Majnusz, K. (2021). A comparative study of the lipophilicity of metformin and phenformin. *Molecules, 26*, 6613.
12. Fanali, S., Haddad, P. R., Poole, C., & Riekkola, M. L. (2017). *Liquid Chromatography Fundamentals and Instrumentation* (2nd ed.). Elsevier-Science. pages-1-808
13. Farràs, M., Miret, J., Camps, M., Román, R., Martínez, Ó., Pujol, X., & Cairó, J. J. (2020). Heavy chain dimers stabilized by disulfide bonds are required to promote in vitro assembly of trastuzumab. *BMC Molecular and Cell Biology, 21*, 2.
14. Farràs, M., Román, R., Camps, M., Miret, J., Martínez, Ó., Pujol, X., & Cairó, J. J. (2020). Homogeneous antibody-drug conjugates: DAR 2 anti-HER2 obtained by conjugation on isolated light chain followed by mAb assembly. *mAbs, 12*, 1702262.
15. Fayed, E. M., Abd-Elgawad, A. M., Elshamy, A. I., El-Halawany, E. S. F., & El-Amier, Y. A. (2021). Essential oil of *Deverra tortuosa* aerial parts: Detailed chemical profile, allelopathic, antimicrobial, and antioxidant activities. *Chemistry & Biodiversity, 18*, e2000914.
16. Folashade, K. O., Omoregie, E. H., & Ochogu, A. P. (2012). Standardization of herbal medicines—A review. *International Journal of Biodiversity & Conservation, 4*, 101–112.
17. Fu, Z. -H., Wu, G., Li, M., Cui, Y. -F., & Wang, L. (2021). Quality study of recombinant anti-interleukin-23 monoclonal antibodies. *Chinese Journal of New Drugs, 30*, 1738–1745.
18. Gagnon, P., Goricar, B., Mencin, N., Zvanut, T., Peljhan, S., Leskovec, M., & Strancar, A. (2021). Multiple-monitor HPLC assays for rapid process development, In-process monitoring, and validation of AAV production and purification. *Pharmaceutics, 13*, 113.
19. Grinberg, N., & Carr, P. W. (2020). *Advances in Chromatography* (Vol. 57). CRC Press. Pages 1-278
20. Guaadaoui, A., Benaicha, S., Elmajdoub, N., Bellaoui, M., & Hamal, A. (2014). What is a bioactive

compound? A combined definition for a preliminary consensus. *International Journal of Food Science & Nutrition, 3*, 174–179.

21. Hassan, M. M., & Nam, S. (2021). Isocratic reverse-phase HPLC method for determination of aspirin, paracetamol, and naproxen. *Preprints,* 2021070229. https://doi.org/10.20944/preprints202107.0229.v1
22. Hassan, M. M., & Nam, S. W. (2021). High-performance liquid chromatography for determining a mixture of nonsteroidal anti-inflammatory drugs. *Electronic Materials Letters, 17*, 414–420.
23. Issaq, H. J. (2001). *A Century of Separation Science*. CRC Press. 1st Edition, Pages 1-776
24. Iwueke, A. V., Ejekwumadu, N. J., Chukwu, E. C., Nwodu, J. A., & Akalonu, C. (2020). Nutritional composition and GC-MS phytochemical analysis of *Thaumatococcus daniellii* leaves. *European Journal of Nutrition & Food Safety, 12*, 81–86.
25. Izuegbuna, O., Otunola, G. A., & Bradley, G. (2021). GC-MS profiling and antineoplastic activity of *Pelargonium inquinans ait* leaves on acute leukemia cell lines U937 and Jurkat. *Nutrition and Cancer*, *3*, 1–23.
26. Jayapala, N., Elavarasan, A. R., Chaudhari, S. R., & Vallikannan, B. (2020). Cytotoxicity and 3T3-L1 cell uptake of lactucaxanthin purified and characterized by LC-MS and NMR from lettuce (*Lactuca sativa*). *Journal of Liquid Chromatography & Related Technologies, 43*, 233–246.
27. Kalala, W. M., Foubert, K., Pieters, L., & Maregesi, S. (2020). HPLC-SPE-NMR analysis of furanosesquiterpenoids from bark exudates of *Commiphora swynnertonii* Burrt. *Phytochemistry Letters, 38*, 128–132.
28. Kupriyanova, O. V., Milyukov, V. A., Shevyrin, V. A., Sadykova, R. G., & Mustafin, R. I. (2020). Development and validation of a gas chromatographic method for quantitative determination of the active ingredient in phenyl salicylate drug substance. *Pharmaceutical Chemistry Journal, 54*, 73–78.
29. Liu, J., Xie, B., Mai, B., Cai, Q., He, R., Guo, D., & Zhang, W. (2021). Development of a sensitive and stable GC-MS/MS method for simultaneous determination of four N-nitrosamine genotoxic impurities in sartan substances. *Journal of Analytical Science & Technology, 12*, 3.
30. Magdy, M. A., & Abdelfatah, R. M. (2020). Green validated HPTLC and HPLC methods for determination of ephedrine hydrochloride and naphazoline nitrate in the presence of methylparaben, in their pure forms and pharmaceutical formulation. *Journal of Planar Chromatography - Modern TLC*, *33*, 141–148.
31. Megawati, D. S., Fasya, A. G., Pratiwi, R. A., & Maghfiroh, N. (2020). Pharmacology potency of thin layer chromatography steroid isolates of *Chlorella sp.* chloroform fraction. *IOP Conference Series: Earth and Environmental Science, 456*, 012012.
32. Moller, A. C., Parra, C., Said, B., Werner, E., Flores, S., Villena, J., & Madrid, A. (2021). Antioxidant and anti-proliferative activity of essential oil and main components from leaves of *Aloysia polystachya* harvested in central Chile. *Molecules, 26*, 131.
33. Morak-Młodawska, B., Pluta, K., & Jeleń, M. (2020). Evaluation of the lipophilicity of new anticancer 1,2,3-triazole-dipyridothiazine hybrids using RP TLC and different computational methods. *Processes*, *8*, 858.
34. Mustafa, G., Arif, R., Atta, A., Sharif, S., & Jamil, A. (2017). Bioactive compounds from medicinal plants and their importance in drug discovery in Pakistan. *Matrix Science Pharma*, *1*, 17–26.

35. Mykhailenko, O., Gudžinskas, Z., Romanova, S., Orlova, T., Kozyra, S., Harna, S., & Volochai, V. (2021). The comparative analysis of carboxylic acid composition of four *Iris* species from Ukraine. *Chemistry & Biodiversity, 18*, e2000969.

36. Nomura, S., Ito, Y., Takegami, S., & Kitade, T. (2020). Development of trace analysis for alkyl methanesulfonates in the delgocitinib drug substance using GC-FID and liquid-liquid extraction with ionic liquid. *Open Chemistry, 18*, 1020–1029.

37. Ovidi, E., Masci, V. L., Taddei, A. R., Paolicelli, P., Petralito, S., Trilli, J., & Giacomello, P. (2020). Chemical investigation and screening of anti-proliferative activity on human cell lines of pure and nano-formulated lavandin essential oil. *Pharmaceuticals, 13*, 352.

38. Parab, M., Shirsat, V. A., Kodgule, Y. M., & Kodgule, M. (2021). A RP-HPLC method for the analysis of neostigmine methylsulfate and process-related impurities, forced degradation studies, in the injection formulation. *International Journal of Analytical Chemistry, 2021*, 5570173. Int J Anal Chem. 2021; 2021: 5570173.

39. Parys, W., Pyka-Pająk, A., & Dołowy, M. (2021). A cost-effective and sensitive TLC-densitometric identification of meloxicam. *Acta Pharmaceutica, 71*, 143–152.

40. Patil, S., Kantikar, G., Koppula, S., & Koppula, P. (2021). Identification and characterization of a new process related impurity in terbutaline sulfate by Accurate-Mass Q-TOF LC/MS/MS and NMR. *Chromatographia, 84*, 381–391.

41. Prajapati, P., & Agrawal, Y. K. (2014). Analysis and impurity identification in pharmaceuticals. *Reviews in Analytical Chemistry, 33*, 123–133.

42. Ramakrishna, R. H., Pratap, S. R., Chandrasekhar, N., & Shamshuddin, S. Z. M. (2021). A simple gas chromatography method for the quantitative determination of related impurity (1,4-butanediol) in busulfan drug. *Rasāyan Journal of Chemistry, 14*, 914–919.

43. Reddy, K., Gurupadayya, B. M., Choezom, L., & Vikram, H. (2021). Determination of phytocomponents and validation of squalene in ethanolic extract of *Clerodendrum serratum* Linn. roots—Using gas chromatography-mass spectroscopy and GC-FID technique. *Journal of Analytical Science & Technology, 12*, 31.

44. Rodrigues, F. N., & Maria, M. O. (2017). Applications of recovered bioactive compounds in cosmetics and health care products. In *Olive Mill Waste, Recent Advances for Sustainable Management* (pp. 255–274). Academic Press.

45. Sahu, A., Balhara, A., Raju, N., Kumar, B. K., Sharma, P., Singh, D. K., & Singh, S. (2021). Characterization of degradation products of celiprolol hydrochloride using hyphenated mass and NMR techniques. *Journal of Pharmaceutical and Biomedical Analysis, 197*, 113953.

46. Santos, A. L., Soares, M. G., de Medeiros, L. S., Ferreira, M. J. P., & Sartorelli, P. (2021). Identification of flavonoid-3-O-glycosides from leaves of *Casearia arborea* (*Salicaceae*) by UHPLC-DAD-ESI-HRMS/MS combined with molecular networking and NMR. *Phytochemical Analysis, 32*, 1–8.

47. Savych, A., Basaraba, R., Muzyka, N., & Ilashchuk, P. (2021). Analysis of fatty acid composition content in the plant components of antidiabetic herbal mixture by GC-MS. *Pharmacia, 68*, 433–439.

48. Savych, A., Marchyshyn, S., & Millan, I. (2021). Determination of carbohydrates in the herbal antidiabetic mixtures by GC-MS. *Acta Pharmaceutica, 71*, 429–443.

49. Savych, A., Marchyshyn, S., Harnyk, M., Kudria, V., & Ocheretniuk, A. (2021). Determination of amino acids content in two samples of the plant mixtures by GC-MS. *Pharmacia, 68*, 283–289.
50. Savych, A., Marchyshyn, S., Kozyr, H., & Yarema, N. (2021). Determination of inulin in the herbal mixtures by GC-MS method. *Pharmacia, 68*, 181–187.
51. Sianipar, N. F., Assidqi, K., Hadisaputri, Y. E., Salam, S., Tarigan, R., & Purnamaningsih, R. (2021). Determination of bioactive compounds of superior mutant rodent tuber (*Typhonium flagelliforme*) in various fractions using GC-MS. *Earth and Environmental Science*, *794*, 012144.
52. Slobodianiuk, L., Budniak, L., Marchyshyn, S., Kostyshyn, L., & Zakharchuk, O. (2021). Analysis of carbohydrates in *Saponaria officinalis* L. using GC/MS method. *Pharmacia, 68*, 339–345.
53. Sulborska, A., Konarska, A., Matysik-Woźniak, A., Dmitruk, M., Weryszko-Chmielewska, E., & Rejdak, R. (2020). Phenolic constituents of *Lamium album L.* subsp. *album* flowers: Anatomical, histochemical, and phytochemical study. *Molecules, 25*, 6025.
54. Teles, A. M., Silva-Silva, J. V., Fernandes, J. M. P., Abreu-Silva, A. L., Calabrese, K. S., & Almeida-Souza, F. (2021). GC-MS characterization of antibacterial, antioxidant, and antitrypanosomal activity of *Syzygium aromaticum* essential oil and eugenol. *Evidence-Based Complementary and Alternative Medicine*, *2021*, 6663255.
55. Tot, K., Lazić, A., & Djaković-Sekulić, T. (2020). A comparative study of chromatographic lipophilicity and bioactivity parameters of selected spirohydantoins. *Journal of Liquid Chromatography & Related Technologies, 43*, 925–933.
56. Ul-Khazir, Z., Yatoo, G. N., Wani, H., Shah, S. A., Zargar, M. I., & Banday, J. A. (2021). Gas chromatographic-mass spectrometric analysis, antibacterial, antioxidant and antiproliferative activities of the needle essential oil of *Abies pindrow* growing wild in Kashmir, India. *Microbial Pathogenesis*, *158*, 105013.
57. Vardhani Devi, D. P. V., Narayanarao, K. M. V., Shyamala, P., Krishna, R. M., & Prasad, K. S. (2020). Determination of 1,2-dibromoethane in tramadol hydrochloride drug substances by head space gas chromatography linked with mass spectrometry. *International Journal of Pharmaceutical Research, 12*, 949–954.
58. Wang, X., Zuo, G. -L., Wang, C. Y., Kim, H. Y., Lim, S. S., & Tong, S. Q. (2020). An off-line DPPH-GC-MS coupling countercurrent chromatography method for screening, identification, and separation of antioxidant compounds in essential oil. *Antioxidants*, *9*, 702.
59. Yang, F., Duan, X., Wang, Z., & Dong, Y. (2022). A gas chromatography flame ionization detector method for rapid simultaneous separation and determination of six active ingredients of anticold drug. *Current Pharmaceutical Analysis, 18*, 71–81.
60. Zakaria Nabti, L., Sahli, F., Laouar, H., Olowo-okere, A., Nkuimi Wandjou, J. G., & Maggi, F. (2020). Chemical composition and antibacterial activity of essential oils from the Algerian endemic *Origanum glandulosum* Desf. against multidrug-resistant uropathogenic *E. coli* Isolates. *Antibiotics*, *9*, 29.
61. Zekič, J., Vovk, I., & Glavnik, V. (2021). Extraction and analyses of flavonoids and phenolic acids from *Canadian Goldenrod* and *Giant Goldenrod*. *Forests, 12*, 40.
62. Zhou, L., Li, J., Kong, Q., Luo, S., Wang, J., Feng, S., & Ding, C. (2021). Chemical composition, antioxidant, antimicrobial, and phytotoxic potential of *Eucalyptus grandis* × *E. urophylla* leaves essential oils. *Molecules, 26*, 1450.

Chapter

REGULATORY AFFAIRS AND DRUG DEVELOPMENT

10

Contents

Introduction

Regulatory affairs (RA) specialists work across the whole drug development lifecycle, from discovery and R&D through commercialization, to guarantee safe, effective, and regulatory-compliant pharmaceutical products. To create and carry out regulatory strategies, they collaborate closely with manufacturers, researchers, and regulatory agencies.

`After a lead compound has been found through the process of drug discovery, the process of developing a new pharmaceutical drug is known as drug development. Preclinical research on microbes and animals is part of it, as is applying for regulatory status—for example, through the US Food and Drug Administration—for an investigational new drug to start human clinical trials. It may also involve the process of getting regulatory approval with a new drug application to commercialize the medication. It usually takes more than ten years to complete the entire process, from conception to preclinical testing in the lab to clinical trial development, including Phase I–III trials, to an approved vaccine or medication.

Orientation and Directional Terms

Term	Definition	Illustration
Drug approval	Drug approval is the process by which a government ruling authority validates a medicinal preparation for a therapeutic use.	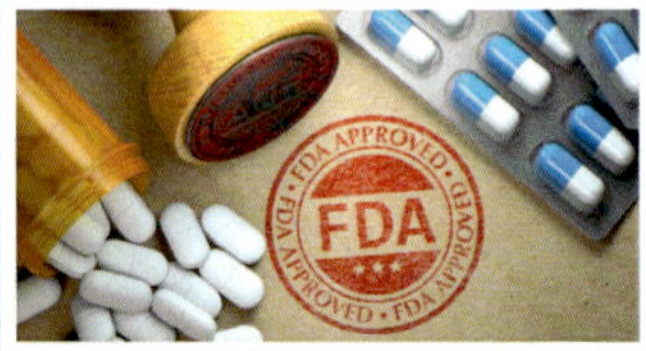
Drug development	Drug development is the process of bringing a new drug or device to market, which involves multiple disciplines.	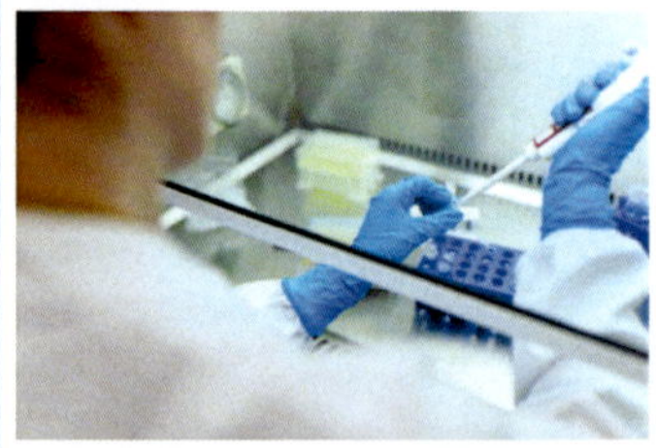
Digital disruption	Digital disruption is represented via digital capabilities, channels, or assets that are also the main causes of digital disruption.	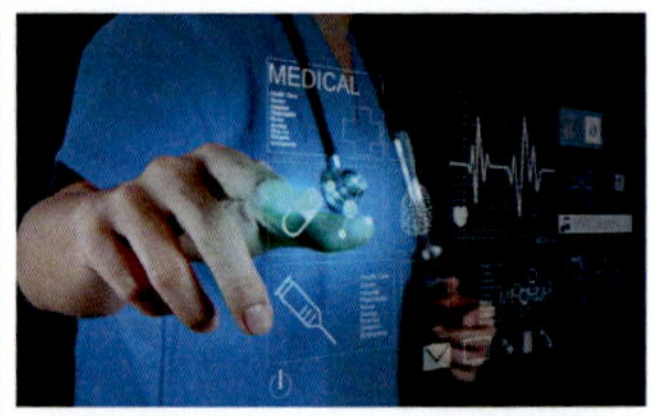
Good Manufacturing Practice	Good Manufacturing Practice (GMP) is a system for ensuring that products are consistently produced and controlled according to quality standards.	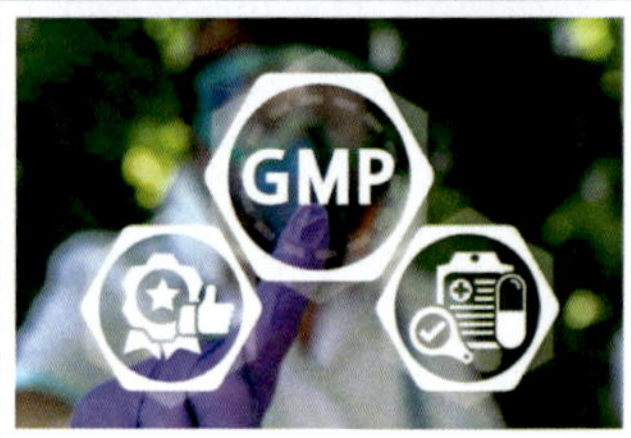
Regulatory Affairs	Regulatory Affairs plays a key role in the pharmaceutical industry: from drug development to commercialization.	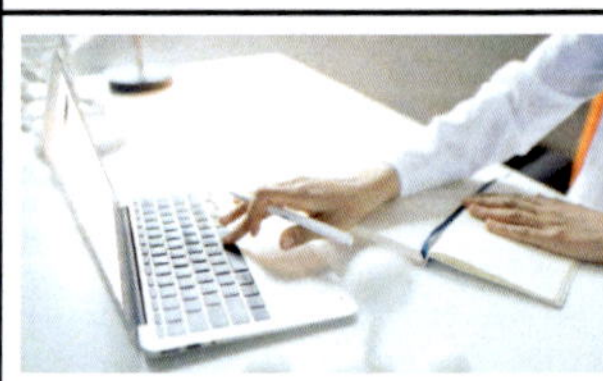
Regulatory science	Regulatory science is a broad term that refers to the scientific methods used to evaluate and approve medical products, including drugs, biologics, and devices.	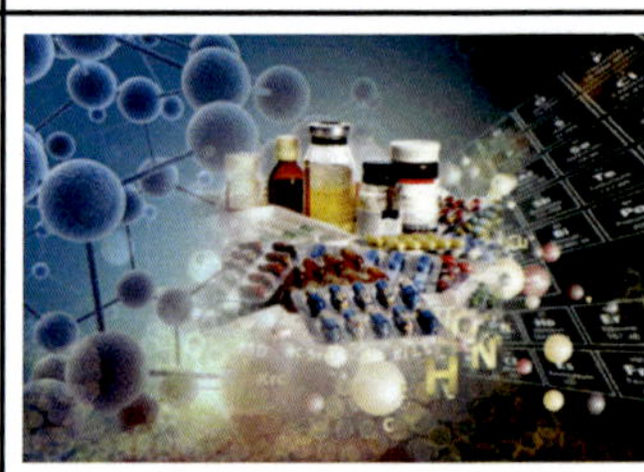

10.1. Regulatory Requirements and Drug Approval Process

The current state of regulatory affairs indicates that different nations must adhere to distinct regulatory standards to approve new drug applications for marketing authorization (MAAs). Every nation has a regulatory body that is in charge of issuing guidelines to control the marketing of pharmaceuticals and enforcing laws and regulations.

To verify a drug's safety and efficacy, nonclinical studies should be carried out once a lead drug molecule has been identified. Clinical trials can then be carried out following the submission of an application to the relevant national authority. Clinical trials are conducted in accordance with protocol during all three phases. When a drug application is reviewed by the appropriate authority and it is determined that the drug addresses quality, safety, and efficacy concerns, the application is approved for marketing. Even after a new drug is approved, the government should conduct post-marketing surveillance, or Phase IV surveillance, to ensure its safety. Even though the drug approval process varies somewhat from nation to nation, there are some commonalities as well.

Currently, approval of a new drug is subject to varying regulatory requirements across different countries. It is nearly impossible to find a single regulatory approach for Marketing Authorization Applications (MAA) that is applicable to multiple countries. As a result, it is essential to understand the legal requirements for MAA in each nation. Every nation has its own set of regulations that must be met in order for a new drug to be approved there.

Adopting a single regulatory strategy for a new drug's approval across national borders is challenging. Therefore, it is necessary to become knowledgeable about the regulatory concerns of different nations. Since the United States of America (USA) and the European Union (EU) are widely recognized as the two largest potential markets for pharmaceutical products worldwide, many businesses concentrate on their pharmaceutical laws. Thus, the US, EU, and Indian regulatory strategies are highlighted in this section.

First and foremost, a lead molecule for a target disease needs to be optimized upon identification. Pre-clinical trials are carried out on animals to verify the safety and effectiveness of newly discovered drugs. To obtain authorization for conducting clinical research, a request for permission should be made to the relevant authority in the relevant nation. To ensure safety and efficacy, clinical trials are conducted in four stages, after which the drug dose is optimized in humans. If the drug satisfies the requirements of safety and efficacy and demonstrates that its benefits outweigh its risks, a Marketing Authorization Application (MAA) is then submitted and approved by the relevant authority (Figure 10.1).

A new drug application (NDA) is a request for permission to market a new drug that is made to the relevant regulatory body, i.e., creative product. A sponsor must submit preclinical and clinical test results, a description of manufacturing trials, and drug information for analysis to be granted permission.

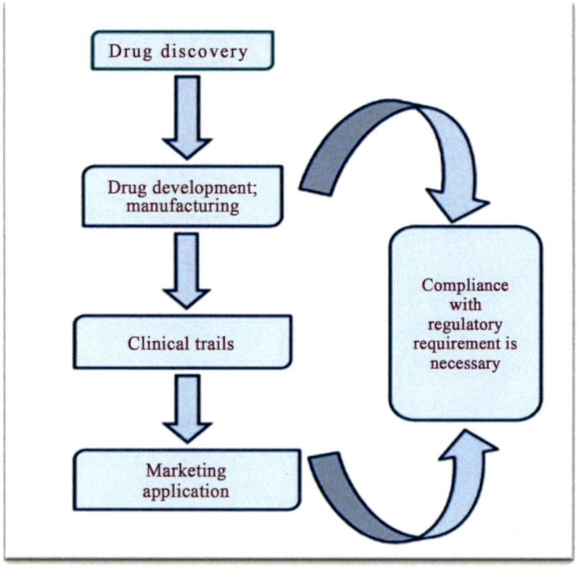

Figure 10.1. *Regulation of drug approval.*

Source: Sawant, A. M., Mali, D. P., & Bhagwat, D. A. (2018). Regulatory requirements and drug approval process in India, Europe and US. Pharmaceut Reg Affairs 7: 210. doi: 10.4172/2167-7689.1000210.

Different phases of clinical trials

- Pre-clinical study
- Phase I – Clinical trial
- Phase II – Exploratory trial
- Phase III – Confirmatory trial
- Phase IV – Post-Marketing trial.

Once the agency receives the NDA, it will be subjected to a technical evaluation to verify that all necessary data and information have been provided in each section to proceed with the application. After the review of the NDA is complete, there are three possible actions that may be taken and communicated to the sponsor.

- Not approvable – list of issues are sent
- Approvable – changes and post-approval studies
- Approval – approved
- Appropriate discussions

10.1.1. Drug Approval Process in India

The Indian parliament established the Drug and Cosmetic Act 1940 and Rules 1945 to control the import, production, distribution, and retailing of pharmaceuticals and cosmetics. It was decided to create the Drugs Controller General (DCGI) office and the Central Drugs Standard Control Organization (CDSCO). The Indian government amended the 1945 Drug and Cosmetics Rules by adding Schedule Y in 1988. The requirements and guidelines for clinical trials are outlined in Schedule Y, which was updated in 2005 to conform to internationally recognized standards. A company in India must apply for permission from the licensing authority (DCGI) by filing Form 44 and providing the information specified in Schedule Y of the Drugs and Cosmetics Act 1940 and Rules 1945 to manufacture or import a new drug. It must conduct clinical trials in compliance with the guidelines outlined in Schedule Y and submit the results of those trials in the format required to demonstrate its efficacy and safety in the Indian population.

10.1.1.1. Rule

According to Section 122A of the Drug and Cosmetics Act, clinical trials may not be required for novel medications that have received approval and have been in use for a number of years in other nations. Schedule Y of the Drugs and Cosmetics Act 1940 and Rules 1945 stipulates in Section 2.4(a) that drug substances found in India must undergo clinical trials through all stages of the process. According to Schedule Y, Drugs and Cosmetics Act 1940 and Rules 1945, Section 2.4(b) states that if a drug substance is found in a country other than India, the applicant must submit the data that is available from those other countries. The licensing authority may then require the applicant to repeat all of the studies or approve the applicant to move forward with Phase III clinical trials. Before the Central Drugs Standard Control Organization (CDSCO) will approve a drug product for import or for the applicant to manufacture a new drug, the drug product must demonstrate its safety and efficacy for use in humans. Regulations 122A, 122B, and 122D of the Drugs and Cosmetics Act 1940 and its rules 1945 outline the data needed to approve an application to import or produce a new drug for commercialization. The DCGI needs the following information:

Generic name

1. Patent status
2. Brief description of physico-chemical/biological
3. Technical information
    i. Stability
    ii. Specifications
    iii. Manufacturing process
    iv. Worldwide regulatory status
    v. Animal pharmacology and toxicity studies
4. Published clinical trial reports
5. Proposed protocol and proforma
6. Trial duration
7. During Masterfile
8. Undertaking to Report Serious or Life-threatening Adverse Drug Reactions.

The status of the drug in other nations determines the necessity of local clinical trials in India. Phase III trials are typically necessary if the medication has previously received approval in another nation. In India, phase I trials are not permitted unless there is international data availability. DCGI gives the go-ahead to carry out Phase I trials in India if the medication has a unique bearing on an Indian health issue, such as tuberculosis or malaria.

Studies on bioavailability and bioequivalency (BABE) ought to be carried out in accordance with BABE guidelines. In addition to safety and efficacy data, detailed information about the drug's marketing status in other nations is also needed. It is also necessary to submit information about the prescription, samples, testing procedures, product monographs, and labels. In India, approval of a clinical trial typically takes three months. Clinical trials can be registered in the Clinical Trials Registry of India (CTRI), which provides information about the trials' subjects and specifics. The rules to be followed under The Drugs and Cosmetics Rules 1945 are:

1. Rule122-A: Application for permission to import new drug
2. Rule122-B: Application for approval to manufacture new drug other than the drugs specified under Schedule C and C (1).
3. Rule122-D: Permission to import or manufacture fixed dose combination.
4. Rule122-DA: Application for permission to conduct clinical trials for New Drug/Investigational New Drug.
5. Rule122-DAB: Compensation in the case of injury or death during the clinical trials.

The Drugs and Cosmetics Act has been amended to define Phase I–IV trials and to clearly outline the roles and responsibilities of sponsors and investigators. In 2006, the clinical trials were further split into two groups. Clinical trials can be carried out in other markets with capable and developed regulatory frameworks under one category (category A), while the remaining ones fall under a different category (category B) Other than A. Category A clinical trials, which are authorized in the U.S. S. Fast tracking is available in India for countries like the United Kingdom, Switzerland, Australia, Canada, Germany, South Africa, Japan, and the European Union. Approval times typically take eight weeks. Category B clinical trials undergo more scrutiny and are approved in 16–18 weeks. DCGI should receive an application for conducting clinical trials in India along with the data from manufacturing, chemistry, control, and animal studies. Attached should be the date of the trial protocol, investigator brochures, and informed consent paperwork. Clinical trials are only carried out with DCGI and ethical committee approval, and a copy of the application must be submitted to them.

Stages of Approval

1. Submission of Clinical Trial application for evaluating safety and efficacy.
2. Requirements for permission of new drugs approval.
3. Post approval changes in biological products: quality, safety and efficacy documents.
4. Preparation of the quality information for drugs mission for new drug approval.

The CTD format is used in the majority of countries. As a result, CDSCO has also chosen to use the CTD format for the technical specifications needed to register pharmaceutical products for use in humans (Figure 10.2).

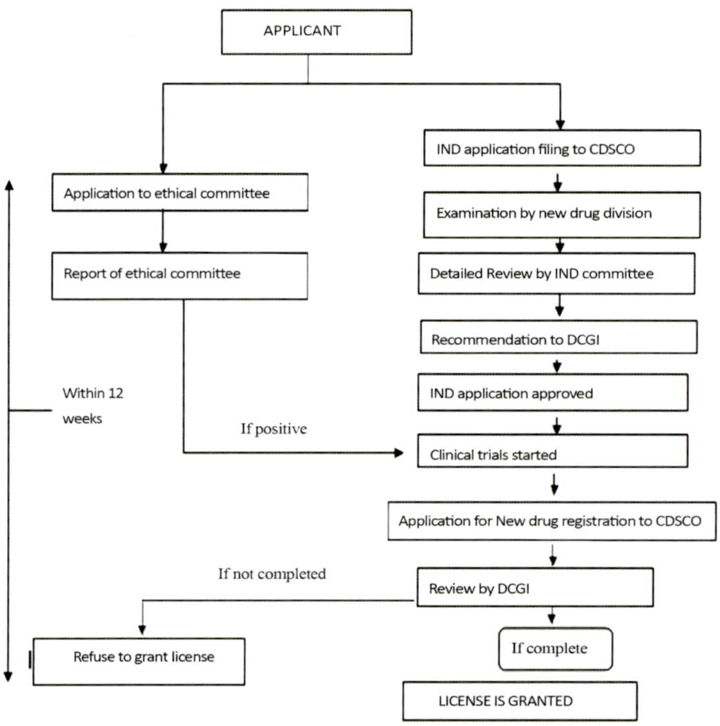

Figure 10.2. *Drug approval process in India.*

Source: Sawant AM, Mali DP, Bhagwat DA (2018). zgulatory requirements and drug approval process in India, Europe and US. Pharmaceut Reg Affairs 7: 210. doi: 10.4172/2167-7689.1000210.

10.1.2. Drug Approval Process in Europe

To coordinate the evaluation and oversight of pharmaceutical products intended for both human and veterinary use among the member states of the European Union (EU), the European Medicines Evaluation Agency (EMEA) was founded in London in 1995. It established an open process for the creation, review, approval, and application of pharmaceutical guidelines. In European countries, there are two stages involved in the drug approval process.

1. Clinical trial.
2. Marketing authorization.

The application for a clinical trial (CTA) is submitted to the state's appropriate authority to carry out the clinical trial inside the European Union (EU). The application is assessed by the relevant body in that member state. Only after approval are the clinical trials carried out. An application for marketing authorization is only submitted once all three clinical trial phases have been finished. The Rules Governing Medicinal Products in the European Union are a series of volumes that contain the European legislation containing the pharmaceutical directives.

- Volume 1: Pharmaceutical Legislation for Medicinal Products for human use
- Volume 2: Notice to Applicants for Medicinal Products for human use
- Volume 3: Scientific Guidelines for Medicinal Products for human use
- Volume 4: Good Manufacturing Practices Guidelines for Medicinal Products for human and veterinary use
- Volume 5: Pharmaceutical Legislation for Medicinal Products for veterinary use
- Volume 6: Notice to Applicants for Medicinal Products for veterinary use.

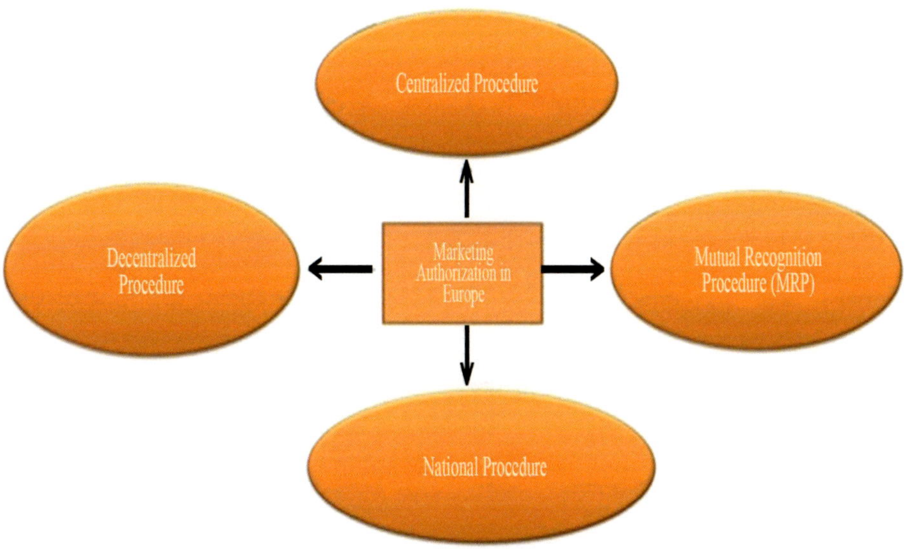

Figure 10.3. *Obtaining marketing approval for pharmaceuticals in the EU.*

Source: Sawant, A. M., Mali, D. P., Bhagwat, D. A. (2018). Regulatory requirements and drug approval process in India, Europe and US. Pharmaceut Reg Affairs 7, 210. doi: 10.4172/2167-7689.1000210.

- Volume 7: Scientific Guidelines for Medicinal Products for veterinary use
- Volume 8: Maximum Residue Limits
- Volume 9: Pharmacovigilance Guidelines for Medicinal Products for human and veterinary use
- Volume 10: Clinical Trials Guidelines.

Pharmaceuticals can be authorized for sale in Europe through a variety of administrative processes and organizational structures. In the European Union, there are four distinct processes for obtaining marketing approval for pharmaceuticals (Figure 10.3).

10.1.2.1. Centralized Procedure

Through the centralized procedure, candidates can get a marketing authorization good for the whole European Union. Applications for new chemical entities (NCEs) and products of the biotechnological sciences are accepted under this procedure. NCEs are grouped as "List B," and all biotechnological products are grouped as "List A.". This process states that a single marketing authorization is good throughout the European Union. After obtaining the Marketing Authorization Approval (MAA), the EMEA staff verifies that the application is accurate and complies with EU regulations. After the application is filed, this appraisal needs to be finished in ten days. The sponsor covers the necessary costs. After that, EMEA has 210 days to review the submission. Reporters are people who evaluate applications and submit reports to the Committee for Medicinal Products for Human Use (CHMP). The European Commission receives the application after CHMP renders a decision on whether to approve or reject it; this process may take up to 90 days. The approval process takes about 300 days total (210+90). With just one application to EMA, this product is recognized by all of the participating nations. Examples include CEP submissions, eDMFs, and CTDs for unique products like pharmaceuticals for all orphans. Everything that is based on biotechnology, including specific medications for cancer and HIV/AIDS, specific antiviral medications, specific medications for neurodegenerative disorders like diabetes, and specific medications for autoimmune diseases and disorders. Rejected applications under these schemes result in EU entry prohibitions.

- Results in a single authorization valid in EU, Norway, Iceland and Liechtenstein
- Application evaluated by assigned Reporters.
- Timeline: EMA opinion issued within 210 days, and submitted to European Commission f or final approval.

Centralized process is compulsory for:

- Those medicines which are derived from any biotechnology processes, such as genetic engineering
- Those medicines which are intended for the treatment of Cancer, HIV/Aids, diabetes, neurodegenerative disorders or autoimmune diseases and other immune dysfunctions.
- Medicines officially designated 'orphan medicines' (medicines used for rare diseases) (Figure 10.4).

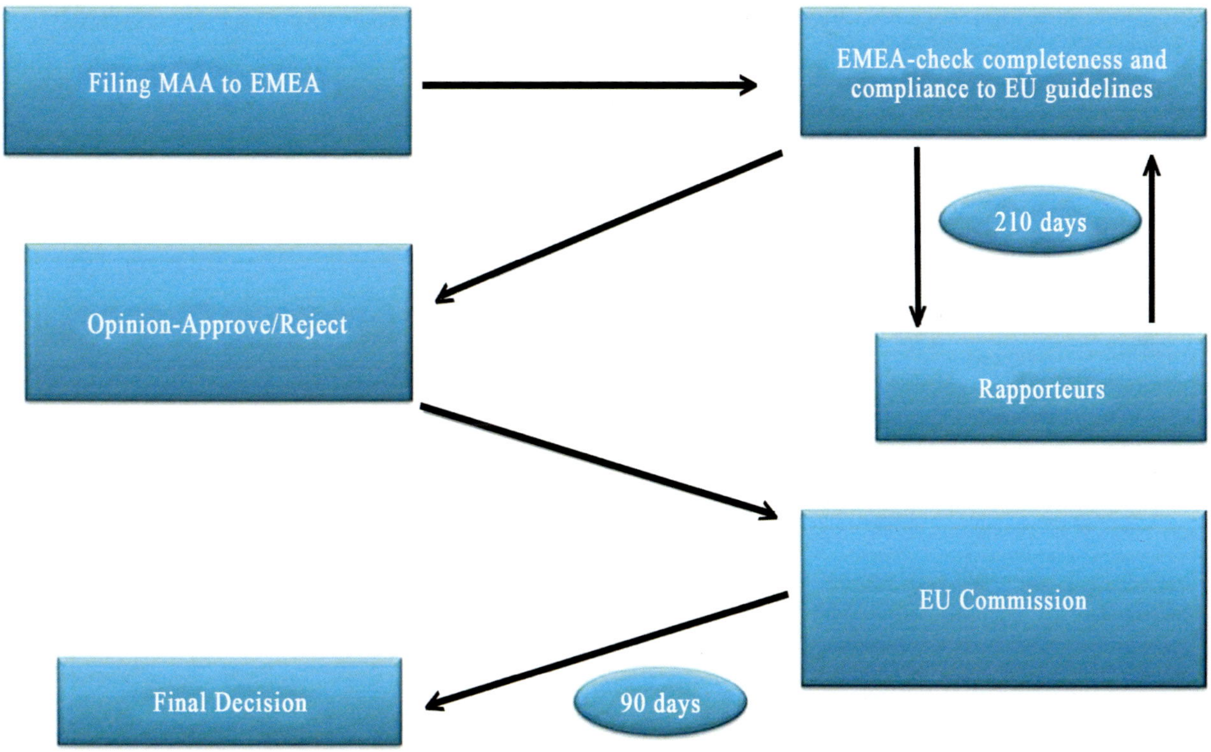

Figure 10.4. *A Centralized procedure.*

Source: Sawant, A. M., Mali, D. P., Bhagwat, D. A. (2018). Regulatory requirements and drug approval process in India, Europe and US. Pharmaceut Reg Affairs 7, 210. doi: 10.4172/2167–7689.1000210.

10.1.2.2. Decentralized Procedure

Under this, a product is concurrently recognized by several member nations. It is regarded as an extremely effective process. In a number of member states, marketing authorizations are obtained through a decentralized process. The application, together with a list of all Concerned Member States (CMSs) that includes a Reference Member State (RMS), are submitted by the sponsor to a national regulatory body. The application and Summary of Product Characteristics (SPCs) must be validated by the RMS. A draft assessment report must be prepared and sent to the CMSs within 210 days, after which it can be approved in 90 days. If a medication is intended to pose a substantial risk to the general public's health. CMSs have 30 days to voice any objections before the CHMP steps in and makes a decision. The following products, however, cannot be registered under this scheme and a negative decision may impact registration in numerous countries: pharmaceuticals for orphans, all biotechnology-based products, specific medications for cancer and HIV/AIDS, specific antiviral medications, specific medications for neurodegenerative disorders, including diabetes, and specific medications for autoimmune diseases or dysfunctions (Figure 10.5).

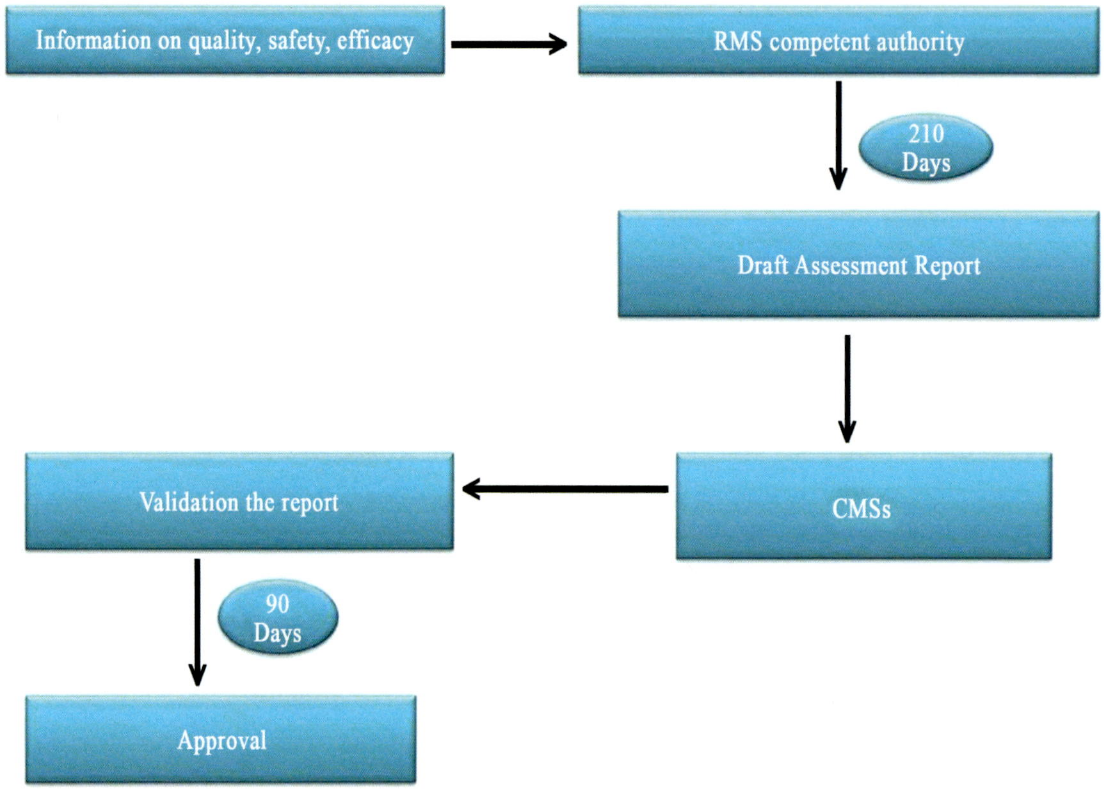

Figure 10.5. *Decentralized procedure.*

Source: Sawant, A. M., Mali, D. P., Bhagwat, D. A. (2018). Regulatory requirements and drug approval process in India, Europe and US. Pharmaceut Reg Affairs 7, 210. doi: 10.4172/2167–7689.1000210.

10.1.2.3. National Procedure

Every country in Europe has its own regulatory body. National procedure is a practice that each country adopts on its own, apart from other countries. Even small businesses can afford the fees. It reduces the expense of translating into regional or English languages. It establishes the foundation for the Mutual Recognition Process.

Biotechnical procedures are not eligible for registration through national channels. For the same, centralized filing through EMA is required. After being examined and approved for marketing, the application is submitted by the sponsor to the national competent authority in accordance with national regulations. Orphan medicinal products, all biotechnology-based products, specific antiviral medications, specific medications for neurodegenerative disorders, including diabetes, and specific medications for autoimmune diseases and dysfunctions are also not eligible for registration under this scheme (Figure 10.6).

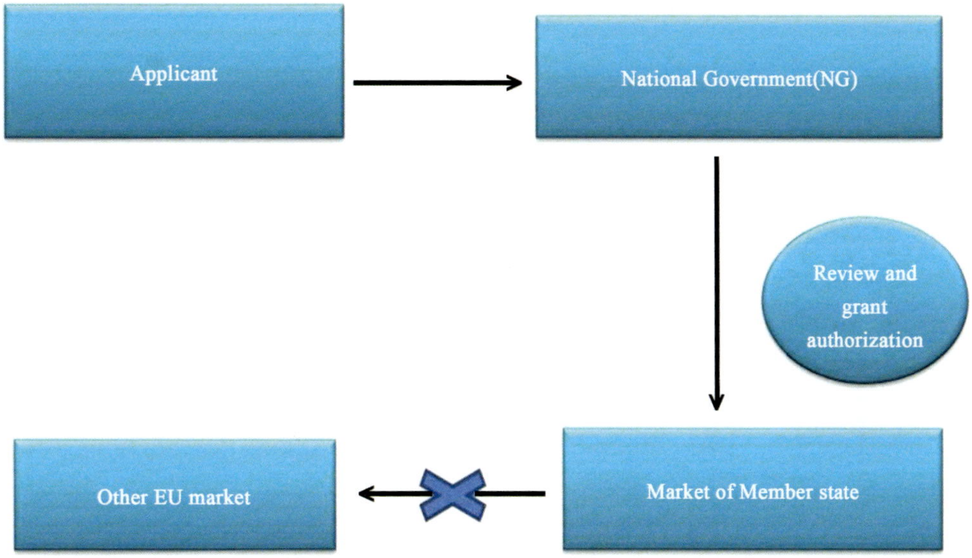

Figure 10.6. *National procedure.*

Source: Sawant, A. M., Mali, D. P., Bhagwat, D. A. (2018). Regulatory requirements and drug approval process in India, Europe and US. Pharmaceut Reg Affairs 7, 210. doi: 10.4172/2167-7689.1000210.

10.1.2.4. Mutual Recognition Procedure (MRP)

According to this, a product registered in one nation is acknowledged by another nation. For the purpose of initial registration, only one application must be submitted. Another member nation accepts the same application with minor modifications related to the region. EU Member States' Assessment Reports on Medicinal Products: Before approval during the Mutual Recognition Process, the Reference Member State's Assessment Report is examined.

The RMS provides a copy of the assessment report to the CMSs, who have 90 days to voice any objections. The submission can be made to any number of the other member states. A national marketing authorization is issued by each CMS with the same SPC. Orphan medicinal products, all biotechnology-based products, specific antiviral medications, specific medications for cancer and HIV/AIDS, specific medications for neurodegenerative disorders, including diabetes, and specific medications for autoimmune diseases or dysfunctions are all prohibited from registration under this scheme (Figure 10.7).

When it comes to approving new drugs, the United States may have the strictest regulations in the world. Many people believe that the requirements for drug approval in the United States are the highest in the world. With the founding of the United States in 1820, a new era of drug regulation in the United States began. The Pharmacopoeia. The original Food and Drugs Act, passed by Congress in 1906, mandated that medications adhere to official standards for potency and purity.

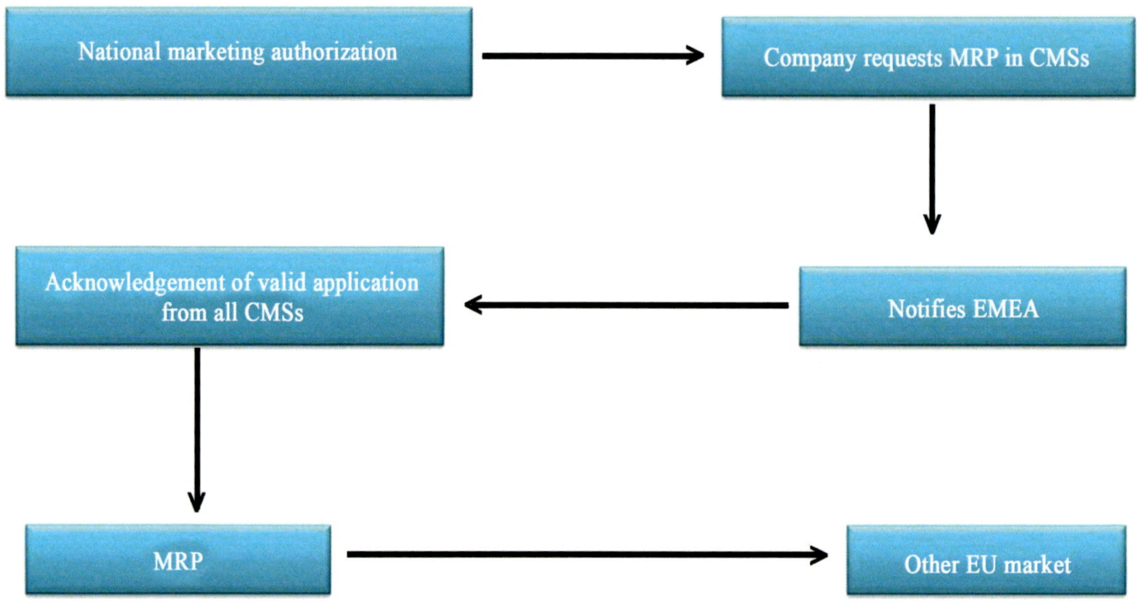

Figure 10.7. *Mutual recognition procedure (MRP).*

Source: Sawant, A. M., Mali, D. P., Bhagwat, D. A. (2018). Regulatory requirements and drug approval process in India, Europe and US. Pharmaceut Reg Affairs 7, 210. doi: 10.4172/2167–7689.1000210.

However, the Federal Food, Drug and Cosmetic Act (of 1938) was passed in 1937 as a result of the sulphanilamide tragedy, which added new requirements requiring new drugs to be proven safe before going on sale. Additionally, the Kefauver-Harris Amendment Act was passed in 1962 and mandates that manufacturers substantiate the safety and efficacy of their drugs (as stated on the label). The protection and promotion of public health falls within the purview of the Food and Drug Administration (FDA). Clinical Trials (CT) and New Drug Application (NDA) approval are the two stages of the FDA's new drug approval process, which is similar to the general drug approval process. A new drug application (NDA) is used to regulate new drug products. These applications are currently accepted in eCTD format for review. The product's efficacy and safety are the main concerns with NDAs. The FDA approval procedure doesn't start until an investigational new drug (IND) application is submitted. To establish guidelines for drug strength and purity, the United States Pharmacopoeia (USP) and its regulations were established in 1820. Key turning points in the development of US drug law include:

- **Food and Drugs Act (1906):** It requires that the drugs must meet official standards of strength and purity.
- **Federal Food, Drug and Cosmetic Act (1938):** It was enacted after sulfanilamide tragedy, to prove the safety of a drug before being marketed.
- **Kefauver- Harris Amendment (1962):** It was passed after the thalidomide disaster. It requires the manufacturers to prove that drug is safe and effective. All the firms should send adverse effect reports to FDA.

- **Orphan Drug Act (1973):** This allows tax deductions for drug companies to develop orphan drugs.
- **Generic Drug Enforcement Act (1992):** It deals with convictions related to ANDA approvals.
- **FDA Modernization Act (1997):** It contains some changes in Federal Food, Drug and Cosmetic Act regarding collection and assessment of user fees and accelerated approval processes.

10.1.2.5. Investigational New Drug Application (INDA)

It is an FDA application that was submitted before any human testing. It provides a thorough explanation of chemistry, information on pharmacology and toxicology, manufacturing and control procedures, and any prior human experience.

- **Types of IND**
  - **An Investigator IND:** It is submitted by a physician who both initiates and conducts an investigation and under whose immediate direction the investigational drug is administered or dispensed. A physician might submit a research IND to propose studying an unapproved drug, or an approved product for a new indication or in a new patient population.
  - **Emergency Use IND:** This allows the FDA to authorize use of an experimental drug in an emergency situation that does not allow time for submission of an IND.
  - **Treatment IND:** It is submitted for experimental drugs showing promise in clinical testing for serious or immediately life-threatening conditions while the final clinical work is conducted and the FDA review takes place.

Commercial and research (noncommercial) types are the two IND categories. The IND application needs to include data in three main areas: (1) studies on animal pharmacology and toxicology; (2) information on manufacturing; and (3) data on clinical protocols and investigators. The sponsor is required to wait 30 calendar days following the submission of the IND before starting any clinical trials. The FDA has the chance to check the IND for safety during this period to ensure that research subjects won't be put at undue risk.

- **IND Content and Format**

Section 312 of the 21st Code of Federal Regulations (CFR) specifies the format and content requirements for IND applications. When submitting an "Investigational New Drug Application," a sponsor (commercial organization) or an investigator planning a clinical study should do so in the following order (Figure 10.8):

1. Form FDA1571
2. Table of contents
3. Introductory statement and investigational plan
4. Investigator's brochure
5. Protocols
6. Chemistry, manufacturing and control (CMC) information
7. Pharmacology and toxicology information
8. Previous human experience
9. Additional information.

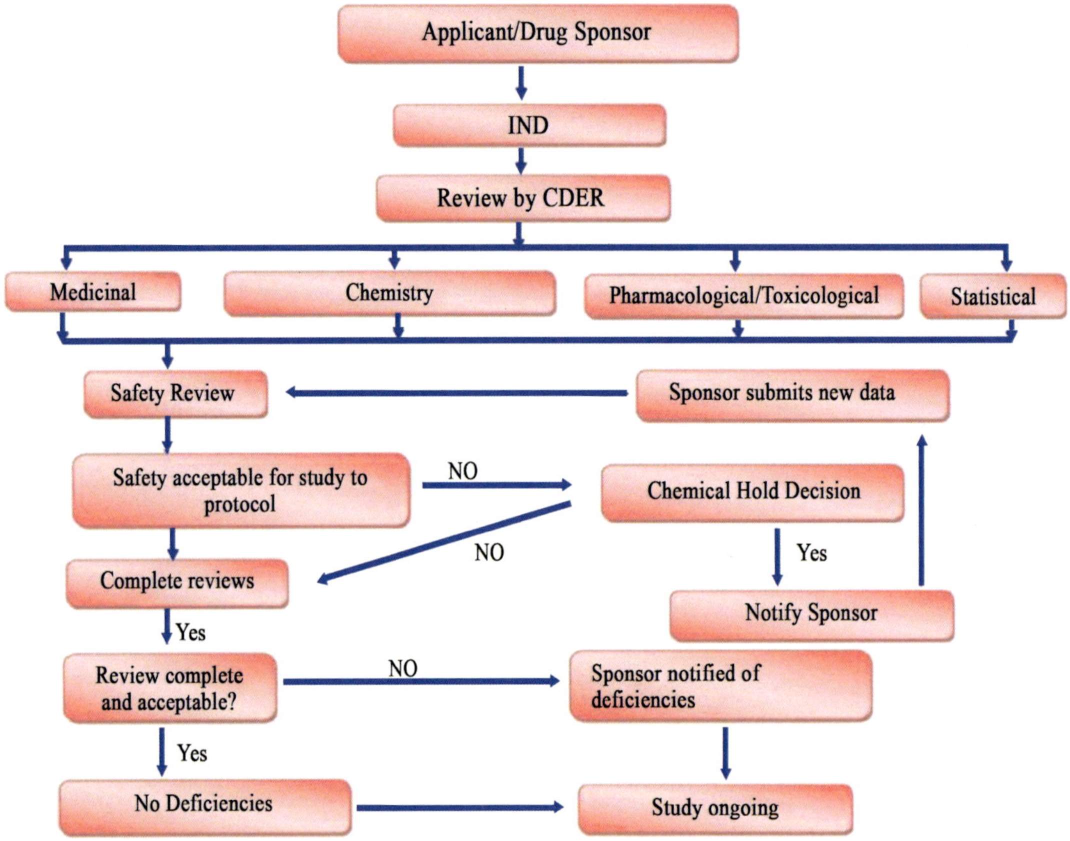

Figure 10.8. *Investigational new drug application.*

Source: Sawant, A. M., Mali, D. P., Bhagwat, D. A. (2018). Regulatory requirements and drug approval process in India, Europe and US. Pharmaceut Reg Affairs 7, 210. doi: 10.4172/2167-7689.1000210.

10.1.2.6. New Drug Application (NDA)

To obtain approval for marketing a new drug in the United States, a New Drug Application is submitted. The information in the IND and the outcomes of clinical trials demonstrating the product's safety and effectiveness are both included in the NDA. The FDA begins the review procedure sixty days after an NDA is submitted. Contents and Format of the NDA: The application is available in two copies: an archival copy and a review copy.

- **Archival Copy:** It includes copies of tabulations and clinical study case report forms, and it acts as a reference source for FDA reviewers to find information not included in the review copy. It is made up of the following components:
  - Application form FDA356
  - Index
  - Summary
  - Technical sections: further typed to

- Chemistry, manufacturing and controls section
- Non-clinical pharmacology and toxicology section
- Human pharmacokinetics and bioavailability section
- Microbiology section
- Clinical data section
- Statistical section
- Pediatric use section
- Samples and Labeling
- Case report forms

• • **Review Copy:** Each technical section is separately bound in each folder. Each technical section should contain:

- Index
- Copy of FDA Form 356h
- Copy of cover letter
- Letters of authorization
- Copy of application n=summary.

Meetings between the sponsor and the FDA are permitted at least twice: once following the conclusion of Phase 2 clinical trials and once before the submission of an NDA, i.e., a pre-NDA conference. After reviewing the study findings, the review panel will decide whether or not to approve the application (Figure 10.9).

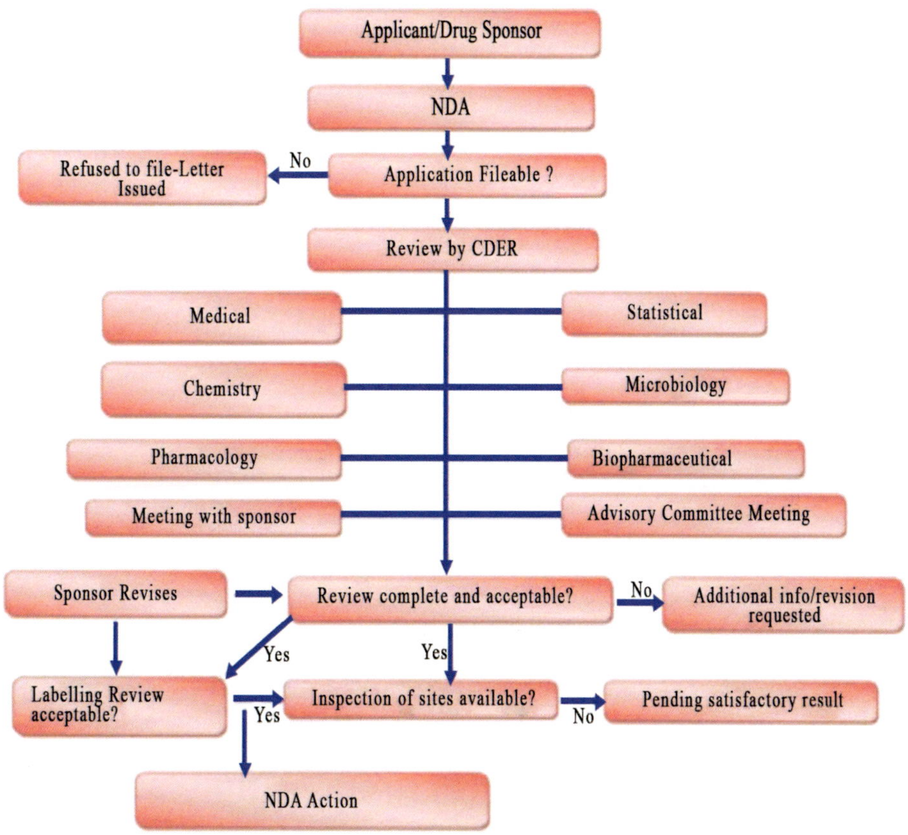

Figure 10.9. *New drug application.*

Source: Sawant AM, Mali DP, Bhagwat DA (2018) Regulatory requirements and drug approval process in India, Europe and US. Pharmaceut. Reg. Affairs 7: 210. doi: 10.4172/2167–7689.1000210.

10.1.2.7. Abbreviated New Drug Application (ANDA)

Products that share or closely resemble the active ingredients, dosage form, strength, administration route, use, and labeling of previously proven safe and effective products are subject to ANDA. It is employed when a business wishes to market a copy of a product whose patent has expired. These medications, known as generics, must adhere to bioequivalency and pharmaceutical standards. An ANDA is sent to the Office of Generic Drugs, Center for Drug Evaluation and Research, for review and approval.

- **Content and Format of ANDA**
  - Application form
  - Table of contents
  - Basis for ANDA submission
  - Conditions of use
  - Active ingredients
  - Route of administration, dosage from, strength, bioequivalence
  - Labeling
  - Chemistry, manufacturing and control
  - Human pharmacokinetics and bioavailability
  - Samples
  - Analytical methods
  - Case report forms and tabulations.

Guidelines on valid statistical analysis for bioequivalence assessment are provided in "Guidance on statistical Procedures for Bioequivalence Studies Using a Standard Two Treatment Crossover Design," published in July 1992 by the Division of Bioequivalence's Office of Generic Drugs of CDER.

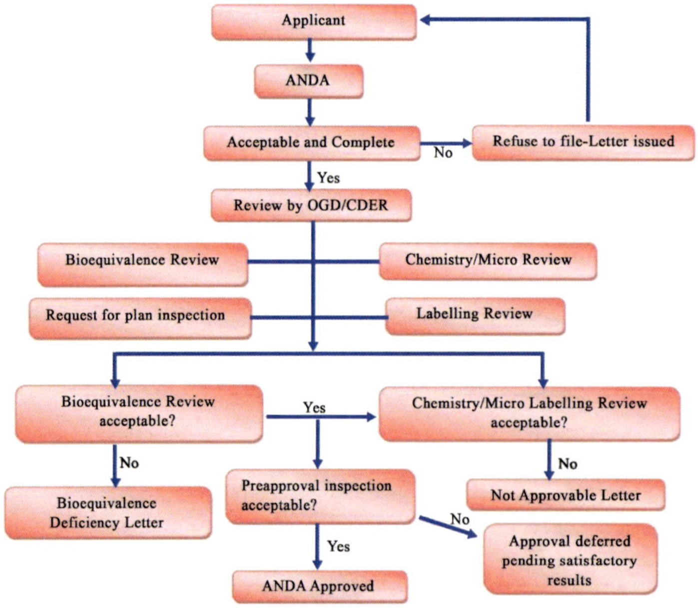

Figure 10.10. *Abbreviated new drug application (ANDA).*

Source: Sawant AM, Mali DP, Bhagwat DA (2018). Sawant AM, Mali DP, Bhagwat DA (2018) regulatory requirements and drug approval process in India, Europe and US. Pharmaceut. Reg. Affairs 7: 210. doi: 10.4172/2167-7689.1000210.

This guarantees the bioequivalency assessment's validity. Sponsors of INDs, NDAs, and ANDAs who plan to conduct studies based on a comparison of pharmacokinetic metrics are advised by the FDA in a draft guidance titled "in vivo bioequivalence studies based on population and bioequivalence." The FDA's "Approved Drug Products with Therapeutic Equivalency Evaluations," or "Orange Book," contains a list of all approved drug products, including both branded and generic medications. It comprises goods for which NDAs or ANDAs have been approved and that the FDA has evaluated for safety and efficacy. Additionally, it offers assessments of therapeutic equivalency for prescription medication products with multiple sources that share the same active ingredients (Figure 10.10).

10.1.2.8. Supplemental New Drug Application (SNDA)

All material modifications to the terms specified in the applications must be approved by filing a supplemental NDA or ANDA after the NDA or ANDA has been approved. Modifications such as those to the ingredients or packaging need to be authorized by the CDER. This category includes drugs that have already received approval for new uses; these approvals are a better innovation because they require fewer resources for review than approvals for original uses (Tables 10.1 and 10.2).

Table 10.1. Differences Between India, the EU and the U.S

Requirements	India	EU	US
Agency	Single agency DCG I (CDSCO)	Multiple agencies ◊ EMEA ◊ CHMP ◊ National health agencies	Single agency USFD A
Registration process	Single registration process	Multiple registration process ◊ Centralised (European community) ◊ Decentralised (at least 2 member states) ◊ Mutual recognition (at least 2 member states) National membe r state)	Single registration process
TSE/BSE study data	Required	Required	Required
Braille co de	Braille code is not required on labelli ng	Braille code is required on labelling	Braille code is not required on labelling
Post approval changes	Post approval chan ges: ◊ Major ◊ Moderate	Post variation in the approved drug: ◊ Type IA ◊ Type IB ◊ Type II	Post approval changes in the approved drug: ◊ Minor ◊ Moderate ◊ major

Source: Sawant, A. M., Mali, D. P., Bhagwat, D. A. (2018). Regulatory requirements and drug approval process in India, Europe and US. Pharmaceut Reg Affairs 7, 210. doi: 10.4172/2167-7689.1000210.

Table 10.2. Manufacturing and Control Requirements

Requirements	India	EU	US
Number of batches	1	3	1
Packaging	Not addressed	Not required	A minimum of 1,00,0000
Process validation	Required	Required	Not required at the time of submission
Batch size	Pilot scale batch	2 pilot scale plus 1 lab batch or minimum of one lakh units whichever is higher	1 pilot scale or minimum of one lakh units whichever is higher

Source: Sawant AM, Mali DP, Bhagwat DA (2018) Regulatory requirements and drug approval process in India, Europe and US. Pharmaceut. Reg. Affairs 7: 210. doi: 10.4172/2167-7689.1000210.

10.2. Good Manufacturing Practices (GMP) In Pharmaceutical Industry

To ensure the highest standards of efficacy, quality, and safety in any process that involves the manufacture of health products, international organizations and institutions, in collaboration with the pharmaceutical industry and several national regulatory authorities in various regions and countries, have developed and issued several guidelines, guidance documents, and directives that are collectively referred to as Good Manufacturing Practices (GMPs). GMPs are regulations that control the manufacture, supply, and distribution of pharmaceuticals. Getting marketing authorization (MA) requires it. Mapping the production, distribution, use, and regulation of pharmaceuticals is the goal of this section.

To achieve, through greater consensus, the continuous evolution of quality assurance, safety, and efficacy, it is intended to show and provide the General/Current State of GMP for Medicinal Products for Human Use, highlighting the significance of a continuous update, regulatory harmonization, its adoption, and monitoring/inspection. This is made possible by the close collaboration of numerous national and international organizations, which results in the regulatory harmonization of GMP for human-use pharmaceuticals and more stringent compliance monitoring by the appropriate authorities. All parties involved in the pharmaceutical and health industries have been working to develop, understand, and apply GMP guidelines since the middle of the first half of the 20th century. This section complies with the most recent EudraLex GMP guidelines for medicinal products intended for human use, which were supplied by the European Commission (EC). The guidelines for GMP for Medicinal Products for Human Use, which are available from regulatory bodies, national and international organizations and institutions, such as the US Food and Drug Administration (FDA), the World Health Organization (WHO), the International Conference on Harmonization of Technical Requirements for Registration of Pharmaceuticals for Human Use (ICH), and Pharmaceutical Inspection Co-Operation Scheme (PIC/S), were consulted when following the EC directives.

10.2.1. National and International Organizations and Institutions

International conference on standardizing technical specifications for pharmaceutical registration intended for human consumption. The International Conference on Harmonization is a global organization whose goal is to promote greater harmonization in the comprehension and application of the guidelines and technical requirements for pharmaceutical product registration. It does this by proposing recommendations and putting the International Organization for Standardization (ISO) standards into practice. The only initiative that unites the pharmaceutical industry in the US, Japan, and Europe with drug regulatory agencies is this organization.

10.2.1.1. Pharmaceutical Inspection Co-Operation Scheme

The Pharmaceutical Inspection Convention (PIC), established by the European Free Trade Association in 1970, served as the foundation for PIC/S, which was developed in 1995. In addition to facilitating communication and collaboration between the relevant authorities, regional and international organizations, and the public at large, it offers constructive cooperation and activity in the field of GMP with multiple goals, including the establishment, development, and upkeep of harmonized GMP standards and quality inspectors systems in the drug industry.

Every decision is made by consensus consists of 43 Participating Authorities at the moment, the majority of whom are European.

10.2.1.2. World Health Organization

For the WHO, pharmaceutical product quality has been a concern. Article 2 of the WHO Constitution, which outlines the obligations to "develop, establish and promote international standards with respect to food, biological, pharmaceutical and similar products," necessitates a definition of global standards."

During the International Conference on Primary Health Care in Alma-Ata in 1978, one of the requirements for the provision of healthcare was recognized as the production and availability of high-quality pharmaceuticals. Similarly, the only way to guarantee the safety and quality of medicinal products is through the efficient operation of national drug regulation and control systems, according to the Conference of Experts on the Rational Use of Drugs, held in Nairobi in 1985, and WHO's Revised Drug Strategy, approved by the World Health Assembly in May 1986. Since then, numerous resolutions have been adopted by the World Health Assembly asking the Organization to create global guidelines, guidelines for action, and tools to ensure the quality of pharmaceuticals, whether they are produced domestically or abroad and traded.

The provisions align perfectly with other internationally accepted GMP texts. The WHO's GMP recommendations should be regarded as advisory guidelines that may need to be modified to account for the unique circumstances of each nation.

10.2.1.3. European Medicines Agency

One of the European Union's (EU) decentralized agencies is the European Medicines Agency (EMA). The Agency is in charge of conducting a scientific review of medications created by EU pharmaceutical companies. EMA has been assigned a wide range of responsibilities, some of which include developing guidelines, establishing standards, and supporting international cooperation with authorities outside the European Union. All rulings are enforceable in all EU member states as well as in Iceland, Liechtenstein, and Norway, which are members of the European Economic Area (EEA). A company is required by law to begin marketing a medication only after receiving an MA.

The European Medicines Agency (EMA) serves as the central point of a network of decentralized EU agencies such as the European Centre for Disease Prevention and Control and the European Monitoring Centre for Drugs and Drug Addiction, as well as over 34 national regulatory bodies, the European Commission, and the European Parliament.

Since September 2003, the EU—including the European Commission and the EMA—has maintained confidentiality agreements with the US—more precisely, with the FDA. As part of their regulatory and scientific procedures, the agreements permit the EU and the FDA to exchange private information. This includes non-public information about guaranteeing the efficacy, safety, and quality of pharmaceuticals intended for human and veterinary use, as well as information on draft laws and regulatory guidance documents. The EMA's office in London has had a permanent FDA representative since 2009, and the FDA's offices have had an EMA representative since early 2010.

Directive 2001/83/EC establishes Community codes for human use pharmaceuticals. 2004 saw the adoption of several amendments (Regulation [EC] No 726/2004 by Regulation [EEC] No 2309/93) by the European Parliament and Council of the EU.

The EU's pharmaceutical industry upholds strict quality management standards in the creation, production, and distribution of pharmaceuticals. A MA system guarantees that all pharmaceuticals are evaluated by an appropriate body to guarantee adherence to current standards for efficacy, quality, and safety. Through the use of quality risk management principles, a manufacturing authorization system guarantees that only authorized manufacturers, whose operations are routinely inspected by the relevant authorities, manufacture or import any goods that are permitted on the European market. Whether their products are sold domestically or abroad, pharmaceutical manufacturers in the EU are obliged to obtain manufacturing authorizations.

10.2.1.4. US Food and Drug Administration

The US Department of Health and Human Services' Food and Drug Administration is an agency tasked with safeguarding the public's health by promoting product innovation and ensuring that pharmaceuticals intended for human use are appropriately regulated. It gives the general public accurate, scientifically supported information about pharmaceuticals. The FDA's duties in the area of pharmaceuticals include safeguarding the public's health by ensuring the efficacy, safety, and quality of pharmaceuticals, vaccines, biological products, and medical devices. The 50 states, the District of Columbia, Puerto Rico, Guam, the Virgin Islands, American Samoa, and other US territories and possessions are all included in the FDA's jurisdiction.

Ensuring the availability of safe and effective medications to enhance public health in the United States is a crucial responsibility of the Center for Drug Evaluation and Research.

The FDA launched a significant initiative in 2002 to enhance product quality and the regulation of the pharmaceutical industry. The initiative covers human medicinal products, including human biological medicinal products like vaccines, and centers on the FDA's current GMP (cGMP) program. With a focus on three main objectives, this initiative seeks to enhance public health promotion and protection. The primary objective is to concentrate cGMP requirements on possible health hazards to the general public by giving manufacturing-related issues more consideration and funding. The second objective is to guarantee that innovation and the introduction of new manufacturing technologies in the pharmaceutical industry are not impeded by the development and implementation of standards for the quality of medicinal products. Enhancing the FDA's approach's predictability and consistency is the third objective, which will ultimately guarantee quality and safety. Title 21 of the Code of Federal Regulations (CFRs) contains the FDA regulations.

10.2.2. Good Manufacturing Practice- The General/Current State

10.2.2.1. Pharmaceutical Quality System

This guideline outlines a thorough model for an efficacy quality system for pharmaceuticals that is based on ISO quality concepts and is applied at every step of the product's life cycle. By following this guideline, technological innovation will increase and the connection between pharmaceutical development and manufacturing activities will be strengthened. Throughout the course of the product's life cycle, the guideline is applicable to supporting the development and manufacturing of pharmaceutical industry substances, active pharmaceutical ingredients, and medicinal products, including biotechnology and biological products.

The term "quality assurance" refers to a broad range of issues that can affect a product's quality either separately or jointly. These issues include managing the quality of raw materials, finished goods and other components, production-related services, and management, production, and inspection procedures. It is used during manufacturing production as well as during pre-production to ensure that the final product satisfies specifications and requirements. Fit for purpose, which states that the product should be appropriate for its intended use, and "right first time" errors should be completely avoided are two concepts that are part of quality assurance. A thorough quality assurance system must be in place and properly implemented to achieve quality. This final concern relates to quality control, quality risk, and GMP management.

10.2.2.2. Personnel

To establish and maintain the Quality Management System and increase effectiveness, the management of an organization must decide which resources—human, financial, material, facility, and equipment—are sufficient and appropriate. For any business to operate properly, efficient human resource management and coordination are essential. To achieve this, enterprise management is responsible for hiring employees and assigning tasks to them.

10.2.2.3. Premises and Equipment

To reduce the chance of errors and to enable efficient cleaning and maintenance, the premises and equipment must abide by all regulations relevant to the tasks to be carried out.

10.2.2.4. Documentation

To function in accordance with GMP regulations, proper documentation is a crucial component of the quality assurance system. The manufacturer's quality management system should contain a detailed definition of all used document and media types. There are various ways that documentation can be found (paper-based, electronic or photographic media). Establishing, tracking, and documenting all activities that have an impact on any aspect of the quality of medicinal products should be the goals of the documentation system.

10.2.2.5. Production

Production activities need to adhere to the protocols explicitly. To ensure high-quality products and to adhere to applicable manufacturing and MA guidelines, they must follow GMP principles. Professionals with the necessary skills should oversee and carry out production. When handling materials and products, it is important to follow written procedures or instructions and, if required, keep records of all handling activities. This includes receiving and placing products under quarantine, sampling, storing, labeling, dispensing, processing, packaging, and distribution.

10.2.2.6. Quality Control

To ensure that the necessary and pertinent tests are conducted and that materials are not released for use or products released for sale or supply until their quality has been deemed satisfactory, quality control is concerned with sampling, specifications, testing, and the organization, documentation, and release procedures. Quality control needs to be a part of every decision that could have an impact on the final product's quality, not just laboratory operations. It is thought that quality control's ability to function satisfactorily depends on its separation from production.

10.2.2.7. Contract Manufacture and Analysis/ Outsourced Activities

Regarding the issuance of MA and manufacturing authorizations, manufacturers' obligations to the member state's competent authorities are outlined in the guidelines governing contract and analysis manufacturing. The purpose of this updated guidance on subcontracting activities governed by GMP, beyond the current scope of operations of the contract manufacture and analysis, is to provide information on activities that fall under the purview of the ICH Q10 document's Pharmaceutical Quality System.

Contract preparation and analysis needs to be properly established, agreed upon, and managed to prevent misunderstandings that could lead to subpar work or products.

10.2.2.8. Complaints and Product Recall

A mechanism for quickly and efficiently recalling products that are known or suspected to be defective from the market should be developed in compliance with the WHO, Article 117 of Directive 2001/83/EC, and Article 84 of Directive 2001/82/EC. Procedures for the Quality Control Unit's evaluation should be included in the procedures.

10.2.2.9. Self-inspection

Self-inspections are intended to evaluate and oversee a manufacturer's adherence to GMP in all areas of production and quality control. It needs to be built with the ability to identify any shortcomings in the way GMP is being applied and suggest solutions.

10.2.2.10. Basic Requirements for Active Substances Used as Starting Materials

An ICH guideline known as Q7A was created by its members. This guideline is meant to offer direction on GMP for producing active ingredients in a system that is suitable for quality control. Ensuring that active substances fulfill the quality and purity requirements that they claim or are represented to possess is another goal of this process.

It is important to remember that neither environmental protection nor worker safety are covered by GMP guidelines. These controls, which are subject to additional legal requirements, are the manufacturer's inherent obligations. The ability of the responsible competent authority to establish specific registration requirements regarding active substances within the framework of manufacturing authorizations and MA is unaffected by these guidelines, which are not meant to define registration requirements or alter pharmacopeia requirements. Every obligation in the registration papers needs to be fulfilled. These guidelines cover the production of sterile active substances only up to the point right before the active substance is rendered sterile, and they do not apply to the production of active substances for human use in pharmaceutical products. Even though the aseptic processing and sterilization of sterile active substances are not covered, those procedures should be carried out in compliance with the GMP guidelines and principles as established by local authorities. This includes the production of active substances made from blood or plasma as raw materials, though whole blood and plasma are not included because there are additional specific technical requirements for the collection and testing of blood. It should be mentioned that medications packaged in bulk are not covered by these guidelines.

10.2.2.11. Manufacture of Medicinal Products

- **Manufacture of Solid and Semi-solid Medicinal Products:** The manufacturer MA holder should prioritize following preventive procedures for this type of medicinal product since it is especially vulnerable to microbial contaminants and other contaminants during manufacturing.
- **Manufacture of Sterile Medicinal Products:** Specific guidelines must be followed during the production of sterile goods to reduce the possibility of microbiological, particulate, and pyrogen contamination. These guidelines heavily rely on the attitudes, knowledge, and training of the personnel involved. Since quality assurance is especially important, this type of manufacturing must strictly adhere to methods and preparation processes that have been carefully established and validated. The production of sterile goods ought to take place in hygienic spaces, to which personnel, equipment, and/or supplies must enter through airlocks.
- **Manufacture of Biological Active Substances and Medicinal Products for Human Use:** Because the production of biological active substances and biological medicinal products for human use involves certain unique considerations arising from the nature of products and manufacturing processes, it is necessary to take some special precautions. These factors play a critical role in shaping the appropriate regulatory control. Biological products are made by processes involving biological processes and materials, such as cell culture or material extraction from living organisms, in contrast to conventional medicinal products, which are typically produced and controlled using repeatable chemical and physical techniques. The range and nature of the byproducts may vary as a result of the inherent variability of these biological processes.
- **Manufacture of Radiopharmaceuticals:** Radiopharmaceuticals need to be produced and handled carefully. The sources and manufacturing processes of radiopharmaceuticals influence the regulatory processes that are required for their control. The kinds of radiation released and the half-lives of radioactive isotopes largely determine the degree of risk. Particular attention must be paid to waste disposal, radioactive isotope contamination, and cross contamination. Owing to their brief half-lives, certain radiopharmaceuticals are produced, released, and given to patients prior to passing all quality control testing. The EC guideline is applied to

manufacturing processes used in the production and quality control of the following products: radiopharmaceuticals, PET radiopharmaceuticals, radioactive precursors for the production of radiopharmaceuticals, and finally radionuclide generators. These manufacturing processes are used by industrial manufacturers, nuclear centers/ institutes, and the PET centers.

The organization in charge of policing radiation safety regulations and radiopharmaceutical transportation is the International Atomic Energy Agency.

- **Manufacture of Pressurized Metered Dose Aerosol Preparations for Inhalation:** According to the EC/EEA's GMP guidelines, the production of pressurized aerosols for inhalation with metering valves calls for extra care because of the unique characteristics of these dosage forms. The manufacturing processes used to produce these medications must reduce the risk of microbiological and particulate contamination. Ensuring the quality of components with valves and the consistency of suspensions is crucial.
- **Manufacture of Medicinal Gases:** In terms of EC/EEA, the gases are defined as medicinal products under Directive 2001/83/EC (designated medicinal gases), and they must adhere to all of the directive's manufacturing specifications, which cover the production of medical gases and active substances gases. In this regard, the production of medicinal gases and active compounds from gases are covered by these guidelines. In every MA dossier, the distinction between the production of medicinal products and active substances should be made explicit. The production of active substances from gases must adhere to any additional guidelines that may be necessary as well as the fundamental specifications for active substances used as starting materials.
- **Investigational Medicinal Products:** The GMP and the guiding principles should be followed when producing this class of pharmaceuticals. When the process grows, procedures must be adaptable and suitable for the product's stage of development. It has been observed that a highly efficient quality system is necessary when manufacturing operations become more complex.
- **Medicinal Products Derived from Human Blood or Plasma:** The rules for gathering, testing, and quality assurance of medical items made from human blood or plasma are established through a quality assurance system. This system is based on a national structure that is independent of manufacturers and adheres to GMP principles and guidelines. These products are classified as biological medicines due to their unique characteristics, with the starting materials being biological substances sourced from humans, such as cells or fluids like blood or plasma. The regulations of the CE also pertain to medical goods made from human blood or plasma that are fractionated within or brought into the EU/EEA. This also includes the starting materials, like human plasma, and stable derivatives of human blood or plasma, like albumin, that are utilized in medical devices. However, these rules do not extend to blood components intended for transfusion.
- **Manufacture of Herbal Medicinal Products:** The methods and processes employed in the production and quality assurance of herbal medicines frequently diverge

significantly from those of conventional pharmaceuticals. The quality of the herbal material should be appropriate. It is necessary to give the manufacturer of the herbal preparation or herbal medicinal product the supporting documentation. More thorough data on the agricultural production of herbal substances is needed for a consistent quality assurance program. These recommendations hold true for any herbal beginning material, including medicinal plants, herbal compounds, and herbal preparations.

- **Ionizing Radiation in the Manufacture of Medicinal Products:** A MA for a product that involves irradiation in its processing should also make reference to the note created by the Committee for Proprietary Medicinal Products, in compliance with the EC/EEA's GMP guidelines.

  Ionizing radiation can be produced by pharmaceutical manufacturers or contracted radiation facility operators, both of whom must possess the necessary manufacturing authorization. Ionizing radiation can be used in the manufacturing process for a variety of purposes.

- **Sampling of Starting and Packaging Materials:** Sampling is the process of taking a small portion of a batch and combining it with other operations to choose a part of a pharmaceutical product for a particular use, following the right protocol. The written and approved procedures that are appropriate for the sample and the type of control that is meant to be applied to the sample and sample material should be followed during this process.

- **Computerized Systems:** Computerized systems, electronic records, and digital signatures must adhere to regulations set forth by the FDA in the US 21 CFR Part 11 and the European Community in Annex 11 of the GMP.

  These rules pertain to any type of computer system utilized in any activity covered by the GMPs. These systems are made up of various hardware and software parts that work together to provide specific functions. When the quality system is replaced by manual operations, there shouldn't be a drop in product quality, process control, or quality assurance.

  The Food and Drug Administration has set standards for what constitutes a trustworthy, dependable, and generally equivalent set of electronic records, handwritten signatures executed on paper, and electronic signatures executed on electronic records.

- **Qualification and Validation:** The EC/EEA's guidelines for GMP qualification and validation outline the principles of qualification and validation that are used in the production of pharmaceuticals. Manufacturers specify what validation work is required in these requirements to demonstrate control over the crucial elements of their specific operations.

- **Certification by a Qualified Person and Batch Release:** For holders of medicinal products with MA or intended for export, the EC/EEA guidelines serve as a GMP guide. It also includes situations where the batch underwent various production or testing phases, were tested at various locations or by various manufacturers, or involved the division of an intermediate or bulk production batch into multiple batches of finished products. In the event that the EC/EEA and third countries have a mutual recognition agreement or not, the release of batches that were imported into the EC/EEA falls under the purview of these guidelines. These regulations also apply to investigational medicinal products.

- **Parametric Release:** A system of release known as parametric release ensures that the product meets the intended quality standards based on data gathered throughout the manufacturing process and in compliance with relevant GMP guidelines, annexes, and requirements. It does not, however, imply that all of the tests listed must be run on the completed product prior to release.

  The EU guidelines specifically focus on the parametric release process for finished products, which does not involve conducting a sterility test. These guidelines align with the standards outlined in the European Pharmacopoeia.

  The PIC/S guidelines aim to reduce or do away with routine testing of finished products, among other things. The purpose of these guidelines is not to impede technological innovation. Although the industry is not required to follow recommendations, it should consider them appropriate.

  When submitting a new medication, the Food and Drug Administration offers suggestions to applicants regarding the data that should be included to support parametric release for sterile products that have been sterilized by moist heat. At the moment, this organization mandates that sterile products fulfill specific sterility standards before being put on the market.

- **Reference and Retention Samples:** The guidelines prepared and supplied by the relevant organisms within this scope provide guidance on the taking and preservation of reference samples of finished products, packaging materials, or starting materials at the EC/EEA level. Guidelines for the gathering and storage of pharmaceutical samples for simultaneous import and distribution are also included in these guidelines. Samples are kept for two reasons: first, to supply a sample for analytical testing; and second, to supply a sample of the final product in its entirety. The samples are separated into two groups: retention samples and reference samples.

- **Quality Risk Management:** Regarding guidance on quality risk management, the ICH Q9 document—which includes GMP guidelines to be adhered to in this situation—was expanded. This guideline provides specific guidelines and tools for risk quality that can be applied to all aspects of pharmaceutical quality, such as the development, manufacture, distribution, and inspection processes, as well as the submission and review of the complete life cycle of substances, medicinal products, biologics, and biotechnology products. It also covers the use of starting materials, solvents, excipients, packaging, and labeling materials, all of which enable regulators and the industry to make more effective and consistent risk-based decisions. It is not meant to raise expectations above and beyond what is necessary at this time. This guideline's objective is to offer a methodical approach to quality risk management. It also acts as an independent foundation or resource, supporting other documents pertaining to ICH quality, and it supplements current quality practices, standards, and guidelines within the context of the pharmaceutical industry and regulatory environment. As such, it is optional in nature.

Risk management for quality can be utilized in various areas, including manufacturing, pharmaceutical development, and creating quality portions of applications for marketing approval. These guidelines also extend to regulatory authorities involved in evaluating pharmaceutical quality, conducting inspections for good manufacturing practices (GMP), and addressing concerns regarding quality issues.

10.3. Future Directions in Regulatory Affairs

The regulatory requirements for therapeutic product marketing authorization are under the purview of regulatory affairs. Numerous factors that affect the development, regulation, and value proposition of new therapeutic products are plaguing this field. Global megatrend shifts, including the emergence of the green economy and changes in geopolitics, have brought attention to the significance of supply chain and manufacturing security, as well as minimizing the environmental effects of product development. The COVID-19 pandemic has accelerated changes brought about by scientific advancements, digital disruption, and a renewed emphasis on the patient's centrality in all stages of therapeutic product development, and increased cooperation between national regulatory authorities.

Every facet of drug development, including the regulation of medicinal products, is being impacted by digital disruption. Simultaneously, scientific advancements have propelled a significant surge in the quantity of cell and gene therapies reaching the market, thereby yielding greater advantages for patients. Regulation of medicinal products has also been affected by the increase in patient involvement in all facets of drug development, including regulatory review. Because clinical trials can move more quickly with the growing integration of real-world evidence, medications will be able to enter the market earlier and post-market regulation will be given more priority by regulators. To increase efficiency at this stage of development, the clinical trial enterprise is incorporating more modeling, updated statistical methodology, and artificial intelligence. Digital twins are being used in manufacturing to test new systems. The industry is getting more integrated as robotics, the Internet of Things, and continuous manufacturing processes become commonplace. Regulatory agencies are also working together more and creating collaborative reviews, work-sharing, and reliance to make it easier to review these cutting-edge products as they enter the regulatory system. Because of all these changes, the workforce needs to be flexible, tech-savvy, and able to pick up new skills and modify existing procedures to fit the new demands.

10.3.1. Megatrends

Regulatory affairs professionals can better navigate the future implications on their roles by having an understanding of how global megatrends are changing. Megatrends are broad, worldwide patterns that could take many years to develop and have the power to fundamentally alter society. The following have been added to the Australian Commonwealth Scientific and Industrial Research Organization's (CSIRO) list of global megatrends: adjusting to a changing environment; becoming leaner, cleaner, and greener; recognizing the importance of health; geopolitical shifts; embracing digital; becoming increasingly autonomous; and recognizing the human dimension (Figure 10.11). These megatrends could have an effect on therapeutic product development, medical advancements, and the work of regulatory professionals. Manufacturing is being impacted by climate change, with a focus on sustainable practices, less environmental impact, and a shift toward a circular manufacturing economy. The growing desire of governments to produce essential pharmaceuticals domestically is a reflection of geopolitical unpredictability, as the COVID-19 pandemic brought attention to supply chain vulnerabilities. Infectious disease risks have been brought to light by the COVID-19 pandemic and are projected to rise in tandem with climate change. The pharmaceutical industry will be impacted by factors such as antibiotic resistance, the aging population's increasing burden of chronic illness, more stress on mental health, and financial restraints on healthcare spending. Positively, future advancements in healthcare and business opportunities will result from the promise of precision medicine, greater digital integration throughout the healthcare system, a shift toward a learning healthcare system, and a focus on wellness and preventative medicine. The three factors that will likely have the biggest effects on regulatory affairs professionals' work processes are digital disruption, artificial intelligence (AI), and human factor. Using big data, artificial intelligence (AI), and machine learning (ML) in regulatory processes, which will enable real-time regulation, utilizing real-world evidence and the growing significance of patient preferences in regulatory decision-making, and a rise in global harmonization, convergence, and reliance between national regulatory authorities are some of the future trends in the regulatory affairs profession that we have identified (Figure 10.11).

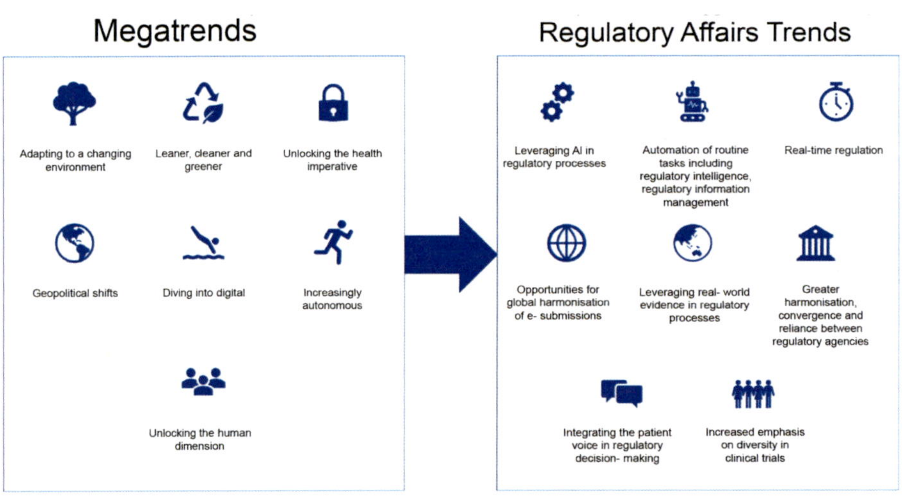

Figure 10.11. *Trends impacting the future of regulatory affairs.*

Source: Orin Chisholm and Helen Critchley. Future directions in regulatory affairs. Frontiers in Medicine. DOI:10.3389/fmed.2022.1082384. https://www.frontiersin.org/articles/10.3389/fmed.2022.1082384/full.

10.3.2. Digital Disruption

All facets of the drug development process, from early-stage target molecule discovery and validation to optimization of the candidate drug structure through the manufacturing process and national regulatory authority approvals, are starting to be impacted by digital disruption. Determining the structure of target proteins and then locating and refining suitable drug candidates that can interact with these proteins to block or modify their function is one of the major challenges in early-stage drug discovery.

Drug discovery is seeing a growing impact from AI and ML. Their use will expedite this stage of the process and lower the failure rate in early-stage drug discovery and development. It ought to lower drug development's expenses and hazards as well. The biannual Critical Assessment of Structure Prediction (CASP) competition saw Alphabet's DeepMind AI predict the three-dimensional (3D) structures of multiple proteins with astounding success in 2018 and 2020. Since then, researchers and drug developers have been able to ascertain the 3D structure of possible targets for drug development by utilizing DeepMind's open-source AlphaFold protein structure database. More recently, the use of AI/ML systems, like Panda Omics and Chemistry 42, has been employed to speed up the identification of lead candidate molecules in addition to finding new targets.

Digital twins are virtual copies of a physical process or asset that can mimic its behavior in real-time. By simulating process flows before they are implemented to ensure process optimization, digital twins can expedite the manufacturing of pharmaceuticals. They can also facilitate technology transfer by allowing the testing of new manufacturing plants prior to construction and requiring staff to complete training on the digital twin environment before entering the actual manufacturing plant. Pharmaceutical companies have previously employed digital twin models. GSK, for instance, optimized its vaccine development and production processes through the use of digital twins.

Digital twins are part of a suite of innovations that will streamline the manufacturing process by greater integration of automation and digitization. As the industry moves toward the new Pharma 4.0, the use of digital twins will increase. Pharma 4.0, or the fourth industrial revolution, includes digitally integrated manufacturing but guarantees data integrity by design and includes organization, culture, and processes, ensuring compliance with current GMP standards and harmonized guidelines like those created by the International Council for Harmonization of Technical Requirements for Pharmaceuticals for Human Use (ICH). Industry 4.0, or the fourth industrial revolution, is the integration of physical and cyber systems. It will make it possible to submit data in real-time to regulatory bodies using cloud-based platforms like Accumulus Synergy. The Accumulus Synergy platform is intended to house company-specific workspaces for businesses to work on their data packages, health authority-specific workspaces for collaboration among NRAs on product data reviews and analysis, and sponsor and regulator communication areas, all safeguarded by cyber-security and data privacy measures.

Digital twins can also be used to model the course of disease. This will allow for the use of digital twin control groups in clinical trials, which will allay concerns about control cohorts' operational and ethical implications. Predicting the effects of medications before they are given to patients will become more feasible as the number of digital twins of individuals rises. As a result, testing the best medication, dosage, timing, and delivery method in an individual's digital twin initially will improve the quality of medicine use while minimizing potential harm to patients. The application of digital twins will expedite the clinical trials enterprise and promote the expansion of precision medicine through increased utilization of "virtual" or "in silico" clinical trials.

The regulatory professional will be impacted by the use of "virtual" or "in silico" clinical trials since data integrity will become crucial. Initiatives like the adoption of the Identification of Medicinal Products (IDMP) standards by the International Organization for Standardization (ISO), which call for the management of substance, product, organization, and referential (SPOR) data, will lead to the digitization of all facets of regulatory operations. This is dependent upon an increasing trend toward structured data formats, which will make it possible to exchange data in real-time via cloud-based platforms like Accumulus Synergy with national regulatory authorities. Therefore, regulatory professionals will need to upskill in digital literacy as they contribute more and more to data flows rather than document flows in the future.

The collection and exchange of data for regulatory compliance requirements will be made easier by the flow of manufacturing information, including in-process release testing, specification testing, and batch release data in a structured format that is collected and stored in data lakes. Automating eCTD compilation enables more effective data transfer into the current eCTD format for regulatory submissions. The portable document format (pdf) used for eCTD writing still necessitates human oversight and interpretation of the data presented in the documents, making automated traceability back to the original data sources or data mining for deeper insights not possible at this time.

Authoring and publishing of regulatory documents, as well as data handling, may be further streamlined with the use of structured content and data management systems. Up until now, businesses have created custom internal structured content management systems, especially for medical records. However, to facilitate quick data and document sharing, industry standards will need to be met by both businesses and regulatory bodies. The shift toward the use of more structured formats for clinical and CMC data packages will be facilitated by the ongoing development of initiatives like Transcelerate's Common Protocol Template, the FDA's Knowledge-Aided Assessment and Structured Application (KASA), standardizing product quality/chemistry-manufacturing-controls (CMC) data, and the widespread adoption of the ICH Q12: Technical and Regulatory Considerations for Pharmaceutical Product Lifecycle Management guideline.

Professionals in regulatory affairs will have more time to devote to data analysis and insight generation, especially concerning the product's benefit-risk profile, thanks to the adoption of structured data formats for regulatory information. Simultaneously, the implementation of more structured benefit-risk analyzes by non-regulatory authorities (NRAs) has the potential to enhance global harmonization of benefit-risk assessment and offer a framework that health authorities can integrate into their benefit-risk algorithms.

The utilization of more dynamic review processes by national regulatory authorities will be necessary to enable real-time data exchange between companies and regulators. This was the case during the COVID-19 pandemic and is reflected in the Real-Time Oncology Review (RTOR) processes developed by the FDA Oncology Center of Excellence. More cooperation and coordination amongst national regulatory authorities (NRAs) are required to support this. Global data standard alignment and harmonization will also make data exchange easier. Data that is "findable, accessible, interoperable, and reusable (FAIR)" will be necessary to facilitate discussions between businesses and health authorities. The Fast Healthcare Interoperability Resources (FHIR) system from Health Level Seven International might end up being the preferred method for exchanging regulatory data. Health information sharing already makes use of it. There would be major advantages to integrating regulatory data with other health information using a common operability system.

For instance, when NRAs approve updates to product safety, physician prescribing software is updated in real-time. Additionally, it will make data mining and the gathering of actual data possible to enhance the quality of medicine and healthcare product use.

The FDA's Emerging Technology Program (ETP), which was created in 2014 as a forum for industry and the FDA to discuss potential regulatory issues surrounding the development and use of novel technologies, is one example of the procedures that regulators are putting in place to make sure they capture new and emerging technologies that are not specifically covered by their legislation. Before regulatory bodies adopt differing views on the use of new technologies, particularly in the manufacturing sector, it is necessary to clearly articulate the benefit: risk balance and international standards.

Examples of these technologies include continuous and modular manufacturing, the development of digital twins, the use of AI models to replace empirical testing, training the model and integrating it with advanced analytics, and active process control. To guarantee a seamless and uniform integration of such technology into therapeutic product development and review, national regulators ought to collaborate.

10.3.3. Evolving Therapeutic Landscape

Innovative new treatments for disease are being developed as a result of the rapid advancements in our knowledge of the molecular causes of disease. This has resulted in a notable surge in the development of novel therapeutics, such as products derived from gene and cell therapy, mRNA-based therapeutics, products derived from CRISPR technology, bi-specific antibodies, nanobodies, 3D printed pharmaceuticals and devices, novel drug-device combination products, and novel delivery routes like pulmonary drug delivery. Data science, digital health, and precision medicine will be the main focuses of future learning healthcare systems.

In its most recent half-year report for 2022, the Alliance for Regenerative Medicine listed 2093 clinical trials for regenerative medicines that are currently in progress. These trials included 32 tissue therapy products, 968 cell therapy, 721 cell-based immune-oncology, and 372 gene therapies. In fact, these products' pipelines are steadily advancing through clinical development and onto the market. The quick development of mRNA-based COVID-19 vaccines and their capacity to be quickly updated when new strains appear have brought RNA therapeutics to light. Beyond mRNA-based vaccines, nucleic acid-based therapeutics encompass aptamers, messenger RNA, small interfering RNAs, microRNAs, antisense oligonucleotides, and DNAzymes.

In 2020, a report was released regarding the first clinical trial utilizing CRISPR-edited T-cells intended to treat non-small-cell lung cancer. Although there was no significant adverse event related to treatment, this trial did not demonstrate an objective response in the treated patients. Gene editing methods like CRISPR, Zinc Finger Nucleases (ZFNs), and Transcription Activator-Like Effector Nucleases (TALENs) are being used in numerous trials today. Regulatory bodies are beginning to observe these products emerging from development, and the US Food and Drug Administration (FDA) has designated several of them as regenerative medicine advanced therapy (RMAT) (e.g., CTX110 from CRISPR Therapeutics) or that the European Medicines Agency (EMA) designated as an orphan drug or as a priority medicine (PRIME) (e.g., RP-L301 from Rocket Pharmaceuticals and CTX001 from CRISPR Therapeutics).

Research and development in the field of digital therapeutics is expanding, which is in line with patients' increasing desire to take an active role in their health and treatment choices. Digital therapeutics are online behavioral treatments that are typically administered through applications to improve patient outcomes. Regulators are creating guidelines on how digital therapeutics will be regulated, through international forums like the International Medical Device Regulators Forum (IMDRF) and through individual regulatory bodies like the Therapeutic Goods Administration (TGA), FDA, and Medicines and Healthcare Products Regulatory Agency (MHRA). Digital therapeutics are most commonly classified as software-as-a-medical-devices (SAMD).

In response to these and other new therapeutics that pose a threat to established regulatory procedures, regulators are employing horizon scanning to stay more aware of emerging technologies and make sure they have the necessary expertise to fill in knowledge gaps in the regulation of these technologies. As an example, the Innovation Observatory is a national horizon scanning facility funded by the National Institute for Health Research in the UK. Independent horizon-scanning groups are also emerging to support regulatory and policy development. We anticipate that, as innovation accelerates, consortia of regulators like the International Coalition of Medicines Regulatory Authorities (ICMRA) as well as individual national regulatory bodies will use horizon-scanning more frequently. The results of these horizon-scanning initiatives should include areas of focus for future regulatory science research, considerations and guidelines for those developing such technologies, and information on regulators' perspectives on identifying and balancing the risks and benefits of these novel therapeutic products.

Health Technology Agencies' (HTA) traditional approaches for calculating the cost-benefit analysis of new treatments are being impacted by the quick development of new treatment types, especially expensive curative treatments. A renewed emphasis on value will influence industry decisions surrounding product development and shift the decision points for value to earlier in the product development lifecycle, even though it won't directly affect the benefit: risk decisions made by NRAs. Additionally, to obtain this data sooner for HTA analysis, it will promote the incorporation of patient-reported outcomes in registration clinical trial designs. The Innovative Licensing and Access Pathway (ILAP) in the UK is a recent illustration of increased cooperation between a health authority and a health technology agency. In collaboration with the National Institute for Health and Care Excellence (NICE), the MHRA and NICE are offering medicine developers an innovation passport designation that grants them early access to support toolkits and assistance in creating a target development profile. The regulatory specialist needs to stay up to date on any modifications at the registration-reimbursement interface.

10.3.4. The Centrality of the Patient

In an effort to better align product development with patient needs, we have witnessed an increase in the importance of the patient over the past few years at every stage of the drug development process. A resolution on improving clinical trials was recently released by the World Health Assembly (WHA) resolution WHA75.8, which recognizes the critical role that trial participants play as well as the necessity of including underrepresented populations in clinical trials. Developed to increase the ability of patients and patient representative groups to meaningfully contribute to medicine development and research, the European Patients' Academy on Therapeutic Innovation (EUPATI) is a pan-European Innovative Medicines Institute (IMI) project of 33 organizations with partners from patient organizations, universities, not-for-profit organizations, and pharmaceutical companies. Guidelines for patient participation in research and development have been published by EUPATI. The patient's opinion is clearly heard when it comes to pricing and reimbursement decisions. To gather data on patient experiences for their evidence-based reviews of healthcare interventions, the US Institute for Clinical and Economic Review (ICER), for instance, offers a patient portal. The National Institute for Health and Care Excellence (NICE) in the UK and the Scottish Medicines Consortium, two other pricing organizations, have both heavily developed formal protocols for incorporating patient experience into their reimbursement decision-making processes.

Additionally, national regulatory bodies are examining the most effective ways to integrate the patient viewpoint into their benefit-risk assessment processes. With a clear focus on "putting the patient first," the delivery plan of MHRA for 2021–2023 includes steps to "embed the needs and expectations of patients.". To improve the methodical gathering of comprehensive patient and caregiver inputs to guide product development and regulatory decision-making, the FDA has published four new guidance documents on "Patient-Focused Drug Development Guidance Series for Enhancing the Incorporation of the Patient's Voice in Medical Product Development and Regulatory Decision Making.". Guidelines for patient participation in regulatory procedures have been developed by EUPATI. The European Medicines Agency (EMA) has a sophisticated procedure for considering patient opinions when making regulatory decisions. They have also updated their guidelines for communicating with patients and patient advocacy organizations. Using structured benefit: risk decision-making processes, like multi-criteria decision analysis, is one structured way that industry and regulators can include patient voice in regulatory decisions.

10.3.5. Global Regulatory Harmonization and Convergence

Paralleling the developments in complex therapeutics, the global COVID-19 pandemic has accelerated regulatory authorities' efforts to collaborate through a variety of mechanisms, including harmonization, convergence, reliance, collaborative review, and work-sharing. They are trying to find areas where they could work together and strategically address safety and regulatory issues by utilizing cooperative forums like the International Pharmaceutical Regulators Program (IPRP), ICMRA, and IMDRF. Greater openness is the cornerstone of these initiatives, as it is one of the fundamental tenets of good regulatory practices. Government-regulatory cooperation (GRP) is also an essential component of GRP. Harmonization is the process of merging national and international standards to promote efficiency in the regulation and development of drugs on a worldwide scale. One example that is widely recognized is how national regulatory bodies have integrated the ICH guidelines. Harmonization was first introduced in the devices domain by the Global Harmonization Task Force (GHTF), which has been replaced by the IMDRF. As a result of the adoption of international standards, documents, and best practices, convergence is the process through which the regulatory requirements of various nations become more similar. The formation of the Asia-Pacific Economic Cooperation (APEC) Regulatory Harmonization Steering Committee in 2008 to promote regulatory requirements convergence and harmonization of registration management amongst APEC member states is an example of regulatory convergence. The Pan American Health Organization (PAHO) and the Pan American Network for Drug Regulatory Harmonization (PANDRH), an initiative of the national regulatory authorities in the Pan-American region, provide support for the pharmaceutical regulatory harmonization processes in the Americas within the framework of national and sub-regional health policies and acknowledge pre-existing asymmetries. That's just one example. As stated by the World Health Organization, "reliance is the process by which a regulatory body in one jurisdiction may consider or give considerable weight to the work done by another regulator, or reputable institution, in reaching its own decision."

Dependency can manifest itself in a variety of ways, indicating differing degrees of recognition or consideration of the judgments, assessments, or other authoritative data that is accessible from other institutions and authorities. To this end, the Australian TGA, for instance, has put the Comparable Overseas Regulator pathways into place. Another illustration of reliance is the recognition of the Certificate of Pharmaceutical Product (CPP) by certain national regulatory bodies. Reliance pathways are being used by some regulatory bodies to facilitate a shortened evaluation process, which expedites the review procedure in those nations. Another example of international regulatory agencies' reliance and cooperation is the EMA's introduction of the "OPEN" pilot project during the COVID-19 pandemic, which allowed other regulatory agencies with whom they had confidentiality agreements to participate internationally in their scientific evaluation process. Participating organizations included Swiss medic, the World Health Organization (WHO), Health Canada (Canada), Japan Ministry of Health, Labor and Welfare/Pharmaceuticals and Medical Devices Agency (MHLW/PMDA), and Swiss medic. Attendance at emergency task force meetings and meetings of the Committee for Human Medicinal Products (CHMP) regarding COVID-19-related treatments and vaccines was permitted for representatives of the participating agencies. It is unclear if, after the pandemic, this effort will be expanded to include additional therapeutic domains.

Project Orbis is a cooperative review program created by the US FDA to expedite regulatory approval of novel oncology medications among member nations. Preliminary data suggests that the initiative is accomplishing its goal and that more nations are joining it.

Following the path of harmonization, convergence, and reliance, the regulators of Australia, Canada, Singapore, Switzerland, and the United Kingdom established the ACCESS Consortium, which is a work-sharing arrangement between several similar mid-sized national regulatory authorities. These nations take part in Project ORBIS as well. To get to the point where participating regulatory authorities divide the Modules for review under confidentiality agreements and memoranda of understanding between the participating authorities, work sharing has evolved over time as a result of extensive information sharing and confidence building between the participating regulators. While the process facilitates the sharing of expertise across geographical boundaries and lessens the regulatory burden on each participant, each participant retains their sovereign decision-making ability. All of these initiatives suggest that national regulatory agencies should work together more closely to address the difficulties of regulating novel, cutting-edge treatments and guaranteeing patients prompt access to them.

10.3.6. Challenges Arising from These Identified Trends

Each of these trends carries many challenges that will need to be addressed because they have an effect on drug development, medical practice, and the regulatory professional's role. The main issues with the development of AI and ML are those of ethics and governance. Protecting human autonomy, well-being, and privacy is one ethical concern. Other ethical concerns include making sure deep learning models used in AI and ML are transparent and explainable, ensuring responsible and accountable use of these technologies, ensuring inclusivity and equity to lessen bias, and promoting responsive and sustainable AI. Data governance issues include sharing, managing, and controlling data, securing informed consent for data used to train AI/ML, protecting individual privacy and de-identifying data, assigning intellectual property rights, and managing and sharing data. To boost trust in the application of AI/ML, robust governance and ethical frameworks will be required, and companies that depend on these systems will need to have well-established quality assurance and auditing procedures. When describing these technologies, making sure they adhere to legal requirements, and communicating with regulators regarding the registration of therapeutic products based on AI and ML, regulatory professionals will need to exude confidence. They must be able to effectively communicate this information both inside their company and to external stakeholders by integrating these systems into their formal benefit-risk decision-making processes.

Organizations face challenges in reskilling and upskilling their workforce due to digital disruption. Developing an agile mindset in workers, bringing all staff members along on the digital transformation journey, and establishing a culture of continuous learning will be the key factors driving effective digital change management within organizations. To effectively transition the organization, organizations must review their leadership styles, staff competency profiles, and incentives for staff members to continue their professional development. To support staff during this transition, it will be necessary to examine and modify ingrained mindsets and infrastructure. An additional obstacle is the accelerating rate of change, which leaves employees exhausted and unable to adjust any further. The possibility and consequences of losing highly skilled personnel who might find it difficult to adjust to their new roles will necessitate the establishment of a solid supportive environment. To develop an organization that guarantees employees have the desire to change and develop to meet future business needs, strong organizational change management will be necessary to create a sustainable workforce that performs well in a hybrid working environment. Some of these problems can be resolved with the aid of a mentorship program in which technically proficient staff members assist less confident staff members during their transition. It will be crucial to assist employees in taking advantage of internal and external learning opportunities to develop their abilities and gain experience with new workflows and systems.

It's a challenge for all of us to stay current with the evolving therapeutic landscape and the creation of novel therapeutics. People can attempt to stay up to date by getting together to exchange knowledge about new treatments and technologies in their field of expertise. Informal on-the-job learning can be enhanced by enrolling in relevant scientific conferences, attending college courses, or earning micro-credentials in particular fields. Management in companies engaged in the discovery and development of therapeutic products must consciously choose to integrate the patient perspective into all phases of drug development. Additionally, it will be necessary for the regulatory professional to remain at the forefront of legislative and regulatory agencies' thinking.

Global harmonization, convergence, and reliance are all expected to rise, but they will do so against a backdrop of heightened nationalism brought on by the COVID-19 pandemic, the war in Ukraine, which has caused energy shockwaves around the world, and climate destabilization. To enable greater equity of access to the advantages of new healthcare technologies and therapies, advanced economies will need to make sure that they guide less developed economies along the path toward greater harmonization, convergence, and reliance. To facilitate information exchange, advanced economies will also need to support changes to the regulatory agencies of developing economies. Last but not least, specialized training and agency-to-agency regulatory staff exchanges will support the development of regulatory best practices internationally.

A Closer Look

Skills for the Future Regulatory Affairs Workforce

These developments in healthcare, medicine and the pharmaceutical and medical device industry will impact the regulatory affairs team. The traditional heavy 'task' based workload will evolve with digital solutions and automation to require broader strategic leadership skills. It is therefore vital that regulatory professionals are equipped with the skills, knowledge, and mindset to develop themselves in order to advance their professional lives.

The current world of work is said to be volatile, uncertain, complex, and ambiguous (VUCA) and the global pandemic has resulted in a "new normal" world of work where these factors are amplified. The World Economic Forum has identified a number of important skills for the future of work including analytical thinking and innovation, active learning, complex problem-solving, critical thinking and analysis, creativity, originality and initiative.

Additional skills identified for the future of work include leadership and social influence, the ability to utilize, design and monitor technology, resilience, an ability to tolerate stress, flexibility and reasoning, problem-solving and ideation. The Institute for the Future identified additional skills in sense-making, cross-cultural competency, virtual collaboration and trans-disciplinarity as essential for the future of work. These skills will all be important in the pursuit of careers in the pharmaceutical and medical technology industry.

Given the major impact of digital transformation, regulatory professionals should focus on their digital literacy skills such as being confident in using dashboards and cloud-based platforms for data visualization, understanding how data are acquired, processed, analyzed and used for predictive purposes, and developing statistical data analysis and data mining skills. Beyond this there is a need to increase competencies in complex reasoning and problem-solving, adaptive thinking, agility, communication and teamwork and leadership and initiative – all elements of what is known as 21st century skills (Figure 10.12).

Generative leaders who strive to leave the world a better place than they found it lead equally with their head, their heart and their hands to unlock the greatest value. This requires a bold vision for the future by reimagining and reinventing ways of working to serve all stakeholders (leading with the head), building a culture that inspires and enables people to do their best work (leading with the heart) and executing through and empowering teams (leading with the hands). These elements together can lead to transformational change, a necessary requirement for thriving in the VUCA world of work. Professionals who take control of their own learning will be able to keep pace with the transformations happening in the industry in general and regulatory affairs specifically and position themselves for future growth opportunities.

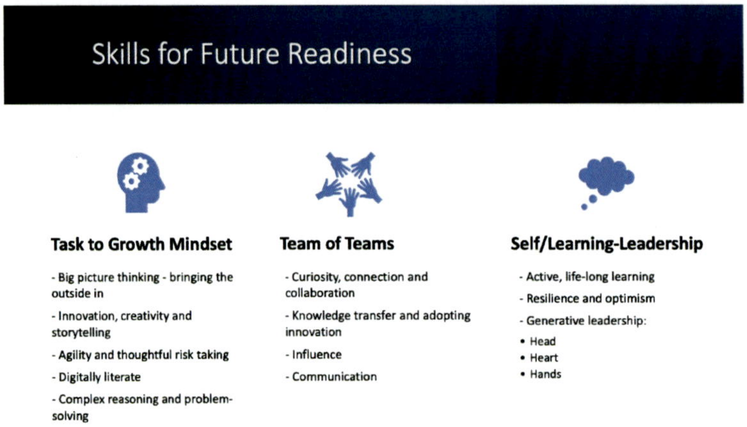

Figure 10.12: *Skills required for future readiness for regulatory affairs professionals.*

Source: Orin Chisholm and Helen Critchley. Future directions in regulatory affairs. Frontiers in Medicine. doi: 10.3389/fmed.2022.1082384. https://www.frontiersin.org/articles/10.3389/fmed.2022.1082384/full.

Regulatory professionals should develop a plan for their continual professional development and learning in conjunction with their managers, after reviewing their individual competencies and identifying gaps. They may seek a mixture of formal education, short courses or micro-credentials or informal learning opportunities to upskill. Short term assignments working in different areas also helps to deepen knowledge and connection and broaden perspectives. This aligns with a growth rather than a task mindset to enable a solution focused way of working. Besides further education and training to develop the necessary skills, regulatory professionals can ensure that they are regularly assessing trends that may impact their work, for example, by regularly reviewing activities and outputs from international regulatory bodies such as ICMRA, IMDRF, IPRP, ICH, and WHO, and keeping up to date on the latest communications from industry bodies in major jurisdictions such as the International Federation of Pharmaceutical Manufacturers and Associations (IFPMA), European Federation of Pharmaceutical Industries and Associations (EFPIA), Pharmaceutical Research and Manufacturers of America (PhRMA), Association of the British Pharmaceutical Industry (ABPI) and other local industry associations. Of course, keeping up to date with what each of the regulators are doing is also vitally important. Regulatory professionals should review updates to strategic plans from regulators to identify future directions for regulatory agencies, as well as updates to legislation. The impacts of major policy changes should be considered, such as the Pharmaceutical Strategy for Europe or updates to country-specific national medicines policies, such as the current update to the National Medicines Policy in Australia. The implementation of such policies may have implications beyond just the country or region involved in the initiative. Reviewing such changes will help regulatory professionals identify international discussions and where various drivers for change are coming from. Finally, regulatory professionals should keep up to date with relevant government reviews that may impact their organizations and industry.

Summary

- Regulatory affairs (RA) professionals are involved in all phases of drug development, from discovery and R&D to commercialization, to ensure that pharmaceutical products are safe, effective, and compliant with regulatory requirements. They work closely with researchers, manufacturers, and regulatory authorities to develop and implement regulatory strategies.
- Drug development is the process of bringing a new pharmaceutical drug to the market once a lead compound has been identified through the process of drug discovery. It includes preclinical research on microorganisms and animals, filing for regulatory status, such as via the United States Food and Drug Administration for an investigational new drug to initiate clinical trials on humans, and may include the step of obtaining regulatory approval with a new drug application to market the drug.
- A New Drug Application (NDA) is an application submitted to the individual regulatory authority for authorization to market a new drug, i.e., innovative product. To gain this permission a sponsor submits preclinical and clinical test data for analyzing the drug information, and description of manufacturing trials.
- Good Manufacturing Practices (GMPs) are a compilation of various guidelines/guidance documents/directives issued and elaborated by international organizations and institutions, in collaboration with the Pharmaceutical Industry and several national regulatory authorities in different regions and countries, to be guaranteed the highest standards of efficacy, quality and safety in any process that involves the manufacture of health products.
- The International Conference on Harmonization is an international organization with the purpose of making recommendations and implementing standards of the International Organization for Standardization (ISO) to achieve greater harmonization in the understanding and application of the guidelines and technical requirements for the registration of pharmaceutical products.
- Quality control is concerned with sampling, specifications and testing as well as the organization, documentation and release procedures which ensure that the required and relevant tests are carried out, and that materials are not released for use, nor products released for sale or supply, until their quality has been judged satisfactory.
- Digital disruption is affecting all aspects of drug development, including the way medicinal products are regulated. At the same time, advances in science have fueled a large increase in the number of cell and gene therapies coming to market and are delivering more benefits for patients. The rise in patient input into all aspects of drug development, including regulatory review, has also impacted medicinal product regulation.

References

1. Ang, K., Saw, E., He, W., Dong, X., & Ramakrishna, S. (2021). Sustainability framework for pharmaceutical manufacturing (PM): a review of research landscape and implementation barriers for circular economy transition. *Journal of Cleaner Production, 280*, 124264. https://doi.org/10.1016/j.jclepro.2020.124264.

2. Cecchini, M., Rubin, E. H., Blumenthal, G. M., Ayalew, K., Burris, H. A., Russell-Einhorn, M., et al. (2019). Challenges with novel clinical trial designs: master protocols. *Clinical Cancer Research, 25*(6), 2049–2057. https://doi.org/10.1158/1078-0432.CCR-18-3544.

3. Chakraborty, R., & Yadav, K. (2018). Drug approval process in US, Europe and India and its regulatory requirements: A Review. *International Journal of Drug Regulatory Affairs, 6*(1), 31–39.

4. Chen, Y., Yang, O., Sampat, C., Bhalode, P., Ramachandran, R., & Ierapetritou, M. (2020). Digital twins in pharmaceutical and biopharmaceutical manufacturing: a literature review. *Processes, 8*(9), 1088. https://doi.org/10.3390/pr8091088.

5. Gupta, N. V., Reddy, C. M., Reddy, K. P., Kulkarni, R. A., & Shivakumar. (2012). Process of Approval of New Drug in India with Emphasis on Clinical trials. *International Journal of Research in Pharmaceutical and Biomedical Sciences, 13*(1), 17–23.

6. Jayatunga, M., Xie, W., Ruder, L., Schulze, U., & Meier, C. (2022). AI in small-molecule drug discovery: a coming wave? *Nature Reviews Drug Discovery, 21*(3), 175–176. https://doi.org/10.1038/d41573-022-00025-1.

7. Mahapatra, A. K., Sameeraja, N. H., & Murthy, P. N. (2014). Drug Approval Process in United States of America, European Union and India: A Review. *AcrcTra, 1*(1), 13–22.

8. Papathanasiou, P., Brassart, L., Blake, P., Hart, A., Whitbread, L., Pembrey, R., et al. (2016). Transparency in drug regulation: public assessment reports in Europe and Australia. *Drug Discovery Today, 21*(11), 1806–1813. https://doi.org/10.1016/j.drudis.2016.06.025.

9. Pombo, M., Porrás, A., Saidon, P., & Cascio, S. (2016). Regulatory convergence and harmonization: barriers to effective use and adoption of common standards. *Revista Panamericana de Salud Pública, 39*(4), 217–225.

10. Smiatek, J., Jung, A., & Bluhmki, E. (2020). Towards a digital bioprocess replica: computational approaches in biopharmaceutical development and manufacturing. *Trends in Biotechnology, 38*(11), 1141–1153. https://doi.org/10.1016/j.tibtech.2020.05.008.

11. Socal, M., Sharfstein, J., & Greene, J. (2021). The pandemic and the supply chain: gaps in pharmaceutical production and distribution. *American Journal of Public Health, 111*(4), 635–639. https://doi.org/10.2105/AJPH.2020.306138.

12. Taylor, D. (2015). The Pharmaceutical Industry and the Future of Drug Development. In R. E. Hester & R. M. Harrison (Eds.), *Issues in Environmental Science and Technology* (pp. 1–33). Royal Society of Chemistry. https://doi.org/10.1039/9781782622345-00001.

13. Van Belkum, S., Brun, N., Cleve, S., McGovern, P., Lumpkin, M., Schaeffer, P., et al. (2022). Artificial intelligence in clinical development and regulatory affairs – preparing for the future. *Regulatory Rapporteur, 15*(3), 17–21.

14. Van Norman, G. A. (2016). Drugs and Devices. *JACC: Basic to Translational Science, 1*(5), 399–412.

INDEX

C

K

L

M

N

O

P

FSC
www.fsc.org
MIX
Papier | Fördert gute Waldnutzung
FSC® C083411

Kolibri 360 GmbH
Ferdinand-Jühlke-Straße 7
99095 Erfurt, Deutschland
produktsicherheit@kolibri360.de